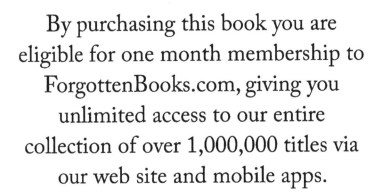

ISBN 978-0-483-37975-6
PIBN 10711133

DOMINION
DENTAL JOURNAL.

(Official Organ of the Ontario Dental Association.)

3158

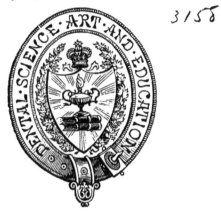

EDITOR:
W. GEORGE BEERS, L.D.S.
MONTREAL, QUE.

CO-EDITORS:

A. C. COGSWELL, D.D.S.   W. B. NESBITT, B.A., M.D.
HALIFAX, N.S.   TORONTO, ONT.

GERMAN EDITOR:
CARL E. KLOTZ, L.D.S.
ST. CATHARINES, ONT.

CORRESPONDING EDITOR:
W. R. PATTON, D.D.S.
COLOGNE, GERMANY.

VOLUME VI.

TORONTO:
OFFICE OF THE DOMINION DENTAL JOURNAL
WESLEY BUILDINGS.
1894.

CONTENTS OF VOL. VI.

ii   CONTENTS

CONTENTS

DOMINION
DENTAL JOURNAL.

VOL. VI.   TORONTO, JANUARY, 1894.   No. 1.

Original Communications.

Dental Dots.

By D. V. BEACOCK, Brockville, Ont.

To repair a broken gum-block, grind out the broken part and fit a plain tooth neatly.

The gas, forceps and vulcanizer are ready oftenest in the hands of the general practitioner. Too many are fast becoming a class of mechanics rather than professionals.

When a gum-block comes off, not broken, but the pins all out, it is sometimes difficult to match them. I have overcome the difficulty by grinding with a disk dove-tails in the block where the pins were, and replacing and vulcanizing.

During each twenty-four hours there is extracted from their respective glands an average of two pounds of saliva, ten pounds of gastric juice, five ounces of pancreatic juice, two pounds of bile, besides a large quantity of other fluids, at least twenty pounds daily in all ; there is as much excreted as secreted.

I have a polishing lathe that has been in use over twenty years, the spindle having worn loose, made a great deal of noise, jumping and rattling, when polishing, especially when running fast with a water motor. To remedy this I took off both caps, filed a little from the under side and replaced. This took up the worn part or lost motion, and it works as well as when first purchased. I may say that I have noticed lathes in several different dental laboratories, that just needed this little necessary attention to steady the spindles, keep them from rattling and make them as good as new

2

It is hard to convince some minds of the value of conserving the teeth. Take, for instance, the fellow who despised the dentist that charged him fifty cents for popping out his tooth so easily, and lauded the tooth carpenter, who charged him only a quarter for dragging him all round the room for half an hour—he could realize the value received. There are unfortunately too many of this class yet. No reasoning has any effect on them ; their minds are too obtuse ; the only way to reach their brains is to give them a large amount of punishment for a small amount of pay; in other words, humbug them.

Brieflets.

By STANLEY BURNS, L.D.S., Smith's Falls.

Often in putting in plastic fillings, especially where objection is taken to the use of the rubber dam or napkins, it is found very difficult to keep the cavities dry. The following method will be found very convenient under such circumstances : First, heat a small piece of impression compound, then dry off the gums surrounding the teeth to be operated on by means of a pellet of cotton saturated with alcohol ; with the thumb and forefingers force the compound over the teeth. It is well to mark on the compound the exact point where the cavities lie. Having done this, while the compound is yet soft, cut out that which overlies the cavities. Carefully remove the *debris*, and it will be found that the lingual or palatine wall (as the case may be) remains intact, in compound. Should any trouble exist in getting the compound to remain in position, better attachment may be had by drying off the gum, and painting it over with copal-ether varnish. This will dry very quickly and adhere firmly.

In the above method the irritation to the sensory nerves is not so great as in the use of either the rubber dam or napkins. Greater freedom is given the patient to swallow the rapidly increasing flow of saliva, and, above all, the advantage in having the palatine wall built up so easily and perfectly, alone repays. If much space exist between the teeth, a portion of compound may be left to act as a matrix between two fillings.

Often after a black rubber plate is polished, it presents a very inferior color—a grayish black. This may be removed by the application of carbon bisulphide. Dampen a cloth with the solution and rub the plate vigorously wherever required. It is well to wash the daubing thoroughly after the use of this solution, as there might otherwise be a tendency to nausea.

Often while grinding down a root for crown or bridge work, it has been found inconvenient to keep the corrundum stone wet. A simple method is as follows : Take the syringe usually found on the operating table, fill it with water ; loop a small rubber band through the ring on the end of the piston, and pass your little finger through the remaining loop ; grasp the syringe well up to the nozzle, and cause pressure to be brought to bear on the piston by drawing forward the finger which is through the loop, thus causing the elastic band to tighten. By this means the operator can cause the water to drop or flow, as desired. By correctly holding the syringe, two fingers will remain free to assist in holding lip, etc.

It may often happen, and too frequently does, in cases where anæsthetics are administered for extracting, that the operator is confronted with a case of hæmorrhage when least prepared for it. A ready and effective method of arresting the unnatural flow is found in tearing off a piece of sponge large enough to fill the wound. Force it into the cavity, and let it remain until such a time as to be thoroughly satisfied that there will not be a recurrence. It is better to dampen sponge in warm water which has been made antiseptic. Owing to its absorbent nature, the free admittance of air through the pores ; together with the ragged edge presented, a clot is immediately formed.

Preliminary Education for Dentistry.

By L. D. S., Toronto.

It does not need much discernment to discover that to-day a high standard of preliminary education is desirable for entrance to the liberal professions. We wish dentistry to rise to this rank. No matter to what extent we extend the curriculum of scientific and practical study, we simply make it ridiculous if we do not exact some much higher preliminary standard than a common school education. It is no reproach to dentistry in the past that we have good operators who could not pass even the examination of a common school, much less that of a university ; but few of these men are prepared to defend such ignorance as a passport to the profession to-day. It is to our credit in Canada that our universities in law and medicine, as well as our boards of examiners in dentistry, require a classical and mathematical course as preliminary ; but in dentistry it did not begin early enough, and some very good men as practitioners graduated as bell-boys and sweepers of the door-step. I say this to their credit in one sense, yet I do not hesitate to declare that it should not be, and that as a rule it will be found, that whatever obstruction and particular annoyance we have had in our progress, can be traced directly to the " beggar on horseback " conceit and crankiness of this class. It was found to be so in other professions until a stiff preliminary was enacted. During some years' residence in the States, I learned this to be the fact in connection also with medicine, and a wonderful social and moral change has occurred by its exaction in the universities of Pennsylvania, Cornell, Yale, Princeton, Lake Forest and North-Western Universities, Johns Hopkins and the University of Wisconsin. The universities of Ontario and Quebec have always had a standard equal to that required of the universities of Oxford, Cambridge, Durham, Edinburgh, Glasgow, and Dublin, even when there was none whatever of a classical and mathematical character in the United States. For instance, the College of Physicians and Surgeons, even of the old Province of Quebec, quite deterred me ten years ago, by sending me in reply to a request, a programme of the preliminary examination, requiring as obligatory subjects three authors in Latin, three in French, first three books of Euclid, also the measurement of the lines, surfaces and volumes of regular geometrical figures; algebra, including fractions and simultaneous equations of the first degree, with English, *Belles Lettres*, history (ancient and modern), geography, and one of the three following as optional subjects— Greek, Physics, Philosophy. A sound knowledge of the grammar of the languages was required. Failure in Latin, arithmetic, or the mother tongue involved rejection. For a time this was the standard required to enter dentistry, but it was somewhat modified.

In Ontario to-day, candidates for the degree of Doctor of Dental Surgery must pass the examinations prescribed for matriculants in the Faculty of Medicine in the University of Toronto, unless they possess a degree in arts from a recognized university, have already matriculated in the Faculty of Arts, or the Faculty of Law, or the Faculty of Medicine, are matriculants in the College of Physicians and Surgeons of Ontario, or have passed the 1st, 2nd or 3rd class departmental non-professional examinations in which the Latin option has been taken.

The facilities for obtaining such preliminary training, especially in Ontario, are better than ever, and I plead for it with all the emphasis possible. The social character of a profession has great weight in a community. I cannot pretend to explain it, but my observation of residence, both in the United States and in Canada, leads me to the conclusion, that if the bell-boys want to be dentists, and there is no reason why they should not so aspire, they should be first compelled to prepare for entrance by a thoroughly good preliminary education.

Furrowed Enamel.

By B.

An interesting case of furrowed enamel came under my observation some time ago. It was that of a boy aged fifteen. From the gingival margin to about half way down to the cutting edge of the six front upper and lower teeth, the enamel was perfect. Beyond that line the grooves ran across each tooth; the cusps of all the cuspids were absent. Throughout the grooves there were pits and notches. The four first permanent molars were entirely devoid of enamel and no appearance of their cusps.

I learned the history of the case as follows: The child was vaccinated by a nurse when two months old, with vaccine from a syphilitic subject. No hereditary taint in either parent. The sore was like that of chancre, ending with secondary syphilis. The child had eruptions for over twelve months. Of course, it is easy to understand how the enamel development would be arrested from lack of nutrition in the enamel organ. Such cases of arrested development from scarlet fever, etc., are not rare. This is the only case I ever met, due to the cause mentioned, and the history of which is so perfectly clear and reliable.

Septic Infection from a Bur.

By W. GEO. BEERS, L.D.S., Montreal.

An illustration of the danger of "dirty dentistry" came within my observation the other day. A young lady in perfect physical health, and whose mouth was as fresh and sweet as a rose in June, was having a lower molar, cervical cavity, prepared by a dentist, who not only used a rickety old engine, but whose burs were so blunt that he had to put on extra pressure to make them cut!

Twice one of the largest burs slipped out of the cavity, tore the gums, and plunging into the mucous folds lying between the tooth and the cheek, revolved there several times before it could be withdrawn. The patient was dismissed after the cavity was filled, without the least attention being paid by the operator to the wound he had inflicted.

Upon questioning the lady, I learned that she had an intelligent appreciation of what to expect from clean and careful treatment; but that quite accidentally she had fallen into the hands of one of the most careless operators, so far as antiseptic precautions were concerned. She remarked that his burs were standing erect out of a small stand, and that she noticed the one which slipped was so covered with white *debris*, evidently of the last tooth in which it had revolved, that its teeth were invisible; that she drew the attention of the operator to this fact before he used it, and that he simply dipped it into cold water and wiped it on a soiled napkin.

About twenty-four hours after the accident the gum in the vicinity became tender and turgid. The face was swollen, the inflammation extending along the inferior maxillary, involving the depressor anguli oris, etc.

The inflammation facilitated the ingress of pathogenic bacteria, which are frequently, if not always, present in the mouth, on the *qui vive* for abrasions and wounds, and the consequences followed. The integrity of the gingival margin had been ruthlessly destroyed by an infected instrument, at a point where the epithelium is composed of more delicate cells than elsewhere. A better invention to infect the muscular folds adjacent could hardly be made than a revolving bur covered with matter for inoculation. The day following I saw the case. To be brief, I made deep incisions directly into and across the place where the bur had entered, with a fine lancet, then syringed fully and freely a four per cent. solution of carbolic acid, as hot as the patient could bear it, and packed the wound with absorbent gauze soaked in the solution. The following day I syringed thoroughly with hydrogen peroxide, which was followed by abundant effervescence. The gauze had kept the wound well open, and the syringing with the peroxide did not, as it might if the orifice was small, distend the tissues and partially close the opening. To accomplish this, the lancing was thoroughly done. The next day I treated the case with pure oil of cinnamon on strips of gauze followed by hot water injection. The patient complained twice of scalding. On the eighth day the normal signs returned; the patient in the meantime had syringed every day with a mild antiseptic wash. What at first appearance seemed to prognosticate a dangerous case of septicæmia disappeared under the treatment. The constitutional disturbances were so severe that the patient lost eleven pounds weight, and though convalescent, is still under the care of the family physician.

There may be pathogenic micro-organisms present in the mouth which do no mischief until the soft tissues are wounded—a simple abrasion may be sufficient. It is a fact that there are foul conditions of the mouth, in spite of which bacteria and the patient thrives. It is not the presence of pathogenic bacteria we have to fear, but the wounds which give them ingress. Vaccine will not inoculate *per se*—the scratch or scrape is needed. It is clear that dirty instruments cannot always be the cause of blood infection in the mouth. We may see displays of dirt on instruments, napkins, headrests spittoons, on the person of the dentist, which one would think the law of self-preservation would alone prevent. Some dirt seems to be healthy. But in spite of the immunity which the power of resistance in the tissues offers to dirt and disease, we never know when dirt may mean death. It is, no doubt, oftener kin to it than we discover. The case I have cited was not one of septic infection from pathogenic bacteria. It was an unmistakable case of direct septic infection from a dirty dental instrument.

Proceedings of Dental Societies.

Odontological Society of Chicago.

At the regular meeting of the Odontological Society of Chicago, held at the Chicago Athletic Club, on Tuesday evening, December 19th, 1893, the following officers were elected for the ensuing year : W. V. B. Ames, President ; C. N. Johnson, Vice-President ; Louis Ottofy, Secretary-Treasurer ; C. S. Case, Curator ; Board of Censors, P. J. Kester, A. W. Harlan, J. W. Wassell.

LOUIS OTTOFY, *Secretary.*

Selections.

"No American Need Apply." Why?

By WILLIAM H. TRUEMAN, D.D.S., Philadelphia.

The subject of the opening paragraph of the editorial in the August number of the *Dental Review* (Vol. VII., 1893, page 692), deserves more than a passing notice. Assuming the statements therein made to be correct, it may, perhaps, tend to a better understanding of the matter to consider, dispassionately, the causes that have led, or that may be leading, to the exclusion from foreign countries of Americans desiring to practise dentistry.

If this exclusion is alone based upon the desire to shut out competition, it is certainly no discredit to the foreign countries adopting it, and equally no reflection upon our system of dental education. We, as Americans, have no reason to complain. It is no more, indeed, than the application and adoption of a national policy, that of protection to home industries, which the United States has always adhered to, and to which it owes much of its prosperity.

As long ago as 1867, a friend and classmate of mine was refused the right to practise dentistry in a town of Switzerland. He was told when he applied to the authorities for the required permission, that a few years before they would have been very glad to have had a well-qualified dentist settle in their midst, but that at that time, several young men, natives of the town, were practising dentistry, after having, at a large expense, qualified themselves therefor by study abroad, and it would be, they felt, an injustice to them to encourage foreign competitors. We see in this incident, I think, the key to the whole matter. There was a time when the American dentist was welcome anywhere and everywhere. He introduced a new industry, or so many improvements upon an old one, that he was welcome to the people who needed his service and equally so to his professional brethren, who found in him an instructor fully equipped and ever ready to communicate.

To the exclusiveness of the Old World he was a stranger. His value as an instructor was evidently appreciated by our British brethren, when in reorganizing their profession in 1878, "for the time being," they decided to recognize the diplomas of two American dental colleges.* This incident is significant when it is remembered that it was done on the representations of British dentists, and that no British subject intending to enter the dental profession could take advantage of it.

Within a comparatively recent period two events have occurred, each having, no doubt, a bearing upon this matter. First, the name, "American dentist," has become the trademark of quacks and charlatans; another instance added to the many, where "the livery of heaven has been stolen to serve the devil in." A second and more important factor is, however, that the American dentist has lost much of his former usefulness to our friends abroad. Largely through his influence foreign dentistry has reached a higher development; natives of these foreign countries have become earnest and apt dental students. They have learned of their American brother many of his practical ways. They have organized, and well organized, too, dental colleges of their own, in their own native lands. They have so well learned from him his practical lessons, that being now prepared to teach they feel able to "go it alone."

Now, it is not natural, right, proper nor just, for any country that has within its borders organized schools where dentistry is

---

*See the report of the General Medical Council, England. *The Journal of the British Dental Association*, Volume XIV. (June 15th, 1893), page 428. Also *British Journal of Dental Science*, Volume XXXVI. (June 15th, 1893), page 562.

taught, schools which have adopted a curriculum satisfactory to the powers that be, the said schools depending largely upon native students for support, to so frame their laws as to encourage, or, if need be, to compel those desiring to qualify for the practice of dentistry in their midst to patronize them ? Patriotism certainly suggests this. American dental colleges have so long had the whole world for their parish, and homage to (so-called) American dentistry has been so general, that it may be to each a rude awakening to find that there are other Richmonds in the field, Richmonds, too, that are likely to stay. We are thus reminded that the world moves.

We thus see that the seed sown by the pioneers who inaugurated a new order of things in dental education at Baltimore in 1839, has been scattered far and wide. That which fell upon a sterile soil and has long lain dormant is beginning to grow, and is likely to produce upon far distant shores abundant fruit. What if it should seem like bread cast upon the waters ? Why complain ? Let us have faith in the promise that in due time it will return unto us again. In the meantime, what matter if it does seem like a little loss of prestige, a little curtailment of business opportunities, are we not a *liberal* profession ? Are we not devoted *solely* to the relief of suffering humanity ? Is not this action of these foreign countries an official recognition of the value of an educated dentist's services ? Let us therefore rejoice and be glad, in that our beloved profession has thus won for itself so prominent a place among peoples that were but a few years ago dental missionary grounds, where the fields were white unto the harvest, and the educated laborers few and far between.

I am firmly impressed that with this exclusion our system of education has absolutely nothing to do. Within a few days, in conversation with an American dentist long resident in Paris, I was informed that throughout continental Europe there has been growing gradually of late a less cordial feeling toward foreign residents, especially those engaged in business, not, however, particularly directed toward Americans. This less cordial feeling toward foreigners is not, however, confined to Europe. It is also present here in the United States. Our far-seeing statesmen are regarding with anxious thought this question of restricting immigration, and it seems to be generally admited that in the near future the national legislator will be compelled to take action upon it. With us at present, so far as the question has developed, we have excluded *absolutely* the more humble subjects of a single nationality only. The idea more generally advanced seems to be, to at first restrict the immigration of the so-called lower or labouring classes ; simply from the fact that with us at present their competition is more markedly felt. But once any nation begins to close its doors to those from other nations whose labor conflicts with native labor, rest assured that if the restriction proves to be profitable and politic, it will be applied to any and every calling where the competition exists. These class distinctions are purely artificial ; any and everyone belongs to the working classes who is leading a useful life, whether wielding a spade, a pen, or a plugger ; by brawn or brain.

The writer of the editorial referred to suggests "our faulty system of education" as a possible cause of this exclusion.

Now, what is the matter with our system of dental education, I would like to know ? I do not agree with the writer of the much discussed circular issued by the World's Congress Auxiliary of the World's Columbian Exposition when he says "that the history of modern dentistry is covered by two generations"; nor yet when he asserts that "scientific dentistry had its birth in the United States of America." He was certainly misinformed, or was indulging in a little questionable " spread-eagleism." I take it that scientific medicine and scientific dentistry are twins ; born of humanity's needs ; they have been nurtured by all civilized races, and in all climes ; the land of their birth, however, it would be difficult at this time to determine. There was, however, inaugurated at Baltimore in 1839, by the organization of a distinct dental college, a new system of dental education that was preëminently American, in that it was preëminently practical. It was really a manual training school, whose scholars were taught the art of dentistry and all that rightly pertains to it. The making of and the use of instruments and appliances used in dental surgery were, in its workshops and operating rooms, practically and systematically taught. This system of dental education, having for its object, and its only object, the making of skilful, practical dentists, commenced in Baltimore in 1839, has been, in every reputable American dental college since organized, adopted, developed and improved, so that it has come to be known as the " American System of Dental Education." Its practical advantages over the older methods then in vogue, were so quickly recognized that within a decade the fame of American dentists began to be world-wide, and in consequence American dental colleges soon drew students from every civilized nation of the globe.

Now, what was the matter with this system ? Can we justly call a system faulty that produces so astounding a result?

The practical success of this system has caused its adoption in whole or in part in perhaps every institution where dentistry is taught. There has, since 1839, been a mighty shaking up of dry bones in the old educational centres of Europe in consequence of this innovation, and in their midst excellent schools have been organized, either as distinct dental schools or in connection with medical institutions. As yet they seem to be, to use a familiar American phrase, " new industries that need government protection from foreign competitors."

Their course of instruction, particularly that of our British brethren, seems to be unnecessarily cumbersome, in that they require a great deal that is not now, and is not likely to be to the average dentist, of the slightest practical value, making the prescribed course inordinately expensive and time-wasting, without adding any corresponding advantage. The only real test of any system of instruction is the result. The real value is not in the cash it costs, nor yet in the time consumed, as the writer of the remarks attached to the memorial sent in to the General Medical Council of England, May 29, 1893, seems to assume ; nor yet in the multiplicity of studies imposed. The real practical question is, which system produces the best dentists ?

Theoretically, a man thoroughly educated, one who has successfully passed the course of studies embraced by the curriculum of a well-appointed college, should make the most promising dental student. That is the ideal towards which the profession seems to be urged. If I understand the question at issue, the supposed faulty part of our dental educational system is, that the American dental colleges do not demand this preliminary education to so great a degree as do those of some other countries.

Now comes the question. Is the theory correct? Have those who, preliminary to entering upon a course of dental instruction, have graduated from a literary college made the best students? Have they, after their professional graduation, made the most skilful dentists? Have they shown their superiority by better work for their patients? Have their greater intellectual attainments made them more useful in advancing professional knowledge, and made them more helpful to their professional brethren ? This is the real practical test.

Without further enlarging upon this, which is merely incidental to the subject under discussion, permit me to say : So long as I find that to the ingenuity and skill of dentists educated in American dental colleges, we, as a profession, are so largely indebted for the most useful of our labor-saving appliances, improved instruments, more successful methods of operating and best examples of individual manipulative ability ; so long as the graduates of American dental colleges continue to be so pronounced a factor, as they have been, in the marvellous advance of dental science in all its departments ; so long as they hold their own so nobly as they now do, as successful and useful original investigators, so long will I most earnestly contend that the colleges and the system of education in vogue therein which has made these men what they are, cannot justly be disparaged by Medical Councils, Dental Societies, or State Dental Examining Boards.

From the fact that the dental journals of Great Britain so largely depend upon writers who are graduates of American colleges, and the further fact that the graduates of the English system, so far, show no evidence that they are to any appreciable extent supplanting their American brethren as leaders of dental thought, I am impressed that a system of dental education in which the students are selected, the course of studies prescribed, and qualifications passed upon by a medical council containing not a single dental practitioner, is not proving so great an improvement that we need hasten to adopt it.

It needs no " reading between the lines," however, to plainly see that the reflections upon the American system of education in the memorial presented to the Medical Council of England and the discussion thereon, were a mere palaver. The resolve to refuse registration to the diplomas of Harvard and Michigan Universities was a simple act of justice too long delayed. They were in a dilemma—they had to either refuse all or admit all; it was a simple business proposition—they had to either shut off this foreign competition or let their own colleges go to the wall, and they chose the wiser course.

The whole matter the world over is simply one of business. It is being considered by business men from a business standpoint, and will be settled on business principles. Business is business—we may denominate our calling " sacred," as does the divine, or contend that *ours* is a highly exalted liberal profession; it is nevertheless a part and parcel of the world's business, resolutions of the dental societies to the contrary notwithstanding.—*Dental Review*.

Correspondence.

A Dominion Dental Association.

To the Editor of the DOMINION DENTAL JOURNAL:

SIR,—In Vol. I. of your journal you gave good reasons, editorially, why your suggestion of a Dental Society for the Dominion should be established, based upon the plan of the Canadian Medical Association, the British Dental Association, and the American Dental Association. I think the time is now ripe, because the dentists of all the provinces are incorporated by provincial acts, and local organizations already existing make it easier to organize one larger body for the Dominion, which would not have power in any way to disturb local legislation, but which would help to harmonize our position. Local societies are valuable; provincial societies are necessary ; but a society embracing all these would broaden our interest, and strengthen us as a body. It would give us a greater pride in our Dominion that we should all meet, say, in Kingston or Toronto, and that the brethren from the Pacific should shake hands with those from the Atlantic. The proceedings would be valuable and important. I would suggest that you issue a card to every dentist in the Dominion soliciting opinions on the subject, and that you publish the result.   PACIFIC.

[We will discuss the matter in a later issue. In the meantime we will be glad to hear from those interested.—ED. D.D.J.]

Reviews.

Surgery. By BERN B. GALLAUDET, M.D., Demonstrator of Anatomy and Clinical Lecturer on Surgery, College of Physicians and Surgeons, New York, Visiting Surgeon, Bellevue Hospital, New York, and CHARLES N. DIXON-JONES, M.D., Assistant Surgeon, Out-Patient Department Presbyterian Hospital, New York. Being the final volume of The Students' Quiz Series, edited by BERN B. GALLAUDET, M.D. Duodecimo, 291 pages, 149 illustrations. Cloth, $1.75. Philadelphia: Lea Brothers & Co., 1893.

This is another of the Students' Quiz Series and one of the most complete in its condensed form. Careful editorial supervision has marked the entire series, of which this is the end.

A Practical Treatise on Mechanical Dentistry. By JOSEPH RICH-ARDSON, M.D., D.D.S. Sixth edition. Edited and revised by GEO. W. WARREN, D.D.S. 600 illustrations. 662 pages. Phila-delphia : P. Blakeston, Son & Co., 1012 Walnut Street. 1893.

This book has become a recognized standard. Dr. Warren has happily undertaken to do for the work of the late Dr. Richardson what Dr. Gorgas has so ably done for that of Chapin Harris. " Useless methods and obsolete theories have been eliminated, thus keeping the dimensions of the book convenient and compact. Much of the text has been re-written, notably the section on crown and bridge work—a volume in itself; it has also been newly illus-trated, bringing the treatise fully up to the time of its publication."

Those who are not acquainted with the work may need to know that the contents are quite up to the mark. Part I. comprises eleven chapters on the metals employed in the laboratory, with observations on fuels and the appliances used in generating and applying heat. Part II. A complete description of artificial dentures, from the treatment of the mouth preparatory to the insertion of plates, etc., to the completion of the most complicated mechanism, in all bases in use, partial, complete, crown and bridge work.

The men who love to boast that they are not theorists, who flatter themselves that practical men need no theory, will discover that even in mechanical dentistry the best practice is based upon sound theory. It is unnecessary to say that the most skilled practical man will find herein much to learn. For students preparing for examination this work is indispensable.

The Hermit of the Nonquon. By Dr. C. N. JOHNSON. Chicago and New York : Rand, McNally & Co., Publishers. Price 50 cents.

We have always believed that, as a general rule, it is the busy men who do the best work. Our readers will be pleased to learn that our friend, Dr. Johnson, has made time, from the western rush of professional life in Chicago, as Professor of Operative Dentistry in the Chicago Dental College, co-editor of the *Dental Review*, active officer of several societies, etc., etc., to give us a story of the Canadian backwoods, true to life and racy of the soil and river. No doubt personal predilection is generally accused of actuating the opinions of a critic. It is a fact, however, that personal knowledge of an author gives a zest to the perusal of anything he writes, and for this reason, if for no other, the story before us should meet a warm welcome from Canadian dentists, and especially from those of Ontario, among whom Dr. Johnson is well known as a brother licentiate and a willing helper.

For the nonce let us forget the doctor's personality, and whether he is a friend or a foe, a white man or a nigger.

Each chapter is a perfect picture in itself, yet the story of Gabrielle, and the other interesting chapters of the Nonquon River are woven into a continuous and picturesque whole, which makes the reader wish the author had made the story longer than the volume of two hundred and thirty-five pages. Those who are familiar with the characteristics of French-Canadian life and character will recognize Dr. Johnson's fidelity in the portrayal of Pierre, whose broken English and *patois* is true to life. It is just such a picture of every-day village and country life as may be met with in the neighborhood described by the author—a mingling of races, each retaining their own idiosyncrasies ; while the curious story of " The Wild Man," which runs throughout the tale, and the strange *denouement* has a touch of originality worthy of any of the best writers of America. Briefly to mention a few of the chapters will perhaps induce our readers to make it one of their

first purchases of the New Year : The Indian and the Fish, The
Villagers, The Wild Man, A Big Catch, A Cradling Match, A
Battle with Turnips, The Deer Hunt, A Horse Trade, Searching
for the Wild Man, Pierre Dufresne, An Old-Time Revival, The
Country Tavern, Hunting for Tamarac Gum, Pierre and the Wild
Man, Back to Life, etc.

And who do you suppose was the wild man? You could never
guess until you had nearly or quite finished the story. The tale
is not only a clever conception, well told and well written, but it
is a positive indication that it is only the first of others to follow,
which will make us as dentists proud of the literary as we are
proud of the professional distinction of our friend and confrere.

Catching's Compendium for 1893. $2.50. Look out for it!
The gist of the practical matter of all the journals for 1893! In
its fourth year. Order it now direct from Dr. B. H. Catching,
Atlanta, Ga., U.S. It will be out early next month.

Editorial.

Didactic Lecturing.

The arguments *pro* and *con* as to the value of purely didactic
lecturing have been well threshed. There are dentists who boast
that they are "practical men," who make cover for their crass
ignorance by pretending to sneer at theory. They fancy they
annihilate a confere when they speak of him as a theorist. It never
occurs to them that however practically skilful they may be, they
are as arrant empirics as a practising physician who knows nothing
of materia medica, but who relies entirely upon the apothecary; or
the surgeon who would undertake to remove a maxillary without
ever having dissected one. Practice without theory is unscientific.
The purely "practical" dentist is nothing but a mechanic, and that
is his proper place. He may be a very respectable mechanic, but
he is only that and nothing more. To call such a man a "doctor"
of dental surgery is to juggle with titles.

What is the matter with didactic teaching? It is difficult to
illuminate scientific lectures so as to keep the attention of the
weary student, and it has often occurred to us that something
might be done, apart from the introduction of clinical and experi-

mental demonstration in the lectures, to secure more co-operative interest.

It is probable that, as a rule, the lectures are too scientific, embrace experience that no student has possessed, and are delivered with such haste or in such a manner as to go in one ear and out of the other. In fact, the subjects often, and the matter always, are sprung upon the students.

We have been trying a change which so far has had very satisfactory results. There is no pretence as to its originality, but we do not know where else it is used. Briefly, it is this : The subject of the lecture having been announced on a previous day, a series of from twenty to thirty questions are first read to the students embracing the lecture to be immediately delivered. The lecture is then given as usual, and at the end the list of questions is given to each student. When the usual " grind " comes on there is no excuse for unpreparedness if the student does his duty half as well as the lecturer. There is deep interest and investigation shown as the result of this system of theoretical teaching. It establishes reciprocity of inquiry between student and lecturer, and in cases where the student has to appear before a separate Board of Examiners to obtain a license to practise—as in Canada—the list of questions of each lecture could be sent to the Board before whom the students must appear. It is a very ancient axiom that any fool can ask questions which wise philosophers cannot answer; but after such a system of mutual study, embracing all the branches demanded, it must be the fault of students themselves if they fail to reach the standard required to pass.

Idle Teeth.

" Everybody knows " that teeth having no antagonists, elongate in course of time, and even loosen and fall out. Teeth which have only half an antagonist are apt to alter their position. Those which are perfectly free of caries and in perfectly healthy histological surroundings not only elongate, but exhibit recession of the gums, and in time all the worst results of caries. Satan finds mischief for idle hands to do. Nature seeks to be rid of idle teeth. Give them something to do and Nature forgives them if the idleness has not become chronic. It is easily possible to fill all gaps in either maxillary. It is important to do so. Teeth which have become tender in the pericementum regain their normal state when they get occupation. As our antagonists in life's struggles strengthen us if we have any pluck, so teeth are helpers when they articulate properly.

" Dental Parlors."

We have " church parlors," " tonsorial parlors," " wine parlors," and " dental parlors." The wine parlors carry a man to the devil more smoothly and speedily than the lowest rum shop. The church would go to the devil, too, if the New York clergymen who want to sell whiskey at cost price under the ægis of the Apostolical Succession, could have their way. Even Judas would have hanged himself rather than have sold wine to the chief priests and elders : but we have ordained apes who seem to have

> " Stolen the livery of the court of Heaven
> To serve the devil in."

However, the " church parlor " is not intended for the " church saloon"; but turn and twist it as you may, the " dental parlor " is the very essence of vulgarity, a pretentious and plausible trap to catch the ignorant and unwary—

> " Will you step into my parlor ? "
> Said the spider to the fly.

It smacks of the saloon, and belongs to the barber. Possibly some men use it, as they put their knives into their mouths and use tooth-picks at the table. They may be saints and go to heaven in spite of bad manners. Ike Walton said he thought it would need more religion to save a gentleman than a beggar at the last day : but pretence and vulgarity and sham on earth can be no sort of preparation for the world to come.

Occasionally a young man beginning practice thinks more of the equipment of his rooms than of his professional knowledge. " All is not gold that glitters " ; yet, it is suggestive of the gullibility of the public, that many people are caught by some extraneous and adventitious " qualification," while perfectly blind to what really constitutes personal and professional ability. We sometimes see large practices built up on a maximum of cheek and a minimum of ability. The " dental parlor " always suggests such a reflection.

The Champion Vulcanizer.

The Champion Vulcanizer was made by Mr. Charles Garth, of Montreal, sixteen years ago, for the late Dr. Webster. We got it from Dr. Webster, with a voluntary guarantee that it was impossible to explode it. Since then several Montreal dentists and quite a number of dentists elsewhere have been nearly killed by explosions, and that of one manufacturer did not differ much from another in their ascension to glory. In various ways they "bust" up by accident, the heat being raised thirty or forty degrees above the vulcanizing point. We have known several blow up at 140°, and carry the top and the flasks through the ceiling. But the Champion of America has been going on steadily for over sixteen years, under the care of a succession of assistants who were fearless of sudden death. At least fifty times we have found the heat up to 210° steam gauge, and the hand only stopped by the pin. Upon one occasion, after fourteen years' service, a boy who was "watching it," noticing that the hand did not move, and not knowing that it had already made the grand tour of 210°, *lifted it over the pin*, and gave it a fresh chance to send him to the happy hunting-grounds. After it had got as far as forty degrees on the second round, it occurred to him that there was something wrong, and having a presentiment of an earthquake, he said a rapid prayer, turned off the gas, and bolted. The Champion was almost red hot with rage, but gradually cooled down. If ever it bursts it will not likely leave a scrap of brass, or copper—or assistant—to tell the tale.

Our Grievance.

People who do a little work ; others who do nothing ; those who are able to work, but who are not willing, as well as those who are willing but not able—everybody seemed to have something to kick about last year. We propose to begin the kicking ourselves for 1894, and we hope that, like a scrimmage in football, it will be taken kindly.

1. As the only dental periodical in Canada, this journal has a prior claim to consideration from Canadian dentists. It would be a reproach to us as a body if we had no such organ of our own. Canadian dentists should subscribe to a Canadian journal first and to any of the others they prefer afterwards.

2. It is the business and duty of secretaries of societies, boards, etc., in each Province to send us prompt reports and the papers of the proceedings, and it should be embodied in the "duties" of these officers. Societies prosper best when these reports are best.

3. We want pithy, practical articles from month to month. If we wanted to insult the poorest dentist in the Dominion, we could not do it better than by accusing him of ignorance of his profession. We know that, as a body, Canadian dentists are eminently practical, many of them quite above the average. One does not need a classical education to contribute a practical fact.

Books.

During the year we receive and review some valuable and interesting works necessary for the wide-awake practitioner. Apart from the purely literary interest which may attract us to books, it is absolutely impossible to know what is going on in the science and art of our profession without them. They save us not only a lot of unnecessary labor, but even a lot of thinking. They do for us what a good many need badly—they teach us the proper use of terms; and they take away the cobwebs from the brain. Even if occasionally they teach error, they stir one to discover truth. The "books for review" which come to us are meant to help students and practitioners. It is impossible for us to do justice to most of them. When only a brief mention is made of such interesting aids as the Quiz Series, it is not to be inferred that they are not as important in their respective line as the larger books specially on dental practice, such as Richardson's Mechanical Dentistry, Miller's Micro-Organism, Mitchell's Dental Chemistry, Gorgas' Dental Medicine, and the valuable works of Tomes, Sexvill, Smale, Salter, etc. We hope that during this year our readers will brush up their libraries, and the older they grow as practitioners the more zealous they will become as students.

"I Guess."

It takes a lot of guessing before one discovers how many beans there are in a quart bottle. But somebody either guesses right, or guesses near it. Still it is pure conjecture.

Sometimes we are disposed to guess that there is a good deal of this random reasoning in our profession : that sometimes very dogmatic opinions are pronounced as to the ætiology, for instance, of pyorrhœa alveolaris, upon no sounder reason or pathology than pure guess-work. Perhaps it does no harm after all, and an ignoramus may blunder upon the truth while a genius is diligently in search of it. Nevertheless, if dentistry and dental pathology are admitted to the rank of scientific professions, we must not imagine that there is a separate and distinct pathology of the teeth and adjacent structures, or that we can ignore the possibility, and indeed the frequent certainty of the constitutional origin of the local diseases we treat. Ætiology and symptomatology need to be more strictly studied in relation to dental disease. The fact is, if we stop to think about it, it is often easier to diagnose upon correct principles, than to guess. Our pathology should not be conducted like a bean-guessing bee.

For "Pillow" read "Pillory."

—

We have long ago despaired of getting every word we write correctly printed. Sometimes the most amusing, and generally the most absurd mistakes occur, and when we look at our own chirography we do not feel like blaming the printer. In the last issue it would appear as if we had invented a new term. Intending to write "pillory us," it appears as "pillow us." May the boyish fun of a good pillow-fight never grow less; but, as between editors over a controversial question, it would be a sight for the gods! It would be more jolly, however, than slinging ink or epithets. The next time we get mad at a contemporary we shall challenge him to immortal combat with solid bolsters.

———

Digging Their Own Graves.

—

The crown and bridge-work fad has put money into the purses of a good many practitioners, but it has dug the graves of some professional reputations. The chief agent of the chief apostle of New York quack advertising, was twice sold out in Montreal by the sheriff, and not only has he decamped, but a large number of pound-foolish people had to eat their Christmas dinners, without the aid of the "unremovable and permanent" bridges which provokingly came to pieces, or loosened, and had to be removed for fear they should be swallowed. But it will not stop the procession. The next humbug will probably find the very same fools to favor it.

———

Our Advertisements.

—

Do you know that the advertisements are in themselves an education? Indeed, a frank friend once told us that he "never bothered himself to read any other part of the journals." He was one of your "practical men," you know. Nevertheless, the advertisements have an important claim upon the interest of every dentist, and they should be carefully examined every month. They comprise a great deal of information which editors cannot supply. We know a dentist who, when having his journals for the year bound, puts the advertisements of all the journals in one separate volume.

Annotations.

A Curious Advertisement.

We are indebted to Mr. Henry Gray, druggist, for the following:

Mr. George Roberts reminds me that I have an old Court and City Register for the year 1752. At the end of the almanack the following curious advertisement appears :—" Artificial Teeth, set in so firm as to eat with them, and so exact, as not to be distinguishable from natural : They are not to be taken out at night, as is by some falsely suggested, but may be worn years together ; yet they are so fitted, that they may be taken out and put in by the Person who wears them at pleasure, and are an Ornament to the Mouth, and greatly help the Speech : Also Teeth are cleaned and drawn by Samuel Rutter and William Green, Operators, who apply themselves wholly to the said Business, and live in Racquet Court, Fleet Street, London." It would be interesting to know what was the price of these teeth, which were " set in so firm as to eat with them, and so exact as not to be distinguishable from natural." The price of the volume was 2s. 6d. with the almanack, and 2s. without it.   WM. SHACKLETON.

The *Western Dental Journal* exposed a fraudulent college in Kansas City, Mo., and asks us to name it. It is the " Kansas City College of Dental Surgery," 1017 Walnut St. The Secretary is J. T. Atkinson. It is a swindle of the first water. We will not charge for this advertisement.

In this connection we have not been asked to draw attention to the fact that the " Kansas City Dental College," of, which Dr. J. D. Patterson is the Secretary, and which has a staff of the best teachers, is one of the colleges recognized by the National Association of Dental Faculties, and in every sense a worthy institution. The little trick of the quack institution in using a name much like the respectable college is an old one. It should be made illegal in any State. Moreover, there is no demand for the multiplication of dental colleges in comparatively small cities. The race of fools who are eager to rush in where angels fear to tread, is not extinct.

It often happens that patients ask us for some temporary remedy to relieve odontalgia. Frequently they need it for children or invalids who cannot be brought to the office. We know very well, too, that the chemists sell a lot of preparations, some of which do more harm than good. It seems, therefore, justifiable for a reliable dentist to supply the public with a reliable preparation. Dr. Henry Ievers, of Quebec city, has prepared a remedy of frankincense and balsam, put up in neat little cases with cotton and a convenient instrument for family use, sold at twenty-five cents. It is supplied to the profession in boxes of half a dozen or more. It is a legitimate and useful thing to have in the house.

We would be grateful if our subscribers would send us such personal items as may interest each other—municipal, legislative, military and other appointments of dentists. Marriages— even if a dentist imitates Dr. W——, and does it four times—will be welcome. Deaths will be unwelcome in one sense, yet necessary in another. A friend once wrote us asking "the present address" of Dr.——, and we stupidly replied by postal card, "Do not know exactly—he is dead."

Without being in any way invidious, we may remark that the leading centre on this continent for practical instruction in prosthetic dentistry is the post-graduate school established by Dr. L. P. Haskell, in Chicago. The Doctor takes hold of college gradu- ates and old practitioners, and after one month's tuition, puts so many new ideas into their heads that they need new hats.

The dentists of Spain met in Madrid, and decided to represent to the Minister of Education, the necessity of reform in dental edu- cation, that the dentists should be accorded by law academic rank, and all the rights and privileges of a profession.

Somebody should bring out a curved needle for the hypodermic syringe. In fact, some other improvements are needed specially for use in the gums.

DOMINION
DENTAL JOURNAL.

| VOL. VI. | TORONTO, FEBRUARY, 1894. | No. 2. |

Original Communications.

Hæmorrhage, Its Ætiology and Treatment.

By W. BELL, L.D.S., Smith's Falls, Ont.

The condition of hæmorrhage is generally described under two heads, viz., that of primary and that of secondary hæmorrhage.

When bleeding takes place from a wound immediately after an operation or injury it is called primary ; when it occurs on reaction from shock or other causes within twenty-four hours, or sometimes longer, it is spoken of as secondary hæmorrhage.

The primary is due to the direct injury to the tissues and vessels; the secondary to the increased force of the circulation during the reaction ; or, perhaps, the most frequent cause met with in the practice of the dentist is the hæmorrhagic diathesis of the patient.

Under ordinary circumstances the free bleeding of a wound or wounds, after the operation of extraction, need not cause any uneasiness. But should the bleeding continue for a prolonged period, there is danger of exhaustion and syncope, and measures should at once be taken to stop the excessive flow of blood.

The effect upon the constitution, of course, varies according to the amount of blood lost ; and is more marked when the blood escapes rapidly than when it flows slowly. When the bleeding is less severe, the face and general surface become blanched and cold, and the lips and mucous membrane pallid, the pulse feeble, fluttering and rapid. These symptoms may end in syncope and convulsions, or the patient may suffer from anæmia or functional disturbances for some lengthened period. Children bear the loss of blood badly, but recover rapidly, while the old stand the loss better, but the effect on their constitution is more permanent.

Sometimes, however, unless the dentist is intimately acquainted with any constitutional idiosyncrasy of his patient, it is extremely difficult to distinguish those subject to hæmorrhagic diathesis from those not so afflicted. In a case of this kind, when there is the slightest suspicion, it is always advisable to inquire whether the patient is subject to excessive bleeding from slight injuries, and thus be able to guard against any trouble. A case in point:

A young man from a neighboring town, a strong, healthy fellow of about twenty-two, was visiting friends here. He called and had a badly decayed superior cuspid and a bicuspid extracted. He bled about the usual amount, and when he left we did not anticipate any trouble. He returned in about two hours so weak that he experienced great difficulty in walking. The face and mucous membrane were pale, head aching, eye languid, and the skin clammy. The wounds had started to bleed shortly after he had left, and had been growing worse all the time. A compress of absorbent cotton saturated with tincture of kramerial and loaded with as much alumen pulv. as would adhere to it, was inserted into each wound. This effectually stopped the hæmorrhage, but the patient was so weakened that it was some hours before he was able to leave the office.

There are a variety of styptics and hæmostatics recommended for the alleviation of hæmorrhage, but our personal experience has been that there is none better than alumen pulv. in combination with some astringent tincture. We consider it superior to the ferri persulph. or the ferri perchlor., for the reason that in nearly every case it accomplishes the desired end, and there is no danger of a slough. In short, it possesses all the good qualities of the iron, without any of its bad ones. Of course we do not mean to say that the tinctures of iron should never be used, for there are cases in which they may be employed very advantageously, but we would use them in the capacity of styptics as a last resort.

Cold is also a powerful styptic. A stream of cold water directed to the bleeding part, or a piece of ice inserted into the wound, is, at times, of great assistance.

Before applying any of these styptics, however, the bleeding part should be wiped out as dry as possible and all coagula removed.

When syncope occurs from loss of blood, do not be too hasty to overcome it, since it is, without doubt, one of the most valuable means Nature employs to check bleeding and assist natural hæmostatics. But the dentist must exercise great caution during the syncope and see that the patient is in no danger.

Beneficial results are obtained from the internal administration of hæmostatics, such as half-grain doses of pil. opii. But opium should never be given when there is any heart trouble. When the hæmorrhagic diathesis exists, iron in full doses is of great service, the tincture of the acetate, or the perchloride in half-drachm doses being the best. Oil of turpentine is likewise a valuable remedy, twenty-minim doses being sufficient for an adult. Gallic acid in ten-grain doses and acetate of lead in one-grain doses are also recommended. All these act upon the blood and dispose it to coagulate.

Reciprocity Between the Dental Boards of the Dominion of Canada.*

By FRANK WOODBURY, D.D.S., Halifax, N.S.

The following statements are only intended to open the question for discussion in this meeting, and do not pretend to be at all complete or exhaustive of the subject, but if our discussion should result in resolutions that will put this association in correspondence with other Dental Societies of the Dominion, my object will be gained.

Every Province now has a Dental Law of some kind, and the profession, from the Atlantic to the Pacific, can be reached officially by correspondence.

Upon examination it will be found that the literary requirements for matriculation as a student of dentistry are very similar in all the Provinces—that the time of studentship does not 'vary much. From three to four years, including college course, is required by every Board in the Dominion.

Ontario and some other Provinces require that students shall be articled to a preceptor under a definite contract. Nova Scotia demands thirty-six months' studentship and requires the certificate of preceptors to prove it.

Nearly all Boards recognize the degrees from a certain number of reputable colleges, which are agreed upon by the Dental Executive Board, and all applicants not possessing these must pass a certain examination, even if holding a degree from a college which is not recognized. This gives the Board practically the power to recognize none, or one, or any number of colleges, yet by not having a common law or reciprocity between the Associations, there are a half dozen other sections of our country where a member of the profession practising in any one, cannot go without undergoing some sort of a professional or matriculation inquisition. Granted that

*Read before the Dental Association of Nova Scotia, September 27th, 1893.

men should be able to meet a certain standard of literary qualification, and the standard should be high enough to guarantee an intelligent professional studentship, and culture enough to provide to
each a mind well trained to think and capable of grasping the profession in its best sense. In no particular lower the standard, but
rather raise it as fast as the facilities for education increase. The
High School is at every young man's door. The State has undertaken to provide the present generation with educational advantages and mental training such as the world has never before seen,
and dental surgery should demand of men now entering it, the
highest necessary preliminary qualifications.

If I am informed correctly, every Board in the Dominion could
agree upon a uniform standard of matriculation without great
change to any curriculum. Now we come to the length and quality
of the term of studentship.

It is my opinion that none of the Provinces exact too long a
period. I thing four years better than three. The physician can
make a greater success on a three years' course than the dental
surgeon can.

There are few occupations that require such continued delicacy
and precision of manipulation, and this can only be acquired by
practice.

Some Boards require that after matriculation the student shall
sign articles with some registered practitioner, and shall by this
ensure attention, and practical tuition in operative and mechanical
dentistry which might not be given him under such a system as
prevails in this province at present. It can readily be seen that
while we require a three years' studentship and ask for proof of it,
in a large number of cases we shall not be able to trace it, and
there will be a great tendency to waste the time between college
terms, with only nominal connection with some dental office. In
Ontario and some other Provinces the student is compelled by his
agreement to spend all his time in either office or college. This
should secure the best results. It gives the college lecture and
clinic and office practice their proper place. We could, with great
benefit to the profession, to students, and satisfaction to ourselves,
adopt this method of articling our young men, and thus securing
the best results obtainable from this branch of student life.

Next comes the college requirements. Nova Scotia recognizes
some thirty dental schools as reputable, and accepts the degrees
from them in lieu of professional examination, but we do not
accept their matriculation examination, because in most cases it is
far below our own standard. Ontario does not recognize *for
practice* the degree from any college, not even Toronto University,
but compels all students to attend a three years' course in the
Royal College of Dental Surgery and confers upon them a license

to practise in Ontario, must produce credentials equivalent to the Ontario standard of matriculation and a diploma from some recognized dental school in order to be admitted, not to practise, but to the senior year of the Royal College of Dental Surgeons of Ontario, and after passing the final examination he may have the title of L.D.S. conferred upon him.

New Brunswick will only admit members of the profession from another Province, after they have been residents of New Brunswick for three months, and have passed an examination before their Board.

These are a few of the distinctive features of some of the provincial laws.

Now, gentlemen, we must not look upon this heap of provincial legislation as selfish means used to save all the patronage for the men in each province. None are intended for offensive warfare, but are walls of protection for the public and profession. They are serving an excellent purpose. This legislation has been indeed a ladder upon which the profession is steadily climbing to its proper position among men. All the Associations have been inspired with the same unselfish motives and noble purposes We understand why our own law exists. Up to this point the various provincial Acts represent a stage in the growth of the profession. Each provincial law has been a centre of crystallization and unification for the individuals in the separate provinces and the amendments from time to time have represented the growth that has taken place. The advance has sounded all along the line, but to make a familiar illustration, these Acts are like the centres of ossification in a molar—fine cusps, good structure, correct in form, but the *sulci* are not complete and show weakness, and are open to attack because not well united. They do not exactly match.

Many of the best colleges have recently extended their course to three years, and *no one* says with truth that their professional training is not excellent. It seems that with proper guards around the matriculation qualifications and office studentship, that graduates from our own or any foreign college should be given the license to practise anywhere they please in the Dominion.

In conclusion, it would seem that if the Associations would rearrange their qualifications for practice that they might agree sufficiently well to be reccgnized throughout the Dominion, it would be a stride in advance, and would give our profession in Canada an *esprit de corps* that would surprise the most sanguine, . and lead to the establishment of colleges of dentistry in various parts of our Dominion, as well as be an object lesson to other countries and some older professions.

Snow and Salt.

By B.

When you have no local anæsthetic convenient, chop up a little ice, or take some snow, mix it with salt, put it in a thin napkin, adapt it to the gums where you want to operate, and after about two minutes' application the gum should be "frozen," and you should be able to extract with little or no pain. In hospital practice, where you want to save poor people pain, this simple application can be used anywhere on the body. I have opened abscesses; I even found it useful in hypersensitiveness of dentine. I constructed a little cup or bowl on the end of a dental instrument for the purpose of carrying the snow-salt and applying it to the gums, but it is easily applied in an ordinary mouth napkin. If a pulp is exposed, close the cavity with cotton before applying the snow-salt.

Why do Vulcanite Upper Plates Crack?

By BREVITY.

1. Because they are too thin.
2. Because they are too thick.
3. Because they are vulcanized too hard.
4. Because they are vulcanized too soft.
5. Because they are badly articulated.
6. Because the *dens sapientiæ* in the process of growth presses too much on the part of the plate which covers the tuberosities of the superior maxillary.
7. Because of the want of lower bicuspids and molars.
8. Because they are not worth a cent at any rate.

Proceedings of Dental Societies.

Dental Association of Nova Scotia.

The third annual meeting was held on the 27th of last September, in Halifax, but owing to various circumstances there were not as many present as at the two previous gatherings. Vice-President, Dr. H. Clay, occupied the chair. The following officers were elected: President, Dr. H. Clay, Pictou; 1st Vice-President, Dr. F. H. Parker, New Glasgow; 2nd Vice-President, Dr. F. W. Stevens, Halifax; Secretary, Dr. Frank Woodbury, Halifax. Executive Committee: Drs. A. C. Cogswell, F. W. Stevens, S. D. Macdonald, J. W. Angwin, J. A. Johnson, Secretary. Auditors: Drs. F. W. Stevens and A. W. Cogswell. The Provincial Board of Nova Scotia consists of Dr. A. C. Cogswell, President; Drs. W. C.

Delaney, J. A. Merrill, H. Woodbury, M. P. Harrington, A. J. McKenna, F. H. Parker.   F. Woodbury, Secretary-Registrar.

The reports of the Board and the Secretary-Registrar were read, which showed seventy-four names on the register.   The deaths of Drs. C. U. Smith, of Halifax ; Jas. E. Crosby, of Yarmouth ; R. W. Macdonald, of Halifax ; and Geo. Hyde, of Truro, were announced, and resolutions of regret and sympathy passed.   Attention was called to a number of dental advertisements in the public prints, which are violations of the Code of Ethics, and a resolution passed disapproving of the same.   Some interesting demonstrations were presented.   The Secretary read a paper on " Reciprocity between the Dental Boards of the Dominion of Canada," which appears among our Original Communications, and after a long and thorough discussion the Association adopted the following resolutions :

Whereas, Believing that the Dental Profession in Canada has arrived at the stage of the development that renders it desirable that the standard of qualification for the practice of dental surgery in each Province should agree sufficiently well to be recognized and endorsed by all other Boards of the Dominion ; and

Whereas, It is the desire of the Dental Association of Nova Scotia to promote this object;

Therefore resolved, That this association hereby recognizes the advantages and necessity of having the qualifications for practice in dentistry in any Province recognized in all other Provinces of the Dominion ; also

Resolved, That the Secretary be instructed to correspond with the Associations of the other Provinces of the Dominion asking them to discuss the question at their next annual meeting and to appoint a representative to meet or correspond with representatives from the other Associations, for the purpose of formulating a standard of qualification to be presented at the next succeeding annual meeting of the Societies for endorsement.

Resolved, That the period of studentship should be increased to four years in this Province, and for the securing of better results and the protection of the students there should be a legal form of articles signed by preceptor and student, and that the Dental Board be authorized to prepare a Bill for presentation at the next session of the Legislature.

Dr. Parker invited the Association to hold the fourth annual meeting at New Glasgow, but Halifax was decided upon.

Vermont State Dental Society.

The next annual meeting will be held the third Wednesday of March, 7.30 p.m., at White River Junction, Vt.   Our Vermont friends always manage to have successful meetings.   A number of Canadian dentists will attend.

Selections.

Teeth Below Medium in Structure.—Their Treatment.*

By Wm. W. Belcher, D.D.S., Seneca Falls, N.Y.

During our last census considerable discussion was had and indignation manifested by certain dentists as to whether or not they should be classed as manufacturers ; whether or not dentistry was a mechanical or a professional calling. The making of a set of teeth is certainly a mechanical operation, likewise the burring out of a simple cavity and the filling thereof with amalgam or gold. But where a careful examination of the mouth is made to determine the best method of constructing a denture ; where the trained eye is called into play to determine the most suitable tooth for the sex and temperament of the patient ; in operative dentistry, where the operation necessitates not only the mechanical act of stopping a cavity, but also calls into play the judgment as to the most suitable filling material for the patient, the tooth, and its position in the dental arch, different cases requiring different treatment, then the mechanical ends and the professional begins. The treatment of teeth below medium in structure, I find, calls for more professional attention than mechanical.

What is the most suitable material for these teeth ? Gold ? How many times in the course of a year you examine mouths studded with soft, frail teeth and find patients completely discouraged ; undecided whether they shall continue to have their teeth filled and refilled, or have them extracted. You examine the mouth and find eighteen or twenty teeth filled with gold in which decay has recommenced around the filling. Of course, they are not *your* fillings ; they were inserted by your competitor down the street. If you are recently graduated, you say, " Fill those teeth with gold, certainly." You talk airily, indiscreetly also, about improper manipulation, and refill with gold. We are sorry for you of course, but more sorry for the patient. If, however, you have been in practice for several years, you have come to the conclusion some time past, that there are other conscientious operators in the world besides yourself, and hesitate for fear of a similar experience. "He who has not discovered cause, has no remedy for effect." To do nothing unless you know what to do, is practice that will be pursued by every judicious practitioner. Can we diagnose the case before us ? I have diagnosed it ; it is a case of incompatibility of tooth structure and filling material. One of the plastic filling materials is called for. What ! not use gold ? Yes, in its proper place ; in

* Read before the VIIth District Dental Society.

teeth above medium in structure nothing compares with gold as a
filling material.   It is as durable when properly manipulated as the
rock on which the man built his house.   Use gold by all means as
a filling material when it is consistent with tooth preservation ; but
in proportion as the teeth fall below the average in density will be
the number of failures with gold, though the greater the skill the
better will be the result.   Our only recourse, then, is a plastic
filling.   We must really descend and become in some degree
" tooth-plasterers."   It is apparent that some are prejudiced against
the use of plastics, to the injury of the teeth, their owners and as
often the claims of the operator.   As the late Dr. Atkinson happily
puts it, " Such a man ought to be prayed with."

The successful utilization of plastic fillings depends as much
upon specific adaptation of means to ends, as does the successful
utilization of gold depend upon manipulative ability.   The plastic
fillings commonly used are amalgam, cement and gutta-percha.
Amalgam is the sheet anchor for the treatment of soft teeth ; it
answers admirably most of the requirements of a filling material,
its color alone making it non-applicable to the anterior teeth.   In
teeth of the lowest scale of density, even amalgam has to take a
second place.   Nearly everyone uses it nowadays more or less.   No
other material has had such a hard struggle for a place in dentistry.
In the early days of amalgam, the better class of dentists waged
war against it on " general principles "—it would lower the manipulative skill and professional standing of dentists.   Time has brought
its own refutation.   Never in the history of dentistry has professional standing and manipulative ability been so high as to-day,
notwithstanding tons of amalgam have been used as a filling
material.   It long ago outlived an inherited prejudice, and we are
now in danger of going to the other extreme of using it when not
indicated.

In filling the teeth with amalgam, the cavity should be prepared
with as much care as with gold ; edges should be beveled and all
angles removed.   When the decay is deep seated and the removal
of the decomposed dentine would expose the pulp, it is excellent
practice to thoroughly carbolize the cavity, cap with gutta-percha
or cement, using great care to have the edges of the cavity free from
decay.   The enamel should be cut away until the edges become
thick and strong.   Always have your patient return in three or four
days that you may polish the fillings with sand-paper and cuttle-
fish disks.   This gives the filling a smooth surface and frees it from
any overhanging edges.   It also adds not a little to its appearance,
as it will not tarnish to the same degree as if left rough.   Another
consideration not to be overlooked is the opportunity to examine
your work at your own leisure.   Now and then you will find a little
fissure you had excavated and in your hurry had forgotten to fill.

Quite as frequently you find in spite of all your warnings and the care of the patient, that while in a plastic condition the filling has been fractured. You now have an opportunity of rectifying all this. It is impossible to properly fill and polish an amalgam filling at one sitting.

A new amalgam which has received considerable attention during the past few years is composed of pure copper and mercury. I have experimented with it during the past four years, and in my estimation it is a material of considerable value. It cannot be used in places in teeth that appeal to the eye, as it discolors badly ; but in soft teeth, where everything else has failed, I have found it invaluable. It is particularly useful in deciduous teeth, being very plastic, and not affected by moisture as other amalgams. I know it is the fashion to condemn this material—" the blackest sheep of them all "—but it has done so well for me, in cases where I had despaired of ever putting in anything more permanent than cement, and had begun to doubt whether the fault was with the material or myself, that I must say a good word for it. One case was that of a young lady for whom I refilled with silver a dozen or more cavities that had been filled a short time before, only to find on her return for professional services six months later thirteen additional places that needed attention, this time not only cavities that had been filled by her former dentist, but also a goodly number of those I had so carefully re-treated. I refilled her teeth, using copper amalgam. A few months ago she was in my office and I had the pleasure of again examining her teeth. Two years had passed since the introduction of the copper ; meanwhile she married and had a child, passing through one of the most trying periods for the teeth. Her health, if anything, was not as good as when I had last seen her, and yet I found but *three new* cavities. Comment is unnecessary.

Another case was that of a lady who had come to the conclusion that nothing could save her teeth, unless perhaps having them filled every year with cement. I found her mouth in a deplorable condition ; decay had taken place around the gold and amalgam fillings ; one of the worst cases I ever saw. I filled several of the worst cases with this material, the others with cement. The result was gratifying in the extreme. At the end of the year I replaced a number of the cement fillings that had worn away with the copper. She returned on a visit to her old home in New Hampshire, and while there had her teeth examined by her former dentist, who had obstinately refused to use the copper amalgam in his practice. The copper amalgam fillings in her mouth convinced him of its value. I received a letter from him some time ago, in which he stated that the amalgam in soft, frail teeth had more than exceeded his expectations. I have used the copper only in teeth far down in the scale, structurally, and am sure that I save many teeth permanently, which I could only hope to temporarily repair with any other material. I am confident that many of the failures in using this material are due to the fact that it is not mixed thoroughly. There is generally enough mercury, and to spare, in the material as it comes from the depots. It is not enough to heat the amalgam until the mercury appears—the mortar and pestal should be thoroughly warmed. Amalgam so treated is plastic in a surprisingly short time.

Cement, as a tooth preserver, stands at the head of the list. As it lasts only from one to three years, it loses much of its value ; still, we occasionally find fillings of this material that have lasted longer, many times in teeth below medium in structure outwearing gold fillings. Great care should be exercised in the use of the phosphoric acid to keep it pure, as it easily absorbs water and deteriorates. The powder, if long exposed, may bring about the same result. It absorbs moisture from the air, like plaster of Paris, and becomes unfit for use. Cement requires the most careful manipulation to obtain the best results ; in fact, next to gold, it requires the most skill of any material used in dentistry. I find a six-sided mixing block very handy when in a hurry, six mixing surfaces instead of the two on the ordinary block.

It is a fact that a given amount of acid only can unite with a quantity of powder sufficient to satisfy its affinity, and if there is an excess of powder, the compound formed is brittle, crumbles and admits moisture freely. Apply the rubber dam, mix the powder and acid until you have a creamy mass, trim as much as possible before it sets, and if you are particular, let your patient read the paper for thirty minutes or more, before removing the dam. Many coat the filling with sandarach or shellac varnish ; but the alcoholic constitutent penetrates deeper than could the saliva and does more harm than good.

Dr. Bonwill has suggested coating the filling with heated paraffine which melts at a temperature lower than wax when heated. He claims to get very good results from its use, saying that it renders the filling and interstices around it impervious to the action of acids. Dr. Flagg suggests a mixture of one part white wax to five parts resin. This simply acts as a protective covering for twenty-four hours. I have tried Dr. Bonwill's method, but have not used it long enough to vouch for its preventing the decomposition of the oxyphosphate. Either method seems preferable to the varnishing process.

One of the most satisfactory methods of filling frail or soft teeth is found in gold inlays set with cement. The work requires time and considerable skill, and is necessarily expensive. By this means, contours can be restored, having all the appearances of gold, with the advantages of cement. For exposed positions, where appearance is an object, this method is *par excellence.* Never attempt to insert and polish an inlay at one sitting. Let the cement harden thoroughly, then make a second appointment for the final smoothing and finishing. Occasionally you find teeth which from the moment of their eruption seem marked for destruction. This is particularly true of the six-year molars, decay often commencing at a dozen different points. The surface of the enamel seems pitted in every direction. I find it easier and less expensive to the patient in the end, to immediately adjust a gold shell covering the whole tooth.

Combination fillings are quite the fad nowadays—combinations of gold and amalgam, cement and gutta-percha, etc. I have found the latter a very satisfactory method. How often we examine an oxyphosphate filling and find it to all appearances perfect, until we discover a pocket along the cervical border, leading directly to the pulp. Gutta-percha is especially valuable here. Place a small pellet at the cervical border of the cavity, finishing with cement. A chlora-percha lining is recommended for the entire cavity before filling with cement, though I have not tried it. Gutta-percha as a permanent filling has a limited field, but it is almost indispensable in cervical or buccal cavities, those exquisitely sensitive points of decay next to the gum. Where it is properly protected, I find it more valuable than gold or amalgam in low grade teeth. In using gutta-percha it is essential that the largest possible portion of both enamel and dentine should be carefully conserved. It is not important that the walls of the cavity should possess thickness or strength—every portion of enamel should be saved. Gutta-percha should always be finished from the centre toward the edges of the cavity. As a final finish, use a moderate amount of pressure to consolidate the filling.—*Odontographic Journal.*

Dental Education.

A large part of the union meeting of the Pennsylvania and New Jersey State Dental Societies was occupied with the important question of education. Dr. Jack's address was scholarly and practical, and we regret that we must merely outline it. Speaking of the professional functions of men, and the high educational requirements for entrance upon a professional career, he shows that the absence of this training is principally responsible for the existence of the pettifogger in law, the quack in medicine, and the fanatic in theology.

"Up to a recent period, nearly all applicants for matriculation were received, and since a preliminary examination has been required, the standard has been of too elementary a degree, and unfortunately is conducted by those who have had the interest to make up as large a class of matriculants as possible."

" The complaint is being made to me, that young men who have been taken as laboratory and office-helpers, without more than the commonest school education, are, after two years of pupilage, entering the ranks of the dental profession. This is one of the degrading influences which have been keeping low the standard of dental education, and have been launching too large a number of poorly fitted novitiates upon the public. If one may, from a common workman with a little knowledge of English, be relegated, in the short period of eighteen months, or, as now, thirty months, to the performance of one of the most difficult and responsible functions, what must be thought by the intelligent members of the community which requires five years for its members to learn properly to do the work of ordinary trades, of a pretended profession which has no higher preliminary standard than the majority of the schools require? How different the result would be in case each student had been required to have, at least, an academic education, or have been subjected to the most rigid tests, by an academic board, *independent of the dental schools."*

Dr. Chas. J. Essig criticized the fairness of State Examining Boards, demanding further examination before practice from holders of dental diplomas, and very clearly exposed the inferiority of such examination to that demanded by the college faculties. He maintained that it required just as high a degree of knowledge to examine students as to teach them ; and the question arose as to the qualifications of some of these examiners. "The present method of examining by state boards is as arbitrary as it is slipshod and superficial. It will not be long before it will become apparent to all who are interested in this phase of dental education, that such examinations should be written ; questions and answers should be in writing, and be placed on record for reference when occasion requires. The questions should be in the handwriting of the examiners, and the answers in that of the candidate."

[It may interest the worthy Doctor to know that this has been the invariable rule in Ontario and Quebec ever since the organization in 1868, and has never been departed from.—ED.]

Dr. Essig stood up bravely for the work of the colleges, and showed that in spite of many difficulties, their faculties, through the National Board of Dental Examiners, and the National Board of Dental Faculties, had lengthened the terms and generally raised the standard of teaching. He deprecated any effort to antagonize the schools and teachers : favored the extension of the time to five years—but " how many students do you think we would have ? " " The commercial side of the question could not be ignored."

Dr. Essig doubted if " any subject in the curriculum can be presented to dental students in a more practical way by well-posted and well-educated dentists than by a medical practitioner. There is a very attractive sentiment embodied in the idea of having the entire faculty of a dental school composed of dentists ; but take chemistry, anatomy and physiology—can these positions be filled with dentists? No. How many of your dental examiners are really competent to examine in these branches. A man cannot take up the study of chemistry successfully in a year, and the same is true of anatomy. He cannot learn anatomy from books ; he cannot take Gray and read it over at sight, and make himself proficient in that branch. You must study anatomy from the cadaver and that takes a long time. One of the leading professors in the chair of anatomy in a dental college, has stated that after he graduated in dentistry he spent seven years in the study of anatomy."

For the Teeth—Some Excellent Rules to Follow in the Care of Them.

One of the most skilful dentists in New York gives these rules for the care of the teeth : Use a soft brush and water the temperature of the mouth. Brush the teeth up and down in the morning, before going to bed, and after eating, whether it is three or six times a day. Use a good tooth powder twice a week, not oftener, except in case of sickness, when the acids from a disordered stomach are apt to have an unwholesome effect upon the dentine. Avoid all tooth pastes and dentifrices that foam in the mouth; the lather is a sure sign of soap, and soap injures the gums, without in any way cleansing the teeth. The very best powder is of precipitated chalk ; it is absolutely harmless, and will clean the enamel without affecting the gums. Orris root or a little wintergreen added gives a pleasant flavor, but in no way improves the chalk. At least a quart of tepid water should be used in rinsing the mouth. A teaspoonful of Listerine in half a glass of water used as a wash and gargle after meals is excellent ; it is good for sore or loose gums; it sweetens the mouth, and is a valuable antiseptic, destroying promptly all odors emanating from diseased gums and teeth, Coarse, hard brushes and soapy dentifrices cause the gums to recede, leaving the dentine exposed. Use a quill pick if necessary after eating, but a piece of waxed foss is better. These rules are worth heeding.

Correspondence.

Friendly Criticism.

To the Editor of the DOMINION DENTAL JOURNAL :

SIR,—I believe much of the reading matter, especially the papers, of our dental journals would be made more interesting and profitable if they were criticized by the readers of the journals.

An essay read before a society often does more good by the discussion it evokes than by the information it may contain.

Many are deterred from writing for their professional journals because they feel that they have nothing new to offer ; while if they would write what they do know, and their papers were criticized in a friendly way, by readers of the journal, the essayist would often profit by it.

These criticisms should not refer to the literary get-up of the papers, for many of us know more than we can properly express.

I have often gained many practical ideas from reading the details of some very commonplace operation. On the other hand, I have often noticed where many of the details of operation described, could be very much simplified.

It would be in such cases where much benefit could be afforded by drawing attention to the paper, and describing the simpler methods.

Kingston, Ont. R. E. SPARKS.

Fees.

To the Editor of the DOMINION DENTAL JOURNAL:

SIR,—When we were first organized in Ontario we had an Association Fee Bill, if I mistake not. We have still at any rate a pretty-well-understood agreement, which I need not refer to in detail, and when we find a dentist making an upper set on vulcanite for $10 beside men who demand $20 or $25, we have to conclude that one of them is a fool or a rascal. The question which one, and which horn of the dilemma will we place him on, is generally solved by personal knowledge. Last week I had a gentleman from Montreal who came to have me insert a filling put in a week ago, which he brought me in a pill-box. It was a dirty, cheap amalgam. When he asked the dentist his fee, the operator replied, " Are you related to ——," mentioning the name of one of the millionaries of Montreal. " Yes, I'm his son, my own dentist is out of town." " Oh ! well, I'll only charge you $5." I understand the regular fee for amalgam in Montreal is $2, and many insert it for $1. Evidently that dentist was both a fool and a rascal.

Now, is it contrary to ethics to have a provincial fee bill, and to fine men who sign it, and who are convicted of breaking it ? A dentist in my own town freely tells his patients, " Oh ! I'm not dependent upon my practice, and therefore I can afford to work cheaply." And yet he has'nt a cent on earth except what he makes in his practice. Yours,

HURON.

[One of the convictions which maturity has brought to us, is the folly of a fee bill. It was never ethical. Moreover, it is never possible. You can combine to sell coals, butter and cheese, but a professional combine to regulate fees would never work until all men were not only equal but honest. The result of attempting anything of the kind would end like the experiment of Charles XII. who after trying in vain to make twelve watches run together, came to the conclusion that it was as great folly attempting to make everybody think alike on matters of religion.—ED. D.D.J.]

The "Dominion Dental Journal."

To the Editor of the DOMINION DENTAL JOURNAL :

DEAR " JOURNAL,"—You have made your New Year call in the shape of a January number of '94. We always appreciate your visits. You used to come but once a quarter : then your visits became as frequent as six times a year, while now you call upon us every month.

You are growing nicely for your age. You are not yet as corpulent as some of your cousins who come to see us. No doubt you would grow faster if those you call upon would give you more five-o'clock teas—something to fill you up.

However, what you do get is wholesome, independent fodder.

I hope you will grow so big you'll bust your "galluses." By the way, your call reminds me that I must send a New Year card, in the shape of a one dollar bill, to your Pa, to help clothe you and pay your travelling expenses, for another year.

Good bye, come again.

Yours truly,   APPRECIATION.

Reviews.

Dental Metallurgy. A Manual for the use of Dental Students. By CHAS. J. ESSIG, M.D., D.D.S., Professor of Mechanical Dentistry and Metallurgy in Dental Department of University of Pennsylvania. 3rd edition, revised. Philadelphia : S. S. White Dental Manufacturing Co., 1893. Pp. 283.

This is one of the valuable little works which has no rival in dental literature. It needs none ; because Dr. Essig has the rare art of condensing a quart of wine into a pint bottle, or, in other words, of putting necessary knowledge into convenient space. It embodies the recent improvements in the production of amalgam, aluminum, iron and steel, and follows the system of spelling and pronunciation of chemical terms as recommended by the chemical section of

the American Association for the Advancement of Science.   It is
sufficiently illustrated for all practical purposes.   The chapter on
amalgam is very complete, including a table of the composition of
some of the well-known dental alloys.   Every student and practitioner will be better off in every sense after they have bought and
read this work.   Any of our Canadian depots can supply it to order.

Editorial.

The Title of "Doctor."

We have always been averse to the use of this title by dentists
who do not possess a medical degree.   When we were first organized in Ontario and Quebec, a few practitioners wanted the
promoters to ask the Local Legislatures for the title of "Doctor"
instead of "Licentiate," but it was so strenuously opposed by the
good sense of the very large majority that it was destroyed at
conception.   In Canada we cannot be accused of hungering after
the title as a purely dental degree, in spite of the fact that patients
persist in dubbing every dentist a doctor, and that a good many
dentists, who have no right to it, allow it to be assumed that they
have.   In conventions and conversations we carelessly address
each other in the same way : while nothing is more common in the
colleges over the border—and nothing rarer here—than to find the
students using it even to the freshmen, if not to the janitor.   When
it was first established by the Baltimore College of Dental Surgery
there were objections made to its separation from medicine, and in
1851, Dr. E. B. Gardette, proposed the abolition of dental colleges,
and substituting for them lectureships in dentistry in each of the
medical schools.   The fact that a large proportion of the dentists,
fifty or sixty years ago, were mechanics and tradesmen who had
picked up ideas and entered practice without any preliminary or
regular dental training, no doubt prejudiced many respectable
men from the advocacy of the title.

At the annual meeting, a few years ago, of the Irish Branch of
the British Dental Association, Dr. R. Theodore Stack, himself a
D.M.D. of Harvard, and an M.D. of Dublin, condemned the use of
the title "doctor" or "surgeon" by dentists, and proposed that the
title "dentist" be prefixed to one's name, as the title "surgeon" in
England.   We should then speak of one another, and be addressed
by our patients as "Dentist Jones," for instance.   It is a title that
does not run glibly off the tongue : but as a destined professional
title it would be as becoming after awhile as to say "Lawyer
Brown," or "Judge Robinson."   We cannot imagine any better
substitute than Dr. Stack's suggestion.

3

In making dentistry a distinct profession, **Dr. Chapin Harris** and his contemporaries were wise in their generation. It was never intended to make a perfectly definite distinction between the primary studies of anatomy, physiology and chemistry, but the average dental student got a mere sessional smattering of these three branches until the National Association of Dental Faculties increased the period of study to three years. Many who fully appreciate the pioneer work of the early men of Baltimore, are yet free to believe, that dentistry would have attained quite as notable progress, without infringing upon a title which at the time was recognized as the exclusive possession of the profession of the physician. How much better, it seems to us, it would have been to adopt some such title as "Master of Dental Surgery," or as in Britain and Canada, "Licentiate of Dental Surgery," and to have left the degree of "Doctor" undisturbed, as a higher title to which students might aspire.

Imagine the oculists and aurists separating themselves from general medical studies, cutting off from their curriculum all that does not pertain specially to the eye and the ear, and claiming that in such a departure the diseases of these two organs would have more thorough study. It would be simply absurd. When the degree of doctor was created in dentistry, our profession was largely mechanical. There were a few men who contended for its constant affiliation with general medicine, but dental pathology and therapeutics were vaguely understood. There was at the time no reason, why the dentist could enter a claim to share in this title on the basis of the slim education which the dental colleges then gave. Certainly we have made great strides. So have medicine and surgery. Yet we can no more pretend to-day than fifty years ago, that we have an equal claim with the original possessors of the degree of doctor to use that title. The fact that there are doctors of philosophy, of science, and of divinity, is no argument, because neither of these encroach upon any branch of the healing art, and it can never be imagined that they assume to possess the doctorate in medicine. No fair argument can be advanced why the dentist educated exclusively along the lines of dental teaching, even in the best of our colleges, should claim a right to use on equal terms, a title which is widely recognized as involving a medical and surgical education of the most comprehensive character.

Anyone familiar with the course demanded of the surgeon in Britain will not question its thoroughness, yet the British surgeon is a plain "Mr." The course of dental studies in Britain to obtain the right to practise is more comprehensive than that required by the National Association of Dental Faculties, yet the British dentist is a plain "Mr." In Canada, after a course of three and a half or four years of twelve months each year, the Board of Examiners have granted the title of " Licentiate " only, and that of " Doctor " emanates only from the University of Toronto. The Legislature of Quebec, only last month, refused the Dental College of the Province of Quebec the right to grant the doctorate in dentistry as an independent college—ignorant of the fact that so many independent colleges in the United States grant it irrespective of universities.

The effort to obtain this privilege was simply to harmonize the requirements of the Quebec school with those of the colleges under the N.A.D.F., which the school in Quebec desired to join. The fact that the D.D.S. was necessary to the College under existing circumstances, does not affect the general principle we are representing in these remarks.

Let us glance at the past history of most of the colleges which have given the D.D.S., and by way of parenthesis, we hope our criticism will not be construed as applicable to the schools since the organization of the N.A.D.F. We can name men by the score who, without any preliminary examination, without even a knowledge of the language in which the lectures were delivered, without any previous practice, and some with less than twelve months' studentship, obtained the degree in one session under six months, in colleges that to-day would not grant it under three years. What value can be attached to such a title so cheaply obtained? It seems to us that the National Association of Dental Faculties would be glad to rid itself of the title, and inaugurate a new one, free at the outset from any suspicion or reproach. It is true that the degree is, as a rule, worthily won to-day. It is equally true that it was unworthily granted for nearly thirty years, and that even when the most deserving men received it after one session, it could not honor them half as much as they honored it by accepting it.

If the N.A.D.F. would empower the colleges to grant another title under the regime of the three years' requirement, with a higher standard of matriculation and recognize it as a superior degree, students would aspire to obtain it, and we in Canada would follow suit. It is rather hard upon Canadian students who, after passing a classical and mathematical preliminary almost equal to the requirements for B.A., and studying for three and a half or four years, find themselves occupying an inferior rank beside scores of doctors of dental surgery who received their parchments after one session of six months. The law of necessity seems to compel the perpetuation of the doctorate in our profession, unless the N.A.D.F. should take the bull by the horns, and not only recognize another title as constituting a legal right to practise, but as one superior to that so long in use. The title originated in the United States, and it is the prerogative of the N.A.D.F. to continue or to supersede it. The latter would best meet our convictions.

Our Manufacturers.

It seems to be an instinct of humanity to disparage if not to denounce manufacturers. It does not matter whether they are cotton kings, sugar kings or tooth kings, we who are consumers are apt sometimes to believe that they get far too big a bite of the bun. There are two sides to this question, but we only fully know our own. We observe that there have been several millionaires made out of dental manufacturers; and it would need a dozen of the most successful dentists at least to make one millionaire. We must remember, however, that every man has his choice, and if he can get the capital and chooses to run the risk, he can become a manufacturer in a month. We may believe, perhaps, that we pay too high for many of our goods, and it is perfectly natural in this age of depreciation and bad pay, that professional men who, perhaps, suffer more than merchants, and who cannot, or do not, attempt to compromise their obligations, should have consideration shown them, and, that when the cost of platina goes down, the cost of teeth should go down, too ; just as the manufacturer expects when flour goes down that his baker will lower the price of bread. The production of quite a number of the necessities of dental practice does not cost as much to-day as ten years ago ; but the selling price has either been increased or remains the same. If we are wrong in this opinion, we are open to correction.

Now, there are many suggestions practising dentists could, if they would, make to manufacturers, which the latter would be glad to receive. We imagine that a number of articles we daily use were not constructed by men in actual practice. Just to name a few : The joints of all forceps made on this continent have sharp edges, and open and close in one of the most ingenious ways to wound the mouth. The joints of the forceps made in England cannot possibly wound the lips. Dental engines and office lathes are made so that if you turn them the wrong way, a screw comes out, and the whole thing is reduced to chaos. We have a new office-lathe, the pedal of which depends for security upon a small pin of steel, and when the pedal slips out of the pin, which it is perpetually doing, the pedal wobbles and the assistant swears. It is a good thing for that pin that blasphemy has no effect upon it. The head-rests— but now we despair. We have waited twenty years for a sensible head-rest, without all the nonsense which provokes patient and operator to distraction, and it is not yet discovered.

Would it not be a good plan and one by which our manu- facturers might profit, for each of the various societies to appoint a committee to report once a year on "suggested improvements?" It is not all the fault of the manufacturers that we have not every- thing just as we would like it ; but committees such as this would not only help the manufacturers, but they would help ourselves, and very soon, perhaps, the former might find that they had received so much material benefit from the scheme that they could afford to bring about the millennium of supplying us with all we want, just as we want it, and at such low prices that some of the next generation of dentists may also get a chance to become millionaires. What a curiosity a man would be who, by entire devotion to dentistry, had become a millionaire?

Official Zeal and Official Reward.

In every profession a spirit of antagonism against the responsible officers of the representative societies is frequently developed. Quacks and impostors regard these officials as their natural-born enemies. Cranks would assassinate them if it was no more illegal than a breach of the dental law. And a great many others who do not know the vexations with which they have to contend, regard them with distrust.

And yet, what does the zeal of the comparatively few in our ranks mean, who are working on Boards in societies, colleges and journals? Does it mean that individual effort is nothing better than individual selfishness? Or is it true that the workers are actuated by an honest desire to improve the professional and moral tone of dentistry as a whole? One thing is true, as surely as a man takes a leading part in education, and shows open hostility to quackery and ignorance, he becomes a target for the mischief-maker. And not only for the mischief of the ignorant from pure "cussedness," but that of the most malevolent of all mischief-makers—the deep, sly, silent enemy, to whom a confrere's success is a personal insult, and who

> "Damn with faint praise, assert with civil leer,
> And without sneering, teach the rest to sneer;
> Willing to wound, and yet afraid to strike.
> Just hint a fault, and hesitate dislike."

Imagine the shame we would feel as Canadians if our progress in dentistry was not proportionate with that of our neighbors. We believe we have proportionately about the same number of men who help and men who hinder. And if some men in both countries had their way, every dentist would be a hermit in his own office, and label his secrets "poison." Somebody must take the lead in associative work, but after all "the post of honor is the private station," and the men who are zealous in the ranks are the men, all things being equal, who merit promotion. It may not be possible always to agree with the actions of the officials. It ought to be possible to believe that their intentions are honest.

It seems a fatality of prominence in any good work to be exposed to a fire of criticism and suspicion. When a man gets his fingers into the public purse ; when he dabbles as a boodler in such dirty business as the politics of Quebec, he can afford to stand abuse. But there is no boodle in the responsibilities of any dental office. When men are zealous in the educational and legislative work of dentistry, it is fair to believe that they are animated by an honest desire to serve the best interests of the profession, just as surely as when men are zealous in the effort to sneak into the profession through special legislative enactment, that they are moved by a spirit of selfishness and a consciousness of their personal ignorance. Busy and honest men have no time to intrigue. Dishonest men have nothing better to do, for all their hope hangs upon the success of their lying. It is a suggestive reflection which ought to be taken to heart by all respectable dentists, that the zeal of one mendacious quack will frequently outweigh and defeat that of a body of honest officials. When the quacks and impostors of dentistry combine for mischief, it is time for all honest practitioners to combine for self-defence.

Dentists in Politics.

Dr. Ed. Casgrain, of Quebec, suggested the idea that we, as dentists, would never get our rights, or be able to obtain proper legislation to protect the public from empiricism, until we brought our profession as a body into politics. In Quebec, for nearly twenty-five years, we have had proficient experience in this line ; but in such isolated and inconsequential detachments, that nobody in the Legislature seemed to be able to afford the time to study what we were driving at, and unless some of our officials almost made their beds in the lobbies, it was impossible to watch the tricks and intrigues of the obstructionist. The only dentist in Parliament is Dr. Ahrens, member for North Perth, Ont. If we had even one in Quebec, we should not be harassed the way we are with tricksters making false representations, and obtaining special privileges denied to men who are willing to enter dentistry by the front door, instead of sneaking in through a hole in the fence. We do not suppose that our brethren in the sister provinces feel the need as we feel it in Quebec. Some day we will give the history of our efforts. In the meantime let us look out for a candidate in our ranks, familiar with both languages, who can afford to devote the time. If we can get him elected for a constituency as an independent candidate, he would serve his constituents as well and us better than if elected on purely party lines. We do not want any of your boodling Mercierites. The Province had one experience of that iniquitous gang. It will be enough for all time to come.

Reciprocity between the Provinces.

Dr. Woodbury, of Halifax, echoes a sentiment at which this journal has frequently hinted. In the suggestion made editorially in the first number of our first volume for the organization of a Dominion Dental Society, it was mentioned that one of the objects would be "to discuss our provincial positions and endeavor to harmonize them," and we are very glad that the first substantial movement has been made down by the sea, and it seems to us that in no way can the object in view be so thoroughly discussed as in a Dominion Dental Society meeting in Toronto, for instance, represented for organization purposes by any number of delegates sent by each province. The proposition could be referred back to the Provincial Associations, and in course of time something practicable could be accomplished. One of the chief difficulties is the great stretch of territory between the Atlantic and the Pacific. Why should not the Maritime Provinces, first of all, complete some unity of legislation on the subject among themselves? The North-Western Province could do the same. It would make it easier of accomplishment subsequently in Ontario and Quebec.

A Pathetic Appeal.

If love or money will induce anyone to send us the following missing numbers of exchanges, we will also acknowledge them in the JOURNAL. Now that the weather is cool, our readers might poke in their garrets for odd numbers, which may be no use to them, but which will enable us to complete the largest dental library in Canada.

American Journal of Dental Science. Vol. 7, No. 5 ; Vol. 8, Nos. 1, 4, 7, 9.

Johnston's Dental Miscellany. Vol. 1, No. 7 ; Vol. 2, October, November ; Vol. 5, May, July ; Vol. 8, May, June, July, August.

The Independent Practitioner. Vol. 1, Nos. 4, 11 ; Vol. 2, Nos. 2, 3, 4, 5, 6 ; Vol. 3, Nos. 1, 2, 3, 4, 5, 6, 8, 9, 11, 12.

Southern Dental Journal. Vol. 4, Nos. 4, 12 ; Vol. 8, Nos. 4, 5, 6, 7, 8, 9, 10, 11, 12 ; Vol. 9, Nos. 1, 2, 10, 12.

Ohio Journal of Dental Science. Vol. 1, Nos. 6, 7, 8, 9, 10, 11, 12 ; Vol. 4, 1, 2, 3, 5, 6, 7, 8, 9, 10, 11, 12.

New England Dental Journal. Vol. 3, No. 11.

We need others by and by. We have a large lot of duplicates which we will exchange.

Annotations.

HENDERSON—THOMAS.—At the manse, 612 Erie St., Port Huron, Mich., on December 12, by the Rev. T. A. Scott, pastor First Presbyterian Church, G. H. Henderson, L.D.S., Elora, to Lucy, youngest daughter of Rees Thomas, Esq., of Thedford, Ont.

ONE of the best measures of the progress of man is the degree of his ability to stand alone, in thought and action, undisturbed, though he may often profit by the adverse opinions and judgments of others. "When the people are a herd they are easily swayed and ruled by one man ; when they are individualized, the dominion of one is not possible." Let us hold, then, and teach that better than great riches and possessions is a brave heart, an enlightened and well-balanced mind, an appreciative, hopeful and helpful soul. Let our labors be a sort of religion, urging us to elevation, seriousness, and chastity of thought and actions.

To quote from Charles Kingsley : "Men can be as original now as ever, if they had but the courage, even the insight. Heroic souls in old times had no more opportunities than we have ; but they used them. There were daring deeds to be done then ; are there none now? Sacrifices to be made ; are there none now? Wrongs to be redressed ; are there none now?"—*International Dental Journal.*

Dr. F. T. Paul recently presented a case before the Pathological Society of London, Eng., in which the patient, a boy aged 5, was born with an irregular patch of skin on the left cheek, near the nose and beneath the inner corner of the eye. Five months before passing under observation, a tooth came to project from the spot ; this was a left upper lateral incisor, and projected from a little red, gum-like tissue ; beneath the tooth was a second, smaller, corresponding with that of the permanent teeth. Neither of the teeth was connected with the superior maxilla. The proper dental arch was well formed, and all the normal teeth were represented in it.

[Several years ago the late Dr. R. P. Howard, of Montreal, asked us to see a similar case. The tooth was a superior supernumerary bicuspid, not fully developed at the apex ; projected below the orbit on the right side, and had no connection with the jaw. The patient felt a hard growth developing for nearly a year. It would have been interesting to examine the histological and microscopical characteristics of such a tooth—containing dermoid from the face—but the patient would not allow it to be touched, and some time afterwards was drowned at sea.—ED. D. D. J.]

DOMINION
DENTAL JOURNAL.

| VOL. VI. | TORONTO, MARCH, 1894. | No. 3. |

Original Communications.

Soliciting Patients.

By L. D. S., Toronto.

A suggestive article could be written on the solicitation of patients, and if we make claim to be a professional body, it is the duty of society officers to see that no man gains entrance who has resorted to trade methods. At the meeting of the American Dental Association in August of last year, resolutions were adopted refusing representation to societies that did not require its members to live up to the requirements of the Code of Ethics ; and in 1891 a resolution was adopted to prohibit individuals who are violating the code from holding clinics or giving other exhibitions before the Association.

Now, it seems to me we are not careful and watchful enough in this matter, and it may explain one reason why a great many who are thoroughly ethical do not come to our meetings. I have seen some gatherings used by men who break the code, for the open purpose of advertising themselves, and before the members realized how they were being gulled. No matter how interesting these matters may be, we have no choice when they come to be measured by the code. The special interest does not make the breach any more pardonable.

But now let me turn the search-light upon others who flatter themselves that they are thoroughly ethical. Do we not see shrewd men who think it perfectly ethical to solicit the physician,

2

the clergyman, and others to send them patients on commission ? I can point you to a few whose chief art lies in dropping mean criticisms about their superiors, and undermining the reputation of brother-practitioners by slighting' remarks whenever they get the opportunity. A medical friend of mine told me that a very indif- ferent dentist in whose office he was giving ether, endeavored to secure his influence by derogatory remarks about his leading con- freres, especially about one confrere. It appeared that he had never had any dental education outside of what he got in the labora- tory and office of a very poor practitioner, and that his examina- tion before the Board was "the worst of any candidate who had ever passed." The physician retorted as follows : " Dr. —— has had and has kept my family practice for twenty years, and I am more satisfied with him every day. I know he always was and always is a diligent student in his profession. You will permit me to say, that my experience as a medical practitioner enables me to judge what a dentist knows of dentistry, and I don't think you've yet learned the A B C of your profession, in spite of the fact that you pull and fill and make teeth."

Unfortunately everybody will not speak so plainly, and many people easily swallow the falsehoods these men circulate to get patients. I know we are no worse than the physicians and the lawyers. All professions have mean and malicious men in their ranks, and the more ignorant they are, the meaner they are. We cannot be expected to puff up the merits of a confrere, or so to extol him that we will drive our own patients to him, but surely the world is big enough for us all, without resorting to dirty methods of obtaining a practice. And I think the meanest and most dangerous men in the ranks of any profession, are those who assume to be ethical, yet who are not the least bit superior in their methods of soliciting patients, to the distributors of pamphlets from door to door whom they condemn.

[We do not suppose an article like the above will have any more effect on the characters represented, than water on a duck's back. This journal has never had any mercy upon men who degrade the profession. But we have great cause for gratitude, that in most of our cities and towns there exists an undoubted fraternity, such as we find among respectable physicians and barristers. You cannot make a man of inborn manners and malice noble by making him a dentist. He may even enter the ministry, and there exhibit it either by proselytizing among sister congre- gations, or by hypocrisy. There is a bright side to humanity. There may not be more saints than sinners, but for every sneak there are a hundred true men. Don't you think so ?—ED. D.D.J.]

Devitalizing Pulps.

By W. B., Smith's Falls, Ont.

There is, perhaps, no operation that calls for treatment at the hands of the dental surgeon, and which is attended with so much unnecessary pain, as the devitalizing of pulps.

We believe that much of the pain which so many operators complain of, as resulting from the application of arsenious acid to a live pulp, is due to the wretched manner in which the agent is too frequently employed.

There are various reasons for this deplorable state of affairs, but the one that stands out in bold relief, high above all others is—carelessness.

Too often when we find an exposure, which it is necessary to devitalize, we neglect to thoroughly remove all the debris immediately overlying and surrounding the point of exposure, and thus at the very outset we make a mistake.

Then again, perhaps, the saliva has almost unchecked headway into the cavity, or the devitalizing agent is not applied directly to the pulp, but is placed almost anywhere so long as it is in the cavity.

And then the grand finale is realized when a pellet of absorbent cotton, saturated with a solution of sandarach, or some other combination of a similar nature, is inserted to seal the orifice.

And it generally succeeds in sealing up more than the cavity, for in about nine cases in every ten it gums over the point of exposure, and prevents the proper operation of the arsenic and a raging toothache is the immediate result.

This should not be.

There is no duty in life, no matter how simple or insignificant, but the proper performance calls for more or less care and the observance of certain laws, or facts. How much more necessary then is it to have a systematized method in dealing with that minute but complex combination of arteries, veins, and nerves we term the dental pulp?

To properly destroy a pulp, it is absolutely necessary that the agent be placed in immediate contact. All decayed and loose particles should be carefully removed and the cavity thoroughly flooded with warm water. If this is conscientiously performed, it ensures us one great essential, namely, that of a clean point to receive the application.

If possible, the rubber dam should be applied and the cavity dried as much as possible. The exposure should also be enlarged as much as it can be without injuring the tissues. A portion of the paste should be directly applied and covered with a layer of dry cotton, or some other material, and seal with warm compound, wax, or gutta percha, care being taken not to exert pressure.

If a little more time was expended, and a little more trouble taken, we would not have so many patients returning with the story of how they suffered intense agony, for some more or less lengthened period, but the pain would, in nearly every case, be reduced to the minimum.

Proceedings of Dental Societies.

Do not forget meeting of Vermont State Dental Society at White River Junction, beginning Wednesday 21st inst.

Selections.

Dental Boards.

By Prof. J. Foster Flagg.

There is an incentive to pass and graduate men who are utterly unfit. They come to us, they work with us, and they get around us in some way—I don't know how—and the result is that some young men who are utterly incompetent go out from our schools. Do we know it? They work hard; they are present at every lecture; they are in the seats with their eyes wide open and their mouths wide open, drinking it all in, poor as it is; we see them every day, and we get to know those boys, and we hope that when they come up for examination they will pass well. What do they do? They are required to make a set of artificial teeth, and they take an impression, which is a wretchedly poor impression; so they say to some fellow-student who is able to take a good impression, "Here, I am going down-stairs a minute; you just take this impression for me, and I will be right back." So the good man takes the impression. Then the poor man swages up a plate, and it is the poorest kind of work, and he gets another man to swage up the plate for him. He sets it in plaster, and where the single teeth are to go he sets them, but where a few teeth are to be ground up together he finds he can't grind them up, so he gets another man to grind up the gum teeth for him. And that piece of work is finally put in by this fellow as his work. He could not do it to save his soul; but how is the teacher to know that? Do you suppose we are going to watch every student at his work? Then, if a student has to prepare a cavity, and don't know how, he gets somebody to do it for him. He can't put the gold in, so he gets someone else to do that; and perhaps he can't finish the filling, and he gets somebody else to finish it up for him. Finally, he brings it to my good friend here, or to me, and he is asked: "Did you do this work?" and he says, "Yes, sir," and he lays his hand on his heart. Then he comes up for examination, and we ask him questions. I would like to read to you, gentlemen, a list of some of the questions that I have asked the students who pass before me. If it doesn't take in the whole range, from A to Z, then I don't know anything about dentistry—that is, in my branch. I have no idea what they do in the other branches, but in my little branch of dentistry I examine students thoroughly, and I ask them questions that I doubt very much if many of my brother hornets could answer. We have forgotten the things we used to know in school, but we keep up with the procession pretty well in practice, and run dentistry decently well in our office. And so it goes on. This man comes up for examination, and his finger-nails are written all over with the letters that he understands, and he gets beside some fellow that he knows is well posted, and he nudges him when a question is asked, and so, finally, he gets 41. He wants 42. That fellow, with all his cheating and defrauding, gets 41. And then I say, "Well, gentlemen, I voted 5 for that fellow; I think I can go one more. I will give him 6." Would not any one of you do that? I ask you, are you such hard-hearted cusses that you would not do that—particularly for your sons? Of course, you will do it. You say, "He has worked hard, he is a reasonably good fellow, a thundering sight better than I was when I started in practice. I did not know one-tenth part as much when I started, so I can afford to give him one more." Thus he gets 42, and he passes. And he goes out and he says, "I guess I got about 59 out of them 60 votes."

Now, when my friend Dr. Osmun said, in speaking of the gentleman who failed to pass the Examining Board, that he came from a reputable college, where they taught those things *in extenso*, I at once assumed that it must be the Philadelphia College, because I would like to know where they teach things any more *in extenso* than they are taught in that college. If the students who go out from that college knew everything that is taught in it, they might rattle most of you old men.

There should be no controversy between our Examining Boards and the schools. If the students cheat us into believing they are fit to pass, they cheat themselves a hundred times more. What is the incentive? It is simply that, as a result of possessing our diploma, they are enabled in many States to practise. If they could not practise under that diploma—if it only stated that these gentlemen have been sufficiently prepared to come before your Examining Boards and take your examination, that we have examined them and think they are capable of passing your examination easily—if these men, having passed our examination, could not practise till they had passed your Examining Boards, don't you suppose they would embrace the opportunities to learn what we give them? Don't you suppose they would learn how to prepare cavities, and take impressions, and swage plates, and grind teeth? Of course they would, because their right to practise would depend on their ability to demonstrate their knowledge of these things before you.—*Items of Interest.*

Anæsthetics, and the Physiology of the Heart.

At the regular meeting of the Odontological Society of Great Britain, last December, a very concise and scientific paper was read by John W. Pickering, D.Sc. (Lond.), on the "Physiology of the Heart in relation to Anæsthetics," treating the subject from an experimental standpoint. The author showed that the following are some of the possible modes of action on the heart :

(1) The anæsthetic acts on the cardiac muscle itself, and may directly paralyze its contractile power.

(2) That the paralysis of the heart when present, is due to the action of the anæsthetic of the intrinsic cardiac nervous mechanism.

(3) That chloroform syncope is due to a reflex cardiac inhibition caused by irritation of the nerve ending of the vagi in the lungs.

(4) That chloroform primarily paralyzes the respiratory centre in the medulla oblongata, and that the consequent asphyxial condition of the blood secondarily paralyzes the heart.

(5) That cardiac dilation, when present, is due to pulmonary obstruction, and that chloroform has no specific action on the heart.

This last view, however, has been rendered improbable by recent experiments, which have shown that chloroform will produce dilatation of *both sides* of the heart.

Dr. Pickering experimented on the hearts of embryos previous to the development of a functional nervous mechanism—the chick embryo between the fiftieth and eightieth hour of incubation presenting an accessible form of heart or nervous system. Though the embryonic circulation is then very active, there is no complication due to a change of blood-pressure ; also the factor of asphyxia is eliminated, except when purposely introduced, by placing the embryo in an atmosphere of carbonic acid. The experiments were made on hearts *in situ*, and under conditions such that their rhythms were maintained for many hours unchanged, provided that no chemical or physical stimuli were applied to them. Chloroform injected under the blastoderm of the embryo, rapidly reduced its cardiac rhythm, and produced an exaggerated diastole. Ether acted as a powerful stimulant to the embryonic heart. These experiments show that chloroform has a depressor and ether an augumentor action—a conclusion at variance with the view of Claude Bernard, reiterated by the Hyderabad Commission. Nitrous oxide and air has but little depressant effect on the embyronic heart ; pure nitrous oxide stops the embryonic heart in diastole. Dr. Pickering showed that there is apparently less danger of cardiac stoppage with the use of oxygen and chloroform, than with chloroform alone.

As to the vexed question as to whether nitrous oxide forms a compound with any of the constituents of the blood, or whether its action is owing to the formation of reduced hæmoglobin and consequent deprivation of the tissues of oxygen, Dr. Dudley Buxton urged the probable formation of compound of nitrous oxide with hæmoglobin, or with some globulin of the plasma. Recent researches lend much probability to these views. The question, however, is left *sub judice*.

Is it possible pharmacologically to antagonize the depressant action of anæsthetics on the heart?

An application of a 1 per cent. solution of ammonium hydrate directly to the ventricle of a frog's heart, restores it almost to its original power. This is proved in experiments on the embryonic heart.

Dr. Wood, of Philadelphia, failed to get any restoration of rhythm by hypodermic injection of atropine, amyl nitrate, or caffeine, while alcohol increased the cardiac depression. Ammonia had slightly beneficial effects, and digitalis, by raising the blood pressure, often averted death. Strychnine, in doses of .00002 grain, increases both the force and frequency of the embryonic heart rhythm. Large doses are depressant. Chloroformed hearts will, if not too strongly poisoned, respond to electrical stimuli. The direct application of heat will often restore a chloroformed heart when chemical and electrical stimuli fail. Dr. Pickering closed by advising the trial of external heat in form of wet rags over the heart.

Dental Doctors.

During the last year several instances in which persons on the Dentists' Register assumed the title of " Dr." were brought before the Council of the Medical Defence Union. It seems to have been considered as an infringement of the Medical Act, and some of the dentists were written to by the Secretaries of the Union, and cautioned.

This action, says the Annual Report, resulted in the use of the title being discontinued in many instances ; but in one case, where the offence was persisted in, the dentist was reported to the General Medical Council. That body, however, appears to have taken little notice of the matter, and we learn that the Defence Union intends to have the whole subject brought up again at a future session.

It is said that in many cases there is a clear history of medical, or rather surgical, practice being carried on by the dentist in addition to his legitimate occupation. This would seem to raise the question as to the proper limits of dental surgery, a point we hope to touch upon when a suitable occasion offers.—*British Journal of Dental Science*, February, '94.

Dentists as Readers.

It has been a constant source of wonder to journalists, who are in position to observe the fact more than others, that dentists care so little for the literature of their profession. It is a lamentable fact that not one dentist in ten is a regular paid-up subscriber to any dental periodical.

Their entire course of reading during the year consists of a few sample copies which drop into their hands from a gratuitous circulation. How any man can be content with this meagre amount of disconnected information concerning the development and progress of his profession, is beyond conjecture.

Five dollars a year, judiciously expended in subscriptions to dental periodicals, would give any man a course of systematic reading that would not only be wonderfully beneficial by keeping his mind refreshed, but would also keep him posted as to the changes, progress and improvements daily occurring.

Can a man keep posted on the political situation of the day by reading a daily paper once a week? It is just as impossible to keep posted in a profession by reading an occasional sample copy.

Then every dentist needs books of reference. There are times when it would be a pleasure to look back and obtain *data* on some important event that happened in the distant past beyond the stretch of memory. To provide for this, these volumes could be bound year by year, at a small expense, and the result would be, in a few years, a valuable library would be collected without any appreciable cost.

Every professional man who receives money for his services, and does not keep posted on the improvements of his profession, is taking money not justly due him. If you expect to give full value in service, you owe it to your clientele to keep read and fully posted. —*Editorial in Southern Dental Journal and Luminary.*

A New Degree.

At a recent meeting of the Regents of the University of Michigan, at the suggestion of the Faculty of the Dental Department, the degree of Doctor of Dental Science was established, to be conferred upon those who, after completing the regular three years' course in a satisfactory manner and graduating, receiving the degree of Doctor of Dental Surgery, take another year's work, which will embrace advance work and original work as well, on certain prescribed lines.

It will be required in order to do this, that the applicant shall have made well-nigh perfect work in his regular course.

The course indicated for this degree in the scheme presented is work in materia medica, embracing laboratory work in organic chemistry, laboratory work, physiology, original work on these lines, and with special reference to some dental remedy ; also, in pathology, embracing embryology and histology, bacteriology, laboratory course and original research on dental diseases.

This course would add very greatly to the equipment of the dental practitioner ; it would give him attainments and ability much in advance of the general graduate in dental surgery.

Those who have given attention to the ordinary practitioners of dentistry as they go out from the usual course of instruction, cannot help being impressed with the great want that is so frequently experienced by the beginner when he is confronted by many of the more severe and obscure cases of diseases of the teeth and mouth.

The object in establishing this course is, if possible, to increase the ability of the beginner in dental practice. That something more is required in this respect than is obtained, not only in dental but in medical colleges as well, in the ordinary course is fully demonstrated by the establishment of Post-Graduate Departments, especially in medicine in nearly all our larger cities, and there seems to be a call for such schools in dentistry.

The efforts as yet, however, have been quite circumscribed, having reference only to some particular line of instruction, as, for example, Prosthetic Dentistry, or the more practical departments of work.

Lubricate. Your Disks and Strips.

We see so many dentists still using sandpaper disks and strips in finishing fillings without vaseline or oil to lubricate them, that we feel like once more calling attention to this matter. It is a censurable species of inhumanity to run a disk dry on a gold filling, or to see-saw a strip back and forth between teeth without using a lubricant. A disk or strip will not heat up so rapidly if covered with vaseline, and contrary to prevalent opinion, the cutting properties will be improved. Quite often the question is asked by those who never use a lubricant : "But will not the vaseline or oil prevent the sandpaper from cutting?" A careful test of the matter will prove to these men that their impressions are wrong. If there were no other recommendations for the use of lubricants than the one of increased cutting power, this would be a sufficient inducement to always employ them. When disks are used with the rubber dam in place, it is extremely difficult to prevent a dry disk from catching up the dam in its revolutions and tearing it, but a disk well lubricated will play over the dam with little danger of a mishap. Another recommendation lies in the fact that when well smeared with vaseline, a disk becomes flexible and can be pressed into depressions and be made to cut at any desired point by guiding it with an instrument. This is well-nigh impossible when a dry disk is used.

This latter consideration is very important wherever a disk is employed between teeth for finishing a filling. If a proper contour is to be left to the filling, it is necessary that the disk shall cut only at the cervical portion of the filling and not at the contact point. A flexible disk may be pressed against the neck of the tooth if desired and all the cutting confined to that region, but a dry disk will almost invariably cut away the contact point and make a flat filling. The variety of curves to be given a flexible disk in cutting is limited only by the dexterity of the operator. Another argument in favor of lubricating the disk or strip is one of economy. In this condition it will hold the fine particles of gold on its surface, and the dentist who preserves his old disks and strips for a time and then turns them over to a refiner for melting, will be surprised at the result.—C. N. JOHNSON, in *Dental Review.*

A Few Things to be Remembered.

By L. P. HASKELL.

In ninety-nine per cent. of mouths the centre of the palate is hard and unyielding, in fact the only portion of the upper jaw which does not change from absorption or yield to pressure. Unless provision is made for it, the plate will, sooner or later, rock This should be remedied by a "relief" in metal plates, of a thin film of wax on the model, extending well up on the anterior portion to near the margin of the process, and to within a quarter of an inch of the rear of plate. In a rubber plate the relief can be made by burring or scraping the plate.

There are more failures in artificial dentures from *faulty articulation* than from any other cause. To guard against this, in adjusting a denture in the mouth, see to it that none of the six anterior teeth touch,—in fact leave a margin of space. This will prevent the tilting of the plate from the rear. Be sure the bicuspids and first molars on both sides meet uniformly ; have no pressure on the second molar, and especially if the lower occluding molar leans forward, as it would crowd the denture forward.

In arranging the *lower* teeth, commence with the second bicuspid so as to ensure a perfect interlocking of the cusps. The fronts must be accommodated to the space allotted to them by crowding or overlapping, if needed.

In ordering teeth from the dealer, see that bicuspids and molars are provided that have a good length of porcelain *above* the pins, so that if necessary to grind, in articulating, the porcelain will not be ground away. The teeth will also present a more natural appearance, Insist upon this from your dealer.

If you desire to restore the expression of the mouth which has been sacrificed by the extraction of the cuspid teeth, remember this invariable rule, viz.: the plate can and should be worn higher over these teeth than elsewhere, and the artificial gum made fuller.

Leave the necks of the cuspids slightly fuller than the other teeth.

Finish the rubber with a festoon around the necks of the teeth.

In selecting teeth for metal plate and crown work, if you desire *strength*, use the perpendicular rather than the cross-pins, and they are less liable to crack in soldering, and do not let your dealer give you anything else.

In polishing metal work, use *oil* with your pumice both on the felt and the brush. To reach all the depressions and interstices, drive a pine stick into the lathe chuck made for it and with sharp knife turn it to a blunt point.—*Ohio Dental Journal.*

Selecting and Keeping Dental Medicines.

While there may be many other things to modify the action of drugs, or the result of their application, we believe that many times negative results come through the use of inferior medicaments.

In the first place there are many impure drugs in the market, especially in the smaller towns ; drugs that are either adulterated or have undergone a change from exposure or long keeping.

On the other hand, we may obtain pure drugs, but allow them to deteriorate through improper care, so that their efficacy is greatly modified.

Some of the dental medicaments that have been found adulterated are :—

Arsenious Acid, adulterated with lime salts, chalk and other substances.

Creasote. It is very difficult to obtain a pure beechwood creasote. Much of the so-called creasote has been found to consist of crude carbolic acid to which has been added creasole and phosole.

Essential Oils; often adulterated with fixed oils, oil of turpentine, chloroform, alcohol, or essential oils of an inferior grade mixed with those of a better quality.

Aconite tincture. This is one of the most uncertain remedies in regard to strength that we use. The commercial article may be strong, weak, or sometimes almost inert. This variation is due to varying quantities of the alkaloid used in its preparation. That prepared from the root is many times more powerful than that prepared from the leaves. The officinal tincture U. S. P. contains 40 per cent. aconite strength ; Fleming's tincture has 79 per cent.; the German, 10 per cent.; the British, 16 per cent.; the French, 20 per cent.; so that care should be used in selection and use of this remedy.

Terebene, as found in the shops, is often contaminated with resin, turpentine, etc.

Cocain salts, may contain organic or other impurities.

Zinc salts. These may contain impurities of lead, copper, iron, aluminum or alkaline earths.

Hydrogen peroxid has been found to contain varying quantities of sulphuric or hydrochloric acids, some samples contain also boric acid and barium.

Prof. H. E. Smith, of Yale College, made a test of some fifty samples of peroxid of hydrogen obtained from as many different stores in New York, New Haven, Hartford and Bridgeport, to determine the quality of this article as dispensed in small amounts. The samples were collected in one ounce glass-stoppered bottles and tested within twenty-four hours after purchasing.

The commercial is supposed to be a 15 volume solution ; that is one which yields fifteen times its own volume of oxygen gas.

The results of these experiments was that 56 per cent. of the samples contained from 7 to 9 volumes of oxygen, 8 per cent. contained no hydrogen peroxid, and the remaining 36 per cent. were regarded deficient inasmuch as they contained less than two per cent.

Regarding acidity, a good reaction for hydrochloric acid was obtained in thirty-three samples, and for sulphuric acid in twelve. Sometimes one only was present, sometimes both. Boric acid was present in small amounts in eighteen cases, and barium in two. These acids are either residues from the process of manufacture or they are added with a view of giving greater stability to the preparations. From whatever cause, they are objectionable impurities.

To obtain the best results from medication it is necessary to have the purest drugs ; hence the necessity of securing those of the most reliable makes, and in original packages from the manufacturer, unless they can be secured fresh from a reliable druggist.

Now, while it is important to obtain pure drugs, it is equally important to preserve them in this state. Many drugs deteriorate in quality if proper precautions are not used for their preservation. Dental medicines are particularly prone to do so, for the dentist uses the majority of drugs so slowly that a supply will last him much longer than the physician. So the care of drugs is a very important factor in their preservation. In way of illustration, we will enumerate a few that deteriorate if not properly cared for.

From the above analysis of hydrogen peroxid we see that there is a considerable and variable difference in the quality of the solutions, even in those of the same make at different times, and the quality is roughly indicated by the differing tendency to spontaneous decomposition in different bottles.

The purer the solution the less liable is it to decompose, and this is, in a degree, independent of the strength of the solution and the temperature at which it is kept.

Solutions of the commercial article, however, are very unstable and should be kept in glass-stoppered bottles, protected from light and heat. Hydrogen peroxid, ordinarily obtained, gives up a part of its oxygen at a temperature of about 34° F. and the amount is increased in proportion as the temperature is raised. Hence the necessity of keeping in a cool place, such as an ice-chest or water cooler.

Among other drugs used in dentistry that are affected by light, heat or exposure may be mentioned :

Bichlorid of mercury solutions.—They are gradually decomposed on exposure to light or in contact with organic matter.

Aristol is decomposed by exposure to light and moisture.

Europhen is affected in the same manner.

Dialyzed iron is affected by age ; thickens, etc.; the solution not remaining potent after being kept for five or six months.

Amyl nitrate is a very volatile liquid, and its alcoholic solutions rapidly deteriorate.

Myrtol evaporates at ordinary temperatures.

Iodine slowly volatilizes at ordinary temperatures if exposed to light and air.

Eugenol, exposed to the air, becomes darker in color and resinous.

Terebene, if exposed to the air, absorbs oxygen and is changed.

Cocain solutions are unstable and soon decompose on exposure to light.

Tannic acid, exposed to moist air, gradually changes ; and aqueous solutions, when exposed to air, mould, ferment and are converted into gallic acid.

Permanganate of potassium, in the presence of moisture, gives up the oxygen it contains and becomes binoxid of manganese.

Essential oils, if pure, are not affected by exposure, but those ordinarily obtained thicken and become resinous on exposure to air.

Ethyl chlorid is volatile at the ordinary temperature.

Nitrate of silver is somewhat affected by exposure to light and air.

Glacial phosphoric acid, if exposed to air, absorbs moisture and is changed in consistency.

Sulphate of zinc is slowly effervescent in dry air.

Aqua ammonia, if exposed to air, readily deteriorates.

Thus we realize the necessity of keeping medicaments in well-stoppered bottles and in a dark, dry and cool place to preserve them. If we are careless in this matter and allow our drugs to deteriorate, we cannot expect satisfactory results from their use.—*Editorial, Ohio Dental Journal.*

Correspondence.

Shall We Be Called "Doctor"?

To the Editor of the DOMINION DENTAL JOURNAL :

SIR,—I am in perfect harmony with the sentiments expressed in your editorial, "The Title of 'Doctor,'" and I have always regarded it as an infringement upon the purely medical title. I would go further and abolish it as applied to any branch of the healing art unless the possessor had obtained an M.D. But if it is wrong to apply it to a branch of medicine and surgery such as dentistry, which devotes its efforts to the treatment of important organs of the human body, why is it right to apply it to the veterinary surgeons, who devote their efforts exclusively to the treatment of the lower animals? I recognize the importance to the material interests of the country, in the better education of the veterinarians, and I rejoice in what they have done for the prevention and treatment of disease among cattle. But I do not see why they have a claim to a title you would deny to the dentists. The importance given to dentistry, as a branch of the healing art, by the "Royal College of Surgeons," and the Medical Council of Great Britain, the knighting by Her Majesty the Queen, of two of the representative men of our profession, are sufficient to show that dentistry occupies a social and professional position only second to general medicine and surgery.

I am fully in favor of the abolition of the title of "Doctor" as applied to dentists, but it will not be easy of accomplishment while it is given to our friends the Vets., who do not take the full medical course. It is no more necessary for the "Vet." than the dentist to take the full medical course, and it is no more necessary for them to be called "Doctor." I am rather in favor of Dr. Stack's proposal to call us by the prefix "Dentist," as "Dentist Jones." The veterinarian might be called "Veterinary Brown."

Whatever the future may bring forth, let us remember that to-day the profession of dentistry in Great Britain, at least, has the very highest social and professional recognition. I cannot see that it is any more necessary in America than in Europe, in order to attain this, that a "Dentist" should be called a "Doctor."

Yours, etc.,

PACIFIC OCEAN.

Reviews.

Diseases and Injuries of the Teeth, Including Pathology and Treatment. A Manual of Practical Dentistry for Students and Practitioners. By MORTON SMALE, M.R.C.S., L.S.A., L.D.S., and J. F. COLYER, L.R.C.P., M.R.C.S., L.D.S. London : Longman, Green & Co., 1893.

It is rather a curious comment on dental science and art, that it is hardly possible for distinguished teachers on either side of the ocean, to produce a work that will fully satisfy the convictions and requirements of the profession in both Europe and America. While it can hardly be denied that in the higher branches of scientific investigation, the best men in the profession in England have been for a long time, and yet remain, the leaders of opinion, it is equally true that in the purely practical they always were, and still remain, in the background. The solution of this fact may be traced partly to the difference in the curriculum of study, and we are free to confess that we have always held the opinion, with the greatest respect for our colleagues in the United States, that of the two systems the former would prove to be the best in the long run. In reviewing contributions to our literature, it is but fair to remember this fact, as a suggestion in tolerance ; and it is an unpardonable folly for either side to introduce national predilections and personal satire—as has been done by some of our contemporaries—in judging the merits or demerits of a scientific work.

From the standpoint of practice on this continent, the volume before us may, in several respects, be questioned as an authority ; but as a model of concise yet sometimes hasty description, stripped of the verbiage which disfigures so many text-books on dentistry ; as a clear and explicit *multum in parvo* one must candidly allow that it is a welcome addition to our literature. We could mention books recognized in our colleges as authorities, so full of literary flatulence, as to remind one of the *savant* mentioned in Moore's Diary, who wrote several folio volumes on the "Digestion of a Flea." One will be struck with the almost laconic style of the authors of this valuable work. There is no *flux de mos*. One has not to blow off a lot of froth before one can drink. There is no inflated nonsense or circumlocution. Perhaps the chief fault is in the other direction. Of the two evils we can spare best the latter.

The authors have adopted the following terms in anatomy—mandible, for inferior maxilla, maxilla being restricted to the upper jaw ; temporo-mandilenlas, as articulation for temporo-maxillary joint ; stylo-mandibular ligament, as mandibular artery and nerve respectively, for the stylo-maxillary ligament and inferior dental artery and nerve. The illustrations are mostly original and are beautiful. The list of contents comprises concise chapters on "First Dentition," "Abnormalities and Diseases of the Temporary Teeth," "Second Dentition," "Abnormalities of the Permanent Teeth," "Concussion, Dislocation and Fracture of the Teeth," "Caries," "Treatment of Caries," "The Dental Pulp and Its Treatment in Health and Disease," "Diseases of the Dental Periosteum," "Erosion," "Attrition," "Abrasion," "Diseases of the Gums," "Saliva and Salivary Calculus," "Odontomes," "Replantation, Transplantation and Implantation of the Teeth," "Extraction, Odontalgia and Neuralgia," "Fractures of the Jaws," "Necrosis of the Jaws," "Empyæma of the Antrum," "Trismus, Diseases Due to the Presence of Diseased Teeth," "Affections of the Tongue Met With in Dental Practice," "Diagnosis of Swelling About the Jaws."

It will readily be perceived by anyone familiar with the routine of the best practice on this continent, that numerous difficulties presented by the authors are not here recognized as difficulties at all; and that certain suggestions, such as that on page 84, that "the laterals should be removed in those cases when the canine presents immediately above them, or the root of the canine is directed towards the median line, or when the laterals are placed much posterior to the arch, or are decayed," are considered radically wrong. We must, also, take exception to the statement as a general principle on page 49, that, in regulating a tooth, it "swings upon its apex, and does not move bodily." We will take the liberty of sending the authors models to disprove that statement. We doubt very much if the statement that "some practitioners employ excision extensively, cutting away large portions of the tooth" (in treating caries) will find any advocates to-day in America. The authors go on to say, "the spaces thus formed should be V-shaped. In the case of the incisors, the base of the V is towards the lingual surface of the teeth. The operation is extensively employed by Dr. Arthur," etc. Although Dr. Arthur practised the system he advocated; he had few, if any, adherents long before his death, which occurred fourteen years ago.

With minor exceptions of this kind, which, no doubt, will be modified in the next edition, the authors carefully and scientifically discuss the diseases and injuries of the teeth; though, if we have any special fault to find, it is that they have not done justice to the best work by the best men in the United States and even in England. A fair recognition on both sides of the ocean of the work of the best investigators is expected in any book of this character. In spite of this, the volume is decidedly one of the most valuable contributions to our professional literature, extremely useful to the student and the busy practitioner. The index is thorough. The publishers deserve credit for the neatness with which their part of the work is done.

Little Things. By Dr. W. H. WRIGHT, Brandon, Vt. Read before Vermont State Dental Society, March, 1893. This reprint puts in a convenient form a very interesting paper. The author specially refers to the use of phenacetine, from two to four grains, once in three hours, to reduce the temperature and induce sleep in acute alveolar abscess, with the accompanying symptoms.

A Contribution to the Study of the Development of the Enamel
By R. R. ANDREWS, A.M., D.D.S., Cambridge, Mass.

Prehistoric Crania from Central America. By R. R. ANDREWS, A.M., D.D.S.

The former is a reprint from the *International Dental Journal,*

3

of the lecture delivered before the World's Columbian Dental Congress ; the latter, a reprint of a paper read before the American Academy of Dental Science, Boston.

Dr. Andrews has a world-wide reputation as a thorough and unbiassed investigator. Students of microscopy should learn to be charitable to the demonstrations of their colleagues. Dr. Andrews has the genial as well as the scientific spirit. His conclusions on the development of enamel are as follows: " I am led to believe that there probably exists in developing enamel, as has already been found in developing bone and dentine, a fibrous substructure on and between which the enamel is deposited. After the enamel is wholly formed, its existence seems to be wholly blotted out in the dense calcification of the tissue. In sections of wholly-f rmed enamel I have never been able to trace it, although I have tried the methods of those who claim to have seen it. In regard to the beaded protoplasmic reticulum of living matter in formed enamel, I have never been able to find it. I believe with Klein that it is improbable that nucleated protoplasmic masses are contained in the interstitial substance of the enamel of a fully-formed tooth." Six fine photo-micrographs illustrate the paper.

The paper on the Prehistoric Crania, now to be seen at the Peabody Museum, at Cambridge, is of great archæological interest. In 1890, Harvard University sent the late Mr. John G. Owens to Central America, and it was during the expedition that these treasures were obtained. We will publish the paper in full in our next issue, with the illustrations which have been kindly supplied by the Publishers of the *International Dental Journal.*

Editorial.

The Laboratory.

Why do so many dentists consider prosthetic post-graduate schools like Dr. Haskell's, a necessity? What is the matter with education in the purely mechanical branches of our profession, that so many men graduate from our colleges, unfitted to master the ordinary, much less the extraordinary difficulties of the laboratory?

Many young men enter upon the study of dentistry with the idea of being expert operators, and leave with the idea that if they attain the feeblest skill at the chair, they need not be mechanics. In college life it was extremely difficult in the past, and it continues so in a lesser degree, to enforce concentration upon the work of the laboratory, and young men were busily engaged at the chair before they could properly construct, from start to finish, an ordinary set of vulcanite. It is much the same as if the medical student began his first year with obstetrics and pathology, without having learned the first principles of anatomy and physiology. It is not uncommon to find students, in their first six months, dabbling in operative work, when they do not know how to make an articulation, or to polish an ordinary set of teeth. They have no pride in the property in the laboratory ; their tools are dirty and kept in disorder ; the lathes are covered with the debris of a week's polishing material, and yet they are happy. We have watched the career of some of these boys. If they have turned out clean, and careful for themselves, it simply proved that they were dirty and dishonest as students ; but as a rule the habits they displayed in the laboratory when learning, followed them through life. Vulcanite has been in many ways a curse to the profession, and we may add to the list this fact, that it has been the means of developing a generation of careless and dirty students, who are a reproach and an obstruction to the higher ideal of dental practice. In the olden time of gold and continuous gum work, the laboratory was at least as clean as a jeweller's bench. There are model laboratories to-day where vulcanite predominates, but they are few and far between in comparison with the period when vulcanite was unknown. How do we explain this fact? Chiefly because students start out with a low standard of opinion as to the skill required to construct vulcanite, and they are as impatient to run as they are indisposed to creep. The result is that when these boys become practitioners they find themselves handicapped; they meet difficulties they cannot overcome, and they have to begin to learn ! It is in every way wiser and more fitting to get, in the beginning of student life, the ground-work of mechanism in all its branches, theoretical and practical; a knowledge of the use and care of tools and apparatus, and to have a clinical experience of prosthetic dentistry before a thought is given to the work of dental operating and pathology. It would not only be better for the student, but certainly for the dentist in whose office the student may be getting his early tuition.

Even if a dentist intends to delegate the mechanical department to an associate or an assistant, he cannot afford to be indifferent, much less ignorant. We cannot put our patients where we put our models and our dies. The patient who consults a dentist expects his personal advice, and in most cases his personal attention. One may go to a barber and take his choice of half a dozen workmen, but as a rule, the dentist of many chairs and many operative assistants is a quack, or has a quack's instincts, and is keener to make his practice purely mercantile than professional. If dentistry is to descend to that sort of practice, it will degenerate ethically until it is relegated to the rank of a trade. It is foolish for a dentist who desires to do the best for his patients, to place himself at the mercy of mechanical assistants, who may leave him in the lurch on short notice. Personal skill in mechanical dentistry is necessary, even to one who has to direct assistants. It seems to us that, all things being equal, a student who is occupied twelve months of his first year exclusively in the laboratory, should get a better training than where his career begins in a college, in utter ignorance of all the minutiæ of the laboratory.

Dr. A. W. Harlan.

Dr. A. W. Harlan has retired from the chief editorship of the *Dental Review*, after laying its foundations deep and sure, and establishing his reputation as one of the best writers and workers in the profession. The duties pertaining to the position he held in connection with the World's Congress was a severe strain, and the worthy Doctor has earned the right to a good rest. While his many friends will miss his name as the editor of the *Review*, we are sure they will commend his good sense in taking care of his health. He is not the sort of man to lie fallow any longer than is necessary.

Dr. C. N. Johnson, who may be called his editorial pupil, succeeds to the position. As an earnest and honest man, fully alive to the wants of the profession, and enthusiastically devoted to its literature, as well as its science, he will make his mark in this new addition to his list of professional responsibilities. While speeding the parting guest with sincere regret, we welcome the coming one with heartiness as sincere.

Personals.

The profession generally will regret to learn of the death of Dr. Henry Snowden, one of the publishers of the *American Journal of Dental Science*, in the seventy-fourth year of his age.

La grippe fastened its fangs on many of our confreres. One of our Quebec pioneers, Dr. L. W. Dowlin, of Sherbrooke, was seriously affected for some time, but we are glad to know he is convalescent.

A supplementary examination was recently held by the Board of Examiners of the "Dental Association of the Province of Quebec." Messrs. J. H. Springle, of Montreal, and —— Lemieux, of Quebec, received the license to practise. One gentleman was rejected.

Annotations.

The Title of "Doctor."

The *Dental Register* informs us that at a meeting of the Regents of the University of Michigan, at the suggestion of the Faculty of the Dental Department, a new degree was established—that of "Doctor of Dental Science," which can only be obtained after completing the three years' regular course and graduating as "Doctor of Dental Surgery." It is evident that the belief is widespread that the latter degree is unsatisfactory, and that there is a conviction that its possession is, in verity, no proof whatever either of a common school education or of professional skill. The conditions under which it was for many years bestowed, and the number of ignorant and illiterate men who possess it, ought to be argument enough in favor of a higher degree. Educated men who have honestly earned it, and who had to associate with the indifferent and ignorant men in their classes who received it all the same, find it difficult to explain how these lazy and ignorant students obtained it. It does not seem to us that there is as much necessity for a four or a five years' course in college as for that preliminary education which alone can equip a student for a proper career. Any lack of early training should be compensated for before students are admitted to study, and this should decidedly involve at least a good knowledge of Latin and mathematics. We see no way of removing the reproach on the D.D.S. D.D.Sc. is not a whit better, unless it requires a much superior matriculation. In Canada, this matriculation is beyond the jurisdiction of the examining and licensing bodies. The Boards have nothing to do with it, and until a student can produce a certificate of having passed it before the selected authorities—who are invariably school teachers of the highest standing—entrance upon study is denied.

One of our correspondents in British Columbia refers to this subject on another page.

Dentists in Politics.

In our last issue we stated that one of our confrères sits in the Ontario Parliament. We have received seven notifications that the statement is incorrect, that in the bye-election he was defeated. We regret this exceedingly, both for the sake of the electors and the profession.

We would just observe, *en passant*, that we wish there was the same anxiety to supply us with correct news, as to correct our news. These personal items are interesting, and we should receive them by the dozen every month.

Obituary.

DIED.—On Feb. 10th, 1894, aged fifty years, Dr. W. C. Delaney, of Halifax, N.S.

[Dr. Delaney had been in feeble health for some time, but his sudden demise so soon after returning from consulting with one of the leading specialists of Philadelphia, was sooner than anticipated, as his immediate death was caused by the bursting of a blood vessel. The doctor was a native of Colchester County, and practised dentistry in Halifax for over twenty-five years quite successfully. He was an active member of the Provincial Dental Board of Nova Scotia, and represented Ward 2 as an alderman for seven years. He was also a director of N. S. Telephone Co., and an active member and deacon in the First Baptist Church of this city. His family will have the sincere sympathy of the profession, and the breach by his death will not soon be made up.—A. C. G.]

Dr. C. N. Pierce says: " My views are that competent examining boards should thoroughly be prepared to examine, and say whether the applicant is qualified to practise dentistry. If we have these, they are for the purpose of judging of the qualification of applicants. They have no right, in my estimation, *appointed as they are by the Legislature*, to ask the applicant whether he has a diploma, or where he got his education. All they want to do is to ascertain if the applicant is qualified to practise dentistry, and it is not their business to know where that qualification was obtained, as long as he possesses it. The board has no right to ask where the information was gained. It is simply whether the information is possessed by the individual, and I would have our board so educated, and so thoroughly appreciate their position, that they should hold that ground, and not accept a diploma or anything but a thorough qualification, for when we have that the public is protected."

[It is not easy to accept the proposition that a candidate for practice should be now allowed to pick up his knowledge wherever or whenever he likes, without attendance upon the privileges which have been provided for so many years. It may apply fully to men who began practice a quarter of a century or more ago, when the colleges were mostly as wretched as they could well be. But to-day there is no excuse for avoiding the schools. The chief thing to do is to raise the standard of entrance examination, and to make such a system, as described on another page by Dr. Flagg, impossible. We quote Dr. Pierce and Dr. Flagg as we might quote many others, to show that in establishing in Canada twenty-five years ago, boards of examiners before whom all applicants for license to practise must pass, we were not behind the times.— ED. D.D.J.]

UN ORIGINAL.—On vient d'enterrer, un vieux dentiste qui a passé cinquante ans de son existence à arracher les molaires de ses concitoyens, qu'il n'avait jamais su, d'ailleurs, soigner autrement que par ce procédé radical. Dans son testament, il a demandé— idée vraiment bizarre—qu'on enterrât avec lui toutes les dents qu'il avait extraites durant sa vie. Ses exécuteurs testamentaires ont pieusement accompli ses vœux, et, dans son cercueil, ils ont fait placer les trente mille dents que le défunt avait extirpées à ses clients au cours de sa longue carrière. Trente mille dents! Y pense-t-on? De quoi monter près de neuf cent cinquante râteliers complets!— *Le Phare du Littoral.*

Translated:

AN ECCENTRIC CHARACTER.—The other day they carried to his grave an old dentist, who spent fifty years of his life in pulling out the molars of his fellow-citizens, as he knew no better way of treating them than by this radical process. In his will he asked— curious notion, that—to have interred with him all the teeth he had extracted during his lifetime. His executors have religiously complied with his wishes, and have placed in his coffin the 30,000 teeth which the deceased had drawn for his clients in the course of his long practice. Thirty thousand teeth! Just think of it!—enough to supply about 900 complete sets.

Dr. J. S. Latimer, in the *Cosmos*, draws attention to the sometimes forgotten fact that it is not necessary to make undercuts in repairing vulcanite plates; that if the surfaces are freshened and painted over with a solution of the unvulcanized caoutchouc, the new material will unite with it. Someone told him that it would answer as well to wet the freshened (scraped) surfaces with kerosene.

Dr. Day showed a novel method of expediting the packing of cases. First apply shellac varnish to the cast, allow it to harden, then add the vulcanite in pieces of from a half inch square or larger, pressing each down on the cast, and smoothing down prominences with a warm spatula until the whole surface is covered, and the building up around the teeth completed as usual. Then flask at one pouring and vulcanize.

Dr. Latimer, after shellacking, covers the surface of the cast with No. 20 tin foil, burnished smooth. Dip a piece of rubber in chloroform and paint over all the surface of the tin.

When are we to have the second edition in English of Dr. W. D. Miller's work on the "Micro-Organisms of the Mouth"? It was issued in German in Leipzig over a year ago. S. S. W. Co., please answer.

.Prof. J. Foster Flagg, one of the most experienced dental college teachers in the United States, has a blunt and honest way of expressing his convictions. As an authority on college matters his opinions cannot be denied. We call attention to an article by him on " Dental Boards," from the *Items of Interest*, which goes to prove the superiority of the principle governing admission to practise in Canada, where all candidates, even if they have all the degrees under the sun, must pass before the Provincial Boards. It was the twenty years' experience obtained on the Quebec Board of graduates and non-graduates, which led us to express certain convictions as to the inferiority of much of the old system of college training, but, if what Prof. Flagg says to-day be true, it ought to direct attention to the present system as well. Why should not each State authorize the National Association of Dental Faculties to appoint the members of State Boards, before whom every graduate would have to appear for examination for admission to practise? The *personnel* of some of the State Boards elected by the State Governor have been objected to as incompetent. The N. A. D. F. could hardly make a mistake.

INSOMNIA.—The *Universal Medical Journal* for January, among recent suggestions in therapeutics, mentions *Chlorobrom* in doses of 1½ ounces, as recommended by a contributor in the *Lancet.* Sulphonal, morphia, chloral and bromide of potassium had all failed. J. E. Huxley says to try Nature's plan instead of drugs : Lower the supply of oxygen to the blood ; produce a little asphyxia ; limit the quantity of air to the lungs. The heart and circulation becoming quicker, the brain will lose its stimulant and sleep will follow. Cover your head with the bed-clothes and breathe and re-breathe only the respired air. When drowsiness is produced, it is easy to go on sleeping, though you push aside the coverings and get as much fresh air as needed. The cat and dog bury their noses in some soft hollow in their hair or fur and soon drop asleep.

[But cats and dogs have neither rent nor taxes to pay ; nor drafts from dental depots, nor accounts to collect to keep them awake.—ED. D.D.J.]

The *Southern Dental Journal and Luminary*, edited by Dr. H. H. Johnson, has a bright, new face, but we wish the sunshine of its countenance would more regularly illuminate the banks of the St. Lawrence. Last year the following numbers missed fire : February, March, April and November. Up north here we like to hear from "away down south in Dixie."

DOMINION
DENTAL JOURNAL.

| VOL. VI. | TORONTO, APRIL, 1894. | No. 4. |

Translations.

(From Foreign Dental Journals, etc., etc.)

By CARL E. KLOTZ, St. Catharines.

THE USE OF STERESOL IN LOCAL ANÆSTHETICS.—M. Creigner, of Paris, says, " Local anæsthetics of different kinds are used for the painless extraction of teeth. The method of applying them often produces as much pain as the extraction itself. To overcome this difficulty different remedies have been applied, but with little success. Steresol has so far given the best satisfaction; when painted on to the gums it forms a skin or coating, benumbing and protecting them from the cold produced by a spray, or from the insertion of the hypodermic point. I have used it for some time, and have found that I can use Coryl (which is a favorite local anæsthetic in Paris—C. E. K.), without the slightest pain or disagreeable effect to the patient, and have been able to extract teeth, and some very difficult to extract, without the patient showing the slightest indication of pain. Steresol is a new preparation, and permits, under favorable circumstances, to apply antiseptic dressing, which otherwise could not be done. Its use in dentistry is varied, and it can be applied to ulcers or abscesses, wounding of the tongue, lips, and gums, etc. In consequence of its continued antiseptic properties it will destroy all microbes with which it comes in contact. It will also obtund sensitive dentine, applied on a pellet of cotton to the cavity."—*Zahntechniche Reform.*

PULP CAPPING.—It is preferable, before capping with phosphate of zinc, to cover the floor and walls of the cavities. Teeth with soft dentine, with a mixture of oil of cloves and tannic acid. After the phosphate capping is hard, fill cavity with metallic filling. —*Zahntechniche Reform.*

2

To Prevent Nausea in Taking Impressions.—Allow the patient to inhale, before and during taking the impression, spirit of camphor.—*Zahntechniche Reform.*

Enamel for Dentures.—M. Bouls, of Paris, covers vulcanite and metallic plates with a flesh-colored enamel of a peculiar kind, and claims that it will wear well for a number of years, and can be easily renewed. The plates are varnished with three different enamels, and dried in a warm-air chamber made for the purpose, which keeps up a steady temperature at a certain degree. The first coating is the foundation, the second gives it the flesh color, and the third imparts the gloss. The plate, vulcanite or metal, to be enamelled, is trimmed but not polished, is slightly warmed and varnished or coated with preparation No. 1, and placed into the warm-air chamber for five minutes at a temperature of from 110° to 115° C. When taken out, varnish again, but put coating on a little thicker, and leave ten to fifteen minutes in warm-air chamber. After cool the surface is made uneven with a chaser or engraver, so as to produce the light and dark shades in the flesh-colored enamel. It is now painted with preparation No. 2, which is the flesh-colored enamel. If the natural gums are of a light color, one coating will be sufficient, but if dark, it will require two or three coatings. This is placed into the warm-air chamber for fifteen minutes. After cool it is ready for a coating of preparation No. 3, which gives it the gloss, and placed in the warm-air chamber for five minutes. The time occupied for enamelling is from one to one and a half hours. Preparation to be had from the firm of Messrs. Nicoud & Cie., Paris.—*Zahntechniche Reform.*

Nitrate of Silver.—A very convenient way of keeping nitrate of silver ready for use is to soak asbestos fibres in a saturated solution, and allow to dry.—*Zahntechniche Reform.*

Tinct. Capsici. is very good to use in the first stages of Periodontitis, or where it is advisable to hasten suppuration. Paint the gums with it. It is also used in connection with Zingiber Pads placed on the gums.—*Zahntechniche Reform.*

What Next? Dog Dentist Wanted.—The following announcement appeared in the *Müncher Neusten Nachrichten,* January 22nd, 1894: "What dentist is prepared, with a guarantee of success, to undertake the thorough scaling and cleansing of a set of teeth of a small pet dog. Address, L. 12,081, c/o. *Münchner Neusten Nachrichten.*" Must it be a full-fledged dentist? Certainly; as many a dog-fancier would think nothing of paying a good round sum to have the teeth of his pet dog taken care of, and that only by the most skilful, provided it is done with the utmost care, and without the slightest pain to the dear little creature ; at the same time he would think twice before he expended the same amount on his own grinders. What a new field for our young dentists ! Come on, ye heroes of notoriety and renown. Quite new. Dental Polyclinic for dogs of every breed. Kindest treatment assured.—*Zahntechniche Reform.*

To Clean Steel Instruments to Make them Appear as New.—Wash well with wood ashes and water to remove all grease, place them for a few seconds in a weak solution of hydrochloric acid (10 to 15 drops to 30 gm. of water). Wash again in clear water ; place them in a solution of chloride of zinc for from 10 to 24 hours, wash again in clear water and dry carefully. They will then have the appearance of being nickel plated.—*Zahntechniche Reform.*

To Strengthen a Partial Gold Plate.—Dr. Read fits a piece of half-round wire to the model about from bicuspid to bicuspid, and fastens it to its place with wax. This is reproduced on the zinc die and also on the plate after being swedged, greatly strengthening it.—*Zahntechniche Reform.*

The Image of His Pa.—The nurse shows the new-born to the proud father.—"Just like his papa, Herr Baron." "Really ?" "No hair, no teeth ; just your *very* image."—*Zahntechniche Reform.*

Aluminium Crowns.—Dr. Heinman swedges crowns of aluminium and fills cusps with amalgam.—*Zahntechniche Reform.*
(Aluminium being a soft metal, time can only tell how it will withstand the force of mastication.—C. E. K.)

To Reset a Denture.—Dr. Dick's method.—He pours plaster of Paris into the plate for an impression ; after plaster of Paris is hard, imbed the teeth about half-way in impression compound, place in articulator and remove plate from impression, take teeth off plate and put in their place in compound. Make a base plate of tea-lead on model, close articulator ; now attach teeth to base plate with sticky wax and hot spatula. Open the articulator and fill up with wax on base to thickness of desired plate ; trim and vulcanize same as usual. This is done when you have a good articulation of the teeth in the mouth and do not wish to alter or change it.—*Zahntechniche Reform.*

Pulp Capping.—Dr. Anthony uses chlora percha. To a 15 gm. solution he adds 1¼ gm. oil of cloves, 6/10 gm. tannic acid, and 1¼ gm. carbolic acid. Make to the consistency of thick cream. A little dropped into the cavity and the chloroform allowed to evaporate. Fill on top of this.—*Zahntechniche Reform.*

IN PERIODONTITIS—Instead of painting the gums with a solution of aconite and iodine, Dr. Jones injects it under the gums close to the alveolar margin. The effect, he claims, is instantaneous.—*Zahntechniche Reform.*

ALUMINIUM SOLDER.—The *Scientific American* gives the following formula: 45 parts of tin and 11 parts of aluminium are melted separately and poured together in the molten state and poured into ingots. No flux required.—*Zahntechniche Reform.*

MATRIX FOR AMALGAM FILLINGS.—Dr. Mathews uses short pieces of very thin rubber tubing, which he slips over the tooth and allows it to remain about three hours after the tooth is filled. *Zahntechniche Reform.*

TO CLEANSE HYPODERMIC SYRINGE POINTS.—If you cannot pass a fine wire through, heat the points; this will burn out all foreign substances. Should a wire be rusted in, then dip the point into oil and heat—this will enable you to pull out the wire; force oil into the point and heat again, and you can remove all traces of rust. Wash with alcohol.—*Zahntechniche Reform.*

HEMOSTATIC.—Professor Cheever considers sulphate of iron and ammonium as the best hemostatic. It causes the blood to coagulate very rapidly, and forms a hard clot which does not irritate the soft tissues. He prefers it to perchloride of iron or to persulphate of iron.—*Zahntechniche Reform.*

Proceedings of Dental Societies.

Vermont State Dental Society.

There are historical and geographical, not to mention the personal, reasons why Canadian dentists should take a special interest in the conventions in the border States. In the Province of Ontario the profession has been under great obligations to friends like Dr. W. C. Barratt, of Buffalo, and others, and to the State societies of New York especially, members of whom have not only visited and contributed to the meetings of the Ontario Association, but who have hospitably received Canadian visitors to the meetings in their State. Vermont, in many ways, seems like a part of the Province of Quebec, and the eighteenth annual meeting of the State society would have been more largely attended by Canadians had it not been for several circumstances which may not likely occur again. It was one of the most pleasant and profitable ever held. Dr. G. W. Hoffman, of White River Junction, had invited the members to hold the meeting there, and the St. George's Hotel was found to be a delightful and cosy centre. The meeting opened on Wednesday, the 21st of March, at 7.30 p.m., with prayer by the Rev. Dr. Snow. The President, Dr. A. J. Parker, of Bellow's Falls, occupied the chair. Dr. Wright offered a resolution of sympathy with Dr. S. J. Andres, of Quebec city, an honorary member of the Society, which was unanimously carried, and the Society requested to convey the same to the doctor. Dr. Andres has been unwell for some time, and was unable to be among the many friends in Vermont who were always glad to see him.

Dr. Hoffman then read a charming address of welcome, which had the unique feature of having been written by his wife. The papers are to be published in our contemporary, the *Ohio Dental Journal*, and we trust Mrs. Hoffman's tribute to the profession of her husband will appear in full.

Dr. J. N. Collins, of Granville, N.Y., read a paper entitled "Filling Root-Canals with Beeswax," in which he described the careful procedure of thoroughly drying the canals, and then introducing the wax and melting it around the mouths of the tubuli with a hot wire. It is not only cleanly and persistently hermetical in adaptation to the surrounding walls, but it is easily removed in the event of subsequent trouble. Dr. Collins stated that Dr. S. B. Palmer, of Syracuse, approved of it, and had publicly stated his belief that it was the best root-canal filling.

Dr. G. A. Young, of Concord, N.H., believed, after long experience, that it did not much matter what the roots are filled with providing gutta-percha and chloroform is not used. He has never seen a case in which the gutta-percha had not absorbed the fluids, and in fact, if removed, a strong odor was present from the pulp cavity. He approved of wax, if he approved of anything. He removed one gutta-percha filling put in by Dr. W. S. Curtis, of West Randolph. It was sweet and clean, because it was crude gutta-percha. Beeswax withstands acids. Only wish we could satisfactorily fill the crown as well as the canals with beeswax. It would make dental practice fun. However, he declared that he did not believe in putting anything into the canals ; has got over all medicating of canals ; believes that the open canals are safer than if filled. If he feels like it, he puts gold into the roots as far as convenient, but is not bound down to any cast-iron rule.

Dr. G. Lennox Curtis, New York, asked Dr. Young if he ever had alveolar abscess following his treatment of "no treatment." Dr. Young replied that he had not any more, and he did not think he had so much as formerly.

Dr. Curtis said it was new to him, and that he would like it scientifically and statistically investigated. Instinctively, he approved of wax ; it left no odor. Best results he has seen were when chloro-percha used, after thorough cleansing to the apex, sterilization, perfect drying by hot air, paper points, etc. Does not look reasonable to omit filling root-canals, leaving air for decomposition, and if heated, drawing back the fluid elements, which must create inflammation and abscess.

Dr. Hoffman, White River Junction, described cases where canals were left empty and found no odor. Never believed in the air theory before. Since then never filled root canals. Sterilized with hot air ; inserted filling, and did not make any special effort to get it up the canals. The results of this practice have been satisfactory.

Dr. Bowers, of Mashua, N.H., tried the air theory for three years ; does not always adhere to it ; doubts if the apex of roots can always be reached. The only dentists who accomplish miracles like that are recent graduates—they never err or have failures.

Dr. C. K. Gerrish, Ester, N.H., then made some very interesting remarks on " The Unknown Dentistry of the Future." He claimed to be a bit of an old-fashioned dentist, not apt to be carried away by every new fad. Had used one gold foil—Abbey's—for thirty years. Never filled a tooth exclusively with adhesive foil. He showed the wonderful knowledge possessed by the Egyptians in the arts and sciences, and what they knew about dental practice. He read a very quaint advertisement of Josiah F. Flagg, in the early part of the century. With respect to the present rage for hypnotism, fifty years ago it was called mesmeric power. The speaker was associated in early life with Dr. W. L. Johnson, of Newburyport, Mass., and he saw thousands of teeth extracted by Dr. Johnson, after he had " mesmerized " the patients, and in no single instance with bad effects. Bleeding, too, was controlled by hypnotism. Dr. Gerrish covered a great deal of ground in referring to the past, and the prospects of the future dental practice. He saw inlays thirty-two years ago retained by gold foil. All honor to the men of fifty years ago, who showed they were artists, and whose success in the face of great difficulties ought to humiliate those of us who think we " know it all." The doctor concluded by drawing an imaginative and humorous picture of the future dentistry—providing future generations have any teeth.

Dr. G. A. Young was to have read a paper, but in his usual bland way he hypnotized the audience to forgive him, as he had brought several good " trotters " from New Hampshire, including the President, Dr. Bowers, and other officials of the State society. Dr. Young is an institution which the Vermont Society begin to feel they cannot do without. As the founder and head centre of the " Trotters' Club," he is not only possessed of great mines of practical knowledge and skill, but a deep vein of humor which runs like a golden thread through his most serious remarks.

On Thursday morning the members re-assembled. Dr. R. M. Chase, of Bethel, opened a discussion on the subject, " Should

Dentists Administer Secret Drugs and Nostrums?" He contended that it is as unethical as it is unscientific to administer drugs the composition of which we do not know. No local anæsthetic should be used, the formula of which was not published on the label. It had been shown by Dr. Kirke that most, if not all, of these preparations contained cocaine, and it is, moreover, a notorious fact that some dentists are publicly lying in their disgraceful advertisements, and pretending to have the monopoly of the use of some such preparation, ignorant whether or not it contains constituents dangerous to health and even to life. There is a class of men who neither respect themselves nor care for the public, more than as patients, whom they can deceive. It may be, too, that many very honorable men use these nostrums, believing that they are harmless. But how can they believe anything about their effects if they are kept in the dark as to their formula?

Dr. Hoffman said that if any men in any dental society will stultify themselves by subscribing to a code of ethics, and then pretend before the public that they have the monopoly of a nostrum of the kind, they lie, and should be expelled. A *dentist* who does it is a sneak of the first water, and should be treated like any other sneak.

Dr. James Lewis, of Burlington, the oldest practitioner in the State, and one of the honorable and respected "fathers" of dentistry, remarked that we claim to be a branch of medicine, but unless we enforce our ethics we do not merit the claim. When advertisers declare they have something new, when they know no more than their patients what the nostrum contains, and do not know the physiological or toxical effects, they injure the profession and they rob their patients. Their claims are mere ghost stories. In Nashville Medical College, the Faculty erased from the graduates' register the names of those who were using such deceptive advertisements. Dental societies should do as much. Hundreds of good teeth are extracted by these advertisers. He believed, from his experience of active practice of over half a century, that there were fewer teeth saved by filling than thirty years ago.

Dr. George O. Webster believed it was necessary for the honor of the Society and for the protection of the public that some action should be taken. He did not believe in any dictatorial despotism which would force men, by law, to avoid these nostrums; but he believed in cleansing the skirts of State societies even of any silent recognition. The Society should not be used as a cloak to enable anyone to advertise these nostrums. He would prefer to see men repenting and becoming ethical, rather than subjecting themselves, by such conduct, to the reproach of their brethren and possible actions for damages some day from their patients.

Dr. G. L. Curtis said, the worst feature was the deceptive advertising. If men felt they must do it, they should resign their connection with the Society, because their influence was a direct injury and insult to members who believed in being ethical.

Dr. James Lewis recalled the use of arsenic by Spooner, and his contemporaries, for reducing sensitiveness of dentine, and the serious results which frequently followed. Some of these local anæsthetic nostrums contained liquid arsenic.

Dr. George F. Cheney, St. Johnsbury, asked, How shall we educate the public? In the analysis of a medicine recently put upon the market, it was discovered that there was enough arsenic in a few drops to kill! Dr. Kirke in his article in the *Cosmos* had shown that of ten local anæsthetic nostrums, only one was free of cocaine (Barr's). He thought that the public press should publish such facts.

Dr. W. Geo. Beers believed that if the public knew the fact that dentists who used these nostrums were ignorant of their composition, they would be loath to have them injected into their blood. Dr. Kirke deserved the thanks of the profession for exposing the duplicity, not only of the men who manufactured these nostrums, but of the men who ignorantly used them. It was a fact, nevertheless, that the public tolerate, if they do not positively enjoy, being deceived. He suggested that the American Dental Association consider this question and pronounce authoritatively, not only on the ethical question, but as to what preparations can be safely used. It would be well to suggest a reliable preparation, and publish the formula under the official approval of the national representative associations (American Dental and the Southern Dental).

Dr. J. L. Perkins, St. Johnsbury, suggested that attention be drawn to the fact, that the gum tissue has frequently sloughed as the result of the hypodermic use of some of these nostrums.

Dr. W. S. Curtis, West Randolph, agreed with the object proposed, but reminded the members that it did not apply, so far as censure in use was concerned, to preparations the formula of which was known and intelligently approved of by the operator.

On motion of Dr. Chase the following resolution, embodying one passed by the Connecticut Valley Dental Society, was unanimously passed :

" *Whereas*, Several compounds and nostrums, more or less familiar to the dental profession, have been and are being promiscuously advertised as secrets, and those which have been proved either useless or injurious, advertised as wonderful, and

" *Whereas*, Such false and vicious advertising is a detriment to our patients and ourselves, and

" *Whereas*, All known local applications, powerful enough to completely destroy the sensibility, are capable of doing serious injury to tooth and structure, and severely to health, therefore

" *Resolved*, That we hereby condemn the practice of the use of such nostrums by the profession, and recommend that any and all legitimate means be used by the members of our societies to educate the public and guard them against the possible harm which may result from the use of these nostrums."

It was decided that secret compounds and nostrums include all compounds put upon the market without a printed formula furnished to the profession at large.

A paper and a talk on "Alveolar Hæmorrhage," by W. George Beers, followed. The writer explained the physiology of coagulation, the causes of imperfect coagulation, the varieties of hæmorrhage—capillary, venous, and arterial—constitutional and local conditions which predisposed to hæmorrhage. He showed that precaution was necessary in dental practice not to venture upon surgical operations, involving the loss of blood, in marked cases of anæmia, when the fibrin is in a state of inefficient solution, the blood of feeble coagulating power, and the vascular trunk of feeble contractile power. The danger of lancing children's gums in certain constitutional conditions was shown. Also the fact that, where leeches are used, the blood coming from the body as soon as the leech is removed will never coagulate; and that, even in ten minutes after the leech is withdrawn, it will take one hour for the blood to coagulate. It is said that this is due to a secretion in the leech with which it impregnates the wound. Attention was drawn to vicarious bleeding during the menstrual period, and the risk of operating at that time. The writer believed that some such physiological localized concentration, followed by vaso-motor disturbance, especially in neurotic girls, as explained by the so-called miracle of the "Stigmata," was apt to occur when teeth were extracted during the catamenia. The decrease of hæmorrhage was thought to be due to the better blood as the result of better food, abundance and cheapness of fruits; better instruments, the abandonment of the old key of Garengeot, etc. Sir Benjamin Ward Richardson, in a paper read before the Odontological Society of Great Britain recently, attributed the decrease in hæmorrhage in his experience to these facts. It was shown that there need be no anxiety if syncope occurred. It relieved the arterial tention. Stimulants should never be used. They increased it. The various orthodox methods of arresting hæmorrhage were mentioned, and attention drawn to the great value of *Lycoperdon giganteum*, or common puff-ball, which Sir Benj. Ward Richardson introduced nearly forty years ago, before the then existing College of Dentists of England. It had been used for centuries to stupify bees before robbing the hives. Dr. Richardson saw this done, and was led to try it as a narcotic. The writer had it analyzed some years ago, and it was discovered that its styptic property was due to phosphate of soda. It acted chemically and mechanically. When he was a student, Dr. Charles Brewster, of Montreal, was using it in his dental practice, and in 1871, after using it for thirteen years, he brought it before the profession in the *Canada Journal of Dental Science.* Dr. Brewster had, for years, been experimenting with it, and having medicated it, and added greatly to its natural advantages, he was induced to place it in the market for our use. It was unexcelled for hæmorrhage, alveolar or otherwise, and Dr. Beers suggested that the dried and medicated *lycoperdon* be tried in the hæmoptysis, where the divided artery is in the lung and the mineral acids are used.

The paper was discussed by Drs. G. L. Curtis, Lewis, and others.

Dr. Thos. Fillebrown, of Boston, who has distinguished himself for his concentration of interest in suggestive therapeutics and operations applied to dental practice, gave a most fascinating lecture on "The Power of Suggestion." Your reporter is forced to make the confession, which he considers at the same time a compliment to Dr. Fillebrown, that his attention was so concentrated that he forgot he had a note-book in his hand ; and he proposes trusting to his memory to prepare a special report, and submit it to Dr. Fillebrown for revision, and then publish it in the DOMINION DENTAL JOURNAL. Dr. Fillebrown demonstrated the power he described, in the mouths of several patients.

Dr. C. H. Wells, Huntingdon, Que., read a paper illustrative of his mechanical treatment of a number of fractures, which had been caused by the celebrated kicking horses of the Province of Quebec. The paper was well discussed by Dr. G. L. Curtis, who paid the essayist many compliments. It pleased him specially to remark the conservative treatment. General surgeons would not have saved the teeth in the cases mentioned.

In the afternoon Dr. Gustave P. Wicksell, Boston, gave clinics "Richmond, Buckern, Wicksell Crowns." Dr. F. R. Jewett, of Woodstock, on "Crown Work." But the *crême de la crême* was the series of surgical clinics by Dr. G. Lennox Curtis, of 124 West 34th St., New York. We will not say that Dr. Curtis is a rising oral surgeon, He has risen, and shines in full effulgence as a cool, wonderfully rapid, and skilful master of oral surgical science. The doctor exhibited one osteo-sarcoma from the antrum as large as a hen's egg. The case was due to a blow on the malar bone. A portion of the jaw and teeth opened into the antrum ; the growth formed in the antrum, and destroyed portions of the malar and superior maxillary bones, and the hard palate. Dr. Curtis removed the teeth with the slightest ridge of alveolus, with very little effort, and the whole tumor was caught with the forceps and withdrawn from the antrum. The periosteum alone remained over the malar and palatal bones. Hæmorrhage was checked by very hot water ; wound firmly packed, and antiseptic precautions used. No secondary hæmorrhage. Case was dismissed in two weeks. In six weeks the boy, who was sixteen years old, returned to duty entirely cured. An artificial jaw of vulcanite was afterwards fitted. The operation occupied twenty-five minutes. Dr. Curtis exhibited photographs of the case, before and after the operation. No deformity, as there was no incision on the face ; Dr. Curtis using various appliances, most of them of his own invention, on the dental engine. He alluded to an artificial portion of jaw, for a similar case, made by Dr. W. G. Beers, which was fitted to a patient. It included an entire upper set of teeth, and an obturator to close an accidental cleft, and was retained *in situ* by a gold spring attached to an apparatus of gold in the lower maxillary. After wearing for three months, the folds of the cheek accommodated themselves so nicely to the plate that the lower apparatus was discarded.

An interesting osteoma was exhibited, which originated under the first inferior molar, left side. A filling had been inserted over a devitalized pulp, which abscessed the next day ; the face was much swollen for two weeks. Gradually subsiding, and leaving a hardened lump in the region of the root, which increased in size for two years, when it had enlarged to the size of a nutmeg. Dentists and surgeons advised no interference ; said it would " absorb." Dentist finally extracted the tooth ; found no sign of abscess ; pulp of tooth was atrophied. The tumor continued to enlarge for two years more, until it became the size and shape of a large walnut ; face disfigured, and mal-occlusion of the teeth. All the bone was destroyed within three-eighths of an inch of lower ridge. The inferior dental vessels and nerves were atrophied from pressure. The operation consisted of laying open the gum tissue, by incision from the dens-sapientiæ to the cuspid—*never touching the face.* Torsion and hot water were used instead of ligaturing. Then denuding the gum, the tumor was well exposed, and with an elevator it was lifted from its place as a cobble-stone might be lifted from the bed of a stream. The sac in which it was lying was dissected away ; packed with antiseptic gauze, and allowed to fill in by granulation. The operation occupied eight minutes. No deformity, and perfect cure.

Dr. Curtis operated before the members on a case evidently an osteoma, which had caused mal-occlusion of the teeth on one side, owing to the lengthening of the two last molars. After extracting the two teeth, he cut into the cancellous structure with a large burr on the dental engine, and removed the growth. It was his opinion that it might recur.

THE BANQUET.

The host of St. George's Hotel got up a very delightful and appetizing banquet. The menu card was very neat. A number of ladies were present. Dr. A. J. Parker presided with dignity and tact. There was more than enough to eat. As the State is Prohibition there was nothing stronger than coffee to drink.

There were lots of good speeches, and " The Trotters " had lots of fun among themselves.

" THE TROTTERS."

After the banquet, this ancient and mysterious organization, born in the State, met in Room 26, to drink the usual two hundred and forty toasts in their own Club concoction, the formula of which, with all respect to the Code of Ethics, cannot be printed on the label. Candidates, upon initiation, are obliged to swallow the mystic cup " Orangesoapcork." One candidate was initiated fifteen times. It is a specific for constipation. An international contest occurred between the champion trotters of the United States and Canada. The American brought down the house, and the Canuck brought down the bed. Two hundred and forty-two fish stories were told. Dr. Young, of Concord, told two hundred and forty-one. The remaining members told the other one. The meeting then adjourned to breakfast.

THE FINISH.

After the ever-vigilant treasurer, Dr. W. H. Munsell, had brought delinquents to time with their subscriptions, Dr. Parker announced that the election of officers would follow. The result was as follows : President, Dr. W. H. Wright, Brandon ; 1st Vice-President, Dr. E. O. Blanchard, West Randolph ; 2nd Vice-President, Dr. F. P. Mathers, Chester; Secretary, Dr. Thos. Mound, Rutland ; Treasurer, Dr. W. H. Munsell, Wells River ; Executive Committee, Drs. C. W. Staples, Lyndonville ; J. A. Robinson, Morrisville ; G. A. Wheeler, West Randolph ; State Prosecutor, Dr. G. W. Hoffman, White River Junction.

There were two causes for regret ; one was that all the members did not wait until the last event of the last day, the other was that we had to part.

Brandon was fixed upon as the next place of meeting.

Many personal matters crowd upon us, which we regret we have not time to enumerate. It was delightful to meet with Dr. James Lewis, and Dr. J. L. Perkins, who bear well the brunt of life and duty, sturdy as their own green mountains. Dr. Lewis is a young-old man, whose professional reminiscences we would like to see in book form. Dr. Perkins is neither young nor old, but he has the spirit of the one, and the matured sense of the other. But they are all " jolly good fellows,"—" which nobody can deny."

THE EXAMINING BOARD.

The following officers of the Board were present :—

Dr. J. L. Perkins, President, St. Johnsbury; Dr. R. M. Chase, Bethel ; Dr. Jas. Lewis, Burlington ; Dr. Geo. O. Webster, St. Alban's ; Dr. A. J. Parker, Bellow's Falls. The meeting began at 2 p.m. on the 21st March. There were seven applicants for license.

An important feature was the practical examination. Each candidate was obliged to perform various operations in the mouth in presence of the Board, and the offices of Drs. Hoffman and Wheeler were used for the purpose, as well as the chairs in the Dental Exhibit. The advantage of this in economizing time was shown in the case of one candidate who quickly demonstrated his inability to prepare a simple cavity, and who withdrew from the ordeal. The following gentlemen were granted licences to practice: D. J. Harrigan, Bellow's Falls; N. P. Bugbee, North Comfret; H. Burbridge, Windsor; Chas. Sutton, Norton Mills. Four candidates were rejected.

We take special pleasure in congratulating the members of the Society on the *personnel* of the Board. It would be difficult to find five men more faithful and able; and it must be remembered that their personal work and worry, purely in the best interests of the profession and the public, is not confined to the few days of the annual meeting, but extends throughout the year; as any member of the Board may, in the interim of the session, examine a candidate and grant a temporary licence to practise until the next meeting. One of the results is that every member is exposed to this inconvenience at any time in his own office; and, as has repeatedly occurred, when the examiner finds that he cannot conscientiously pass a candidate, he is certain to be assailed, personally and professionally, by the particular friends of the candidate. It is easy to imagine how this may cause direct financial loss to the examiner. The responsibility and annoyance in this respect may be quite serious. Moreover, if it should happen that an examiner showed unfair leniency, he does an injustice to the licensed members as well as to the people.

EXHIBITORS.

The following had very interesting exhibits of their goods, which were closed during the meetings of the Society: T. Hudson, Troy, N.Y.; Wood & Reynolds, Boston; Boston Dental Manufacturing Co.; S. S. White Dental Manufacturing Co., Boston; A. J. Smith, Providence, R.I.; Gideon Sibley, Philadelphia, Pa.; Wilmington Dental Manufacturing Co.; B. L. Knapp & Co., Boston.

Whatever may now and then be said as to the distracting attraction of the exhibits, they are an educational boon to the profession, especially to those who practise where there are no depots in their locality.

The Dental and Surgical Microcosm has suspended publication until October next, owing to the long and severe illness in the family of the editor and subsequent death of his wife and only son. We extend our sympathy to our bereaved contemporary.

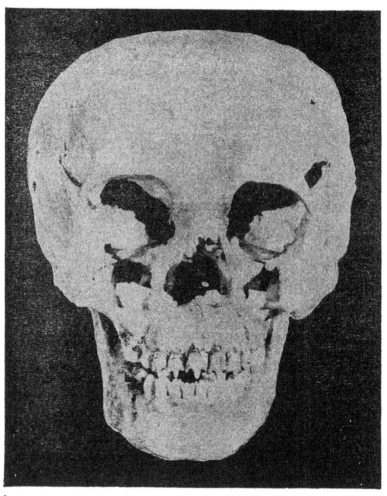

Filed teeth of skull over one thousand years old. Photographed by R. R. Andrews from Central American Exhibit, Peabody Museum, Cambridge. (Skull, grave 14, Labna, Yucatan. Found by M. H. Saville.)

Prehistoric Crania From Central America.*

By R. R. ANDREWS, A.M., D.D.S., Cambridge, Mass.

At the Peabody Museum, at Cambridge, there is a collection of archæological treasures, recently found in Central America, that have especial interest to the dental profession.   These, consisting of crania, parts of the skeleton, a collection of teeth curiously filed and inlaid, with a fine collection of pottery and instruments which were made from bone, stone, and from a volcanic glass (obsidian), together with carvings and statues, are soon to be on public exhibition.   They are being arranged in cases and around the room, while large numbers of photographs, showing the site of the excavations, are arranged within the cabinets upon the walls.

In 1890 the expedition that obtained them was sent to Central America by Harvard University under the charge of Mr. John G. Owens, a young archæologist of great promise, who died at his post of duty after the explorations were about complete.   The expense of this expedition was defrayed by certain wealthy Bostonians.   Most of these archæological treasures were brought from Copan, Honduras, and certain other ruins found in Yucatan. Mr. C. P. Bowditch, of Boston, who has been very much interested in the expedition, has now the charge of the collection.   Mr. M. H. Saville, to whom I am much indebted, and who was with the expedition, states that the site where these things were found was covered by a growth of old trees, and it was necessary for the natives to cut these away before the excavations commenced.   An ancient temple of some kind was long supposed to have existed here, from the fact that carved blocks of stone had been from time to time dug up in the locality, and the excavations proved this supposition to be a fact.   A large temple was unearthed, together with a number of the homes of the former inhabitants, and graves were found under the floors of the rooms of the houses. These graves were either stoned in or cemented, after the bodies had been partly covered with loose earth.   Other graves were found in deep cemented chambers under the level of the ground, these chambers having the triangular arch commonly found in the buildings of this prehistoric people.   The teeth on exhibition were obtained at Copan, Honduras.   The skull, which is here shown, was taken from a grave at Labna, Yucatan, and is probably of a later date than the skeletons found at Copan, although it is undoubtedly pre-

Skeleton 7, Mound 36.
Filed without inlay.

* A Paper read before the American Academy of Dental Science, Boston.

historic.   It was found by Mr. M. H. Saville, in grave No. 14 and in it may be seen how curiously were filed the six anterior upper and lower teeth.   It is undoubtedly a Maya skull, of a person—probably a female—about twenty years of age, judging from the erupting wisdom-teeth.   As no metal of any kind was found in any of the excavations, the teeth were probably ground down with coarse stone instruments.   There is no decay in any of the teeth, all being sound ; but the left superior cuspid is just

GROUP I. (From Copan, Honduras.)

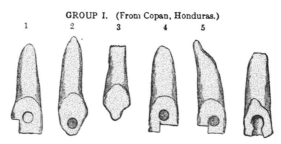

1. Central incisor, inlay lost, filed; 2. Cuspid, beautiful green jade inlay near cutting-edge; 3. Bicuspid, root absorbed, probably by abscess; 4. Central incisor, green jade inlay and filed; 5. Central incisor, green jade inlay and filed; 6. Cuspid, inlay lost, broken through to cutting-edge.

erupting about a quarter of an inch inside the arch.   It would seem as though these early people were flesh-eaters, and perhaps cannibals, and that the teeth may have been filed in this manner for the purpose of better tearing of flesh.   The photograph would imply that the skull was of considerable capacity, but it recedes very perceptibly from the orbits upward, so as to appear as though much flattened.   The teeth that were found at Copan, near by, are perhaps more interesting than the skull.   Many of these have small circular pieces of green jade inlaid in a cavity that has been drilled by a stone or glass instrument in the face of the incisors and cuspids.   These inlays are a little more than an eighth of an inch in diameter, the outer surface is rounded and brightly polished, and as perfectly fitted as it could be by the most skilled operator of to-day, with all the modern instruments at his command.   In a few of the teeth the inlays have loosened so that it can be taken out, and there appears to be a white substance, perhaps a cement, between the inlay and the tooth, used to hold the inlay in place.   It would seem that this inlay might be some mark of distinction, perhaps used in the mouth of a chief or head man of the people.   Some of these teeth are filed and have no inlay.   Some are inlaid and not filed.   And some are both filed and inlaid.   Quite a number of the teeth are badly decayed. Much of this decay appears to be at the cervical border, and in no case does there appear to be any filling of any kind used to stop decay.   None of them were filled for prophylactic purposes.   In the teeth from skeleton 8, mound 36, found at Copan, two of the teeth that may have formerly had an inlay were partially filled with something that seemed like a red cement substance. None of these from this skeleton were filed, but in the lower jaw of the skeleton was found the most interesting curiosity in the whole collection to dentists—a lower, left, lateral incisor that has been carved from some dark stone, and which has been implanted to take the place of one that had been lost. The tartar upon it would seem to show that it had been worn for some time during life. This implantation antedates Dr. Younger's experiments by about fifteen hundred years. Many of the teeth were so completely covered with tartar as to form masses nearly double their original size, and in one case an upper molar had the tartar deposited in

GROUP II. (Skeleton 8, Mound 36, Copan.)

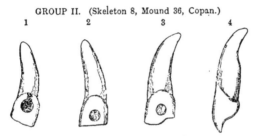

Superior—1. Partially filled with a reddish cement (cuspid); 2. Almost wholly filled with a reddish cement (incisor); 3. Green jade inlay, no filing (incisor); 4. Cuspid, same jaw, no filing and no inlay.

GROUP II.—*Continued.*

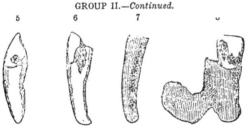

Inferior—5, 6. Cuspids decayed, no inlay, no filing; 7. Stone tooth, carved from a dark stone; 8. Decayed bicuspid and piece of socket.

such a way, and to such a degree, that it formed a shape that articulated on the gum of the lower jaw where the teeth had previously been lost. In one case, at least, the drilling of the tooth to produce a cavity in which to fit the inlay, had encroached upon the pulp, and there is distinct evidence of recalcification of pulp tissue at this point.

The whole collection is one of much interest, perhaps the most interesting evidence of prehistoric dental work that is to be found in any museum, and it is well worth a visit to Cambridge to see.—*International Dental Journal.*

[We are under obligation to the publishers of the *International Dental Journal* for the plates used in Dr. Andrew's paper on " Prehistoric Crania from Central America."—ED. D.D.J.]

Correspondence.

The Title of Doctor.

To the Editor of the DOMINION DENTAL JOURNAL :

DEAR SIR,—During the past few months there has been considerable discussion regarding the title of " doctor," as applied to dentists.   The British Medical Defence Union has taken exception to the title as so used, while your editorial, and a communication from one of your correspondents are evidently also opposed to its use among dentists.

If, as I understand it, the title " doctor " was originally applied to a teacher, and later to one who had acquired a certain amount of knowlege in any particular direction, the title is not misapplied in the case under discussion.   The title was originally applied to those persons making the laws and religion of their country a particular study.   In earlier times there were doctors of law and religion combined, for law and religion were then supposed to be inseparably related.   Later on, when there came a distinction between civil law and ecclesiastical law, there became Doctors of Law and Doctors of Divinity.   When the medical profession emerged from the chaos of witchcraft and sorcery and its concomitant ignorance, its members took to themselves the title of Doctor of Medicine, as designating a certain knowledge of the principles of that science.   There are now Doctors of Law, of Divinity, of Philosophy, of Medicine, of Music and of Dentistry.   One profession has as much right to the title as has another.   The real cause of complaint has arisen from the fact that the common people with their usual ignorance have continually called physicians doctors, until even the physicians themselves have been led to believe that the title is distinctively their own.

Dentistry is a profession, as noble, as difficult, as useful and as aspiring as any other.   Its members have, or should have, as good a general education, and as minute a special education as those of any other profession.

Each profession has its share of " black sheep," its retarding and retrogressive elements ; but dentistry has pre-eminently its share of careful students and conscientious investigators.   The profession of divinity has been in existence for thousands of years, yet its old speculations are speculations still.   It has not advanced one jot on the line of scientific demonstration.

The profession of law is still struggling with the principle of justice, and has never advanced beyond a sort of classified expediency.   Medicine has made great advances during the past century.   It no longer casts out devils, nor charms away disease, it grapples with, relieves and cures many of the most stubborn and fatal conditions. Medicine has taken several hundred years to advance from the barber's pole to its present exalted position. But what shall we say of dentistry?

Its cradle was the blacksmith's shop, and the village cobbler's bench. In less than a century it has grown until it embraces within its domain a chemistry, a materia medica, a metallurgy, a pathology, a bacteriology, an anatomy—a combination of the physician, metallurgist and mechanician. It requires the training of the judgment, the memory, the eye and the hand. It is the connecting link between the philosopher and artisan.

Dentistry requires a greater versatility than does any other profession. No one man ever becomes equally expert in all of its branches, and in like manner few men fail in each and every one of its branches. This last consideration has led some people to suppose that dentistry is an easy profession to practise. Nothing could be more removed from the truth.

The dentist who can, in succession, treat an abscess, extract under chloroform, put in a gold filling, make a gold crown or a plate, and set up a regulating appliance, has been in turn a physician, surgeon, mechanician, moulder, metallurgist, chemist, and engineer.

Is he not entitled to a recognition of his proficiency?

The title "doctor" signifies the attainment of a certain knowledge in some direction. Surely the dentist is as fully entitled to it as are the theologian, the philosopher, the physician, and the musician.

Yours very truly,
MARK G. MCILHINNEY, D.D.S.

Ottawa, March 20th, 1894.

Unlicensed Practitioners.

To the Editor of the DOMINION DENTAL JOURNAL:

DEAR SIR,—A short time ago I received from our friend and professional brother, Dr. Hanna, of Kemptville, Ont., a circular asking for opinions as to how to enforce the law with reference to unlicensed practitioners.

Let me offer my suggestions through your columns, and they will reach Dr. Hanna as well as others.

The difficulty of securing evidence to convict, as well as a magistrate to try any case, is incident to the attempted enforcement of any unpopular law.

The Act in question is supposed to exist for the protection of the public, while it really protects the unlicensed practitioner more than it does any one else.

The aversion to act shown by the necessary witnesses and the indispensable magistrate as representatives of the public, proves that *in their estimation* the Act is not for their benefit, or at least not necessary for their protection, but on the contrary, for the benefit of the dentists.

It is human nature to exercise one's own choice in selecting a tooth-tinker, as in choosing anything else, and it is just as truly human nature to try every imaginable quack remedy first, and the best skill last.

If the object is to protect the public, it seems to me that the most sensible course would be to give warning by public notice that the offending persons are not legally qualified to practise dentistry, then, if the public choose to employ their services, I don't see how you can prevent it. It involves the fundamental fact of ethical impossibility to legislate men into correct living.

It seems impracticable to enforce the Act by conviction and fine, and no one, either in the profession or out of it, cares to be a party to it.

It seems to me that legal notice issued by the proper authority and " posted in conspicuous places " would be an effective weapon, if, indeed, the law has a right to exist at all, which is questionable in my mind, as I do not believe in the theory of protection, and I think it ought to be plain to the most short-sighted that in practice it is a failure. A. STACKHOUSE.

KINGSTON, ONT., *March 19th, 1894.*

Reviews.

Minor Surgery and Bandaging. By HENRY R. WHARTON, M.D., Demonstrator of Surgery in the University of Pennsylvania. In one 12mo. volume of 529 pages, with 416 engravings, many being photographic. Cloth, $3.00. Philadelphia : Lea Brothers & Co. 1893.

In response to the demand for a second edition, the author has revised his work to make it represent in every way the advances of the two years which have elapsed since its first appearance. The exceptionally rich and beautiful series of illustrations, in connection with a singularly clear text, afford the student and practitioner all needed instruction in the many procedures grouped under the title. The pictures of bandaging are photographically reproduced from actual life. The author has construed his title very generously, and has placed within the covers far more information than is usually accredited to Minor Surgery, but readers will scarcely object to such liberality. Antiseptic Surgery is dealt with in accordance with the latest and most approved practice.

Catching's Compendium of Practical Dentistry. Volume IV. B. H. CATCHING, Editor and Publisher, Atlanta, Ga., U.S. Price, $2.50.

Every dentist who wants to keep posted in the practical progress of the profession, must do one of two things—subscribe to all the journals in English, German, French, Italian, Spanish, and Portuguese, at a cost of about $100, or get this compedium of Dr. Catching's, at a cost of $2.50. The editor had the happy thought to secure the co-operation of the following eminent confreres : Dr. A. C. Hugenschmidt, of Paris, as editor and translator of the French journals ; Dr. W. D. Miller, of Berlin, as editor and translator of the German ; Dr. W. Dunn, of Florence, as editor and translator of the Italian ; and Dr. J. R. De Silva, as editor and translator of the Spanish and Portuguese. This gives it a cosmopolitan character : embracing "the condensed practical results of the dental journals of six different nations." By sending a postal order direct to the editor, the book will be forwarded by mail. It is as full of digestible dental ideas as a Canadian egg is full of meat.

A Dictionary of Medical Science. Containing a full explanation of the various subjects and terms of Anatomy, Physiology, Medical Chemistry, Pharmacy, Pharmacology, Therapeutics, Medicine, Hygiene, Dietetics, Pathology, Surgery, Bacteriology, Ophthalmology, Otology, Laryngology, Dermatology, Gynecology, Obstetrics, Pediatrics, Medical Jurisprudence and Dentistry, etc., etc. By ROBLEY DUNGLISON, M.D., LL.D., late Professor of Institutes of Medicine in the Jefferson Medical College of Philadelphia. Edited by RICHARD J. DUNGLISON, A.M., M.D. New (21st) edition, thoroughly revised, greatly enlarged and improved, with the Pronunciation, Accentuation and derivation of the Terms. In one magnificent imperial octavo volume of 1181 pages. Cloth, $7.00 ; leather, $8.00. Philadelphia : Lea Bros. & Co. 1893.

For sixty years *Dunglison's Medical Dictionary* has been the standard authority in medical terminology, and twenty-one editions have been required to meet the ever-increasing demand. In no previous issue have the changes and additions been so great. *Forty-four thousand* new words and phrases have been added to place the work in conformity with the most advanced terminology of the time. Everything obsolete has been excised, yet the work contains about one hundred pages more matter than its predecessor. The page has been enlarged, so that this great work is still comprised in one convenient volume. For the first time, pronunciation has been introduced, being indicated by a simple and clear phonetic spelling. Derivation, an unexcelled aid to remembrance of meanings, is also thoroughly given. The full and explanatory definitions for which "Dunglison" has always been noted, have been expanded to include much valuable and practical information not always easily found elsewhere. Thus, under Diseases are given their symptoms and treatment ; under Drugs, their properties and doses ; under Poisoning, the symptoms, antidotes and treatment. Numerous tables enrich the alphabet and place an immense amount of information clearly and conveniently at hand. Examples may be found in the tables of *Doses* and *Bacteria.* It is safe to call *Dunglison's Medical Dictionary* an indispensable book for students, practitioners, pharmacists, dentists and all concerned with any of the medical sciences.

Anatomy, Descriptive and Surgical. By HENRY GRAY, F.R.S., Lecturer on Anatomy at St. George's Hospital, London. New American from the thirteenth enlarged and improved English edition. Edited by T. PICKERING PICK, F.R.C.S , Examiner in Anatomy, Royal College of Surgeons of England. In one imperial octavo volume of 1100 pages, with 635 large engravings. Price with illustrations in colors : Cloth, $7.00 ; leather, $8.00. Price with illustrations in black : Cloth, $6.00 ; leather, $7.00. Philadelphia : Lea Brothers & Co. 1893.

Since 1857, *Gray's Anatomy* has unquestionably been the standard text-book on its subject among all English-speaking peoples. The demand for thirteen editions has been utilized by subjecting the work to the searching revision of the foremost anatomists of a generation. In no other way is accuracy and completeness to be attained in treating of so complex and detailed a science. The series of illustrations is quite as famous as the text. Their large size not only enables the various parts to be brought into view, but also allows their names to be engraved directly upon them. Thus not only the name, but the extent of a part is indicated at a glance, a matter of obvious importance and convenience. Many new illustrations appear in this edition, and the whole series has been re-engraved wherever clearness could be promoted. The liberal use of colors lends added prominence to the attachments of muscles, to veins, arteries and nerves. The work is also published with illustrations in black alone.

As heretofore, the revision has been most thoroughly performed, so that the work is kept always abreast with the advances of its science. Especial attention has been paid to the application of anatomy to surgery, and the work is therefore indispensable to all who find in the exigencies of practice the need of recalling the details of the dissecting room.

Editorial.

German Translations.

Dr. Carl Klotz, of St. Catharines, Ont., has placed the profession under obligations, by undertaking to give us, periodically, translations from a German exchange.

Matriculation for Dentistry.

When the profession was first organized in the Province of Ontario, and the following year in the Province of Quebec, the political aspect necessarily monopolized attention. Then the proportional educational standard had to be slowly but surely considered ; and in course of time the conviction dawned upon us, that the future social and professional status depended very largely upon a standard of matriculation examination for entrance to study. It was comparatively easy in Ontario, where the system of education has perhaps no superior in any country, to make a decided advance ; but in Quebec, with its racial and legislative peculiarities, we were repeatedly made the shuttlecock of some crank, who succeeded in obtaining special legislation by intrigue, in spite of the protests of an almost united profession. At one time, the examination was that of the College of Physicians and Surgeons, the very highest standard on this continent ; then it was reduced to a mere nothing ; and again it was amended so as to lead to the suspicion that the almighty dollar was more influential than a knowledge even of "the three R's." We do not hesitate to say, that we have the most unbounded distrust of the permanency of any legislation, made for us by any government in the Province of Quebec, since the *regime* of Mr. Mercier opened the eyes of certain members of Parliament to the possibilities of boodle. From personal experience, extending over twenty-four years, of efforts to make a certain element recognize the requirements of the profession and the protection of the public, we are free to declare, that there may always be a sufficient number of members open to bribery to defeat a full measure of justice. It is a humiliating confession ; but the facts in our possession would be still more humiliating to a community which makes any pretence to honesty in its legislation. We may discuss this special matter more fully at another time. Nevertheless, we have been strangely successful, for the time being, in obtaining a further amendment respecting the matriculation examination, which removes it entirely from the jurisdiction of the universities, and places it exclusively in the hands of the Board of Examiners. This change not only enables the Board to select the subjects of examination, but the examiners, and two of the leading educationalists of the Province, one English and one French—Dr. Howe and Abbé Verean—have accepted the appointments. The examination will occupy two days. The following is the present programme of subjects, subject each year to alteration :

PRELIMINARY EXAMINATION FOR ADMISSION TO THE STUDY OF DENTISTRY.

Latin.—Cæsar's Commentaries, Book I., with Virgil's Æneid, Book I. ; questions of Grammar and Construction.

English.—Writing from dictation, Grammar and Analysis, a critical knowledge of one of Shakespeare's plays.

French.—Translation in English of extracts from Fenelon's " Adventures de Telemaque," questions of Grammar.

Literature.—Elements of the subject, with the History of English Literature from the reign of Queen Elizabeth to the present time.

History.—Of Britain, France and Canada.

Geography.—Modern, especially of Britain and France, and of their colonies and possessions.

Arithmetic.—To the end of Square Root, and to include a knowledge of the *Metrical* System.

Algebra.—To Simultaneous Equations of the first degree inclusive.

Geometry.—Euclid, Books I., II., III., and the first twenty Propositions of Book VI. ; also the measurement of the Surfaces and Volumes of the regular geometrical figures.

NOTE.—The above subjects are obligatory. In addition to them, candidates must choose one of the two following:

Philosophy.—Logic, and Intellectual and Moral Philosophy.

Physics.—Elementary Statics and Dynamics of Solids and Fluids, with the chapter on Heat.

The programme for French-speaking candidates will be the same as the foregoing which is for English-speaking candidates, except that the subjects of *English* and *French* will be, so to speak, *reversed* as follows :

French.—Writing from dictation, Grammar and Analysis. A critical knowledge of " Les Fables de La Fontaine."

English.—Translation into French of extracts from Washington Irving's " Life of Columbus," with questions of Grammar.

Literature.—Elements of the Subject, History of French Literature from the reign of Louis XIV. to the present time.

Old Journals.

Many dentists read their journals, and after awhile throw them away. Almost every practitioner in Canada has an accumulation of sample copies of the various journals published, which they may not value more than waste paper. If they would take the trouble to pack them into parcels and address them to us, we would be very grateful. We can make good use of them.

Annotations.

The *Dental Register*, with Dr J. Taft still at the helm, has, every month for many years, issued a complete directory of dental societies in the United States, by which we learn there are thirty-five State and thirty-six local societies, besides the two more representative bodies, the " American Dental Association " and the " Southern Dental Association."

We learn from Dr. P. Dubois, of Paris, France, that the *Revue Internationale* and *D' Odontologie* have been incorporated in one, with Dr. Dubois as editor and administrator. We cordially commend this journal to our confreres in Canada and the United States whose mother-tongue is French. Dr. Dubois is well-known in Europe as one of the most distinguished teachers.

Failures in crown work are often due to the mistake commonly made of using too soft gold. Many operators use ready made seamless crowns of twenty-two and twenty-four karat gold. These golds are not alloyed with metals that would tend to stiffen them from the fact that it would increase the difficulty of stamping them up. A stiff gold of a sufficiently high karat to prevent a discoloration in the mouth, though harder to adjust and fit, will always prove more durable and less liable to stretch during the process of fitting and from the force of mastication after it is finished. When these soft crowns are used it is best to stiffen them well by flowing a thin layer of high karat solder over the outer surface before cementing to place. Where the operator possesses the requisite skill it is generally better and safer to make each individual crown to suit the case. The different solderings of the band and top all have the effect of stiffening and hardening the gold so that by the time the crown is complete it is sufficiently rigid to prevent its being stretched from use.

The good old *American Journal of Dental Science*, now in the twenty-seventh year of its present existence, but in the forty-seventh of its entire career, is always welcome. We can never forget that it was the first dental journal in the world. In three years more it will commemorate its fiftieth anniversary, and we would suggest to its publishers—a little ahead of time, perhaps—to issue a special number, with pictures of its founders, etc. We will gladly send our subscription towards the issue of a journalistic monument to the memories of its founders.

LABOR.—Life to some is drudgery; to some, pain; to others, pleasure; but to *all*, work. Let none feel a sense of sore disappointment that life to them becomes routine. It is a necessary consequence of our nature that our work and our pleasures should tend to become routine. The same wants, the same demands, and similar duties meet us on the threshold of everyday. We look forward to some great occasion on which to give proof of a heroic spirit, and complain of the petty routine of daily life. It is this succession of little duties, little works apparently of no account, which constitute the grand work of life ; and we display true nobility when we cheerfully take these up and go forward, content to " Labor and to wait."—*Editorial in Southern Journal.*

DOMINION
DENTAL JOURNAL.

| VOL. VI. | TORONTO, MAY, 1894. | No. 5. |

Original Communications.

The Power of Suggestion.

By DR. THOMAS FILLEBROWN, Boston, Mass.

At the meeting of the Vermont State Dental Society, in March, Dr. Fillebrown gave an interesting talk on " The Power of Suggestion." The following report will give a fair idea of his remarks, though, of course, it is imperfect as a whole :

Suggestion in the wakeful state and without any attempt to produce hypnosis, had been so successfully used by him as an obtundent for sensitive dentine, during the past six months, that he felt that a few words upon the subject would prove useful to many, and not entirely without interest to all.

The many duties demanding his time was his excuse for presenting remarks so imperfectly prepared ; but he trusted the important points would not seem to be left obscure.

For a good appreciation of the subject he proposed to discuss, it is necessary to understand somewhat fully the results of modern psychical research, especially the newly-discovered fact of a double consciousness or a double layer of mental activity. On the upper plane or layer, so to speak, is the conscious mental activity. In the lower plane or layer, the subconscious or subliminal mental activity resides. For instance, when one passes along the street, the first recognizes what we are conscious of seeing ; the second recognizes all that we do see.

It is in the subliminal consciousness that habits are formed. It is in this that the lasting effects of shock are felt. It is in the subliminal mind that fears become fixed that sometimes so entirely control our being and welfare. This subconsciousness directly

2

controls the physical functions, hence it is through this that the circulation becomes permanently disturbed, and digestion and nutrition disordered.

Neuralgic pains, and very often rheumatic pains, hypersensitiveness of many parts of the system, sensitiveness of the dentine, in most cases depend upon a disordered condition of this subliminal layer of the mind.

The subconsciousness is peculiarly susceptible to suggestion. A very slight suggestion will cause blushing, a little stronger suggestion will produce embarrassment ; also fear, joy; sorrow, and all these emotions are experienced without any circumstance connected with the person to cause them, except the bare suggestion of the idea to the imagination.

Expectant attention has long been recognized as one of the most powerful synergists to the actions of medicines. The patient's knowledge of what the medicine is expected to do, very often decides what the action shall be. This is simply the power of suggestion. It was this power that led a good professor of medicine, who practised in New Hampshire a half century ago, to think that the compound tincture of gum guiac. was all the medicine needed in any physician's practice ; for it was all that he needed. The oft-repeated story of the curative action of brown bread pills, is explained in the same way.

Suggestion is the principal and almost whole power of naboli, and the multitude of more recently manufactured dental obtundents. Unless anæsthesia of the dentine is suggested, very little, or more likely, no effect is produced.

Now, as a matter of fact, suggestion is ordinarily just as effective in inducing anæsthesia of the dentine, without any pretence of using any medicinal agency.

More than two years ago, Dr. Fillebrown demonstrated that, in the hypnotic state, suggestion was sufficient to anæsthetize the dentine of the most sensitive teeth. He has lately found that suggestion, in the ordinary wakeful state, is quite equal to the necessities of most cases, and now seldom induces hypnosis to increase suggestibility.

He never urges suggestion upon patients. It is to only a portion that he applied it ; many do not need it, others do not desire it, some object to it. In the last four weeks he had used suggestion for fifteen patients, and, as many of these had several sittings each, it made almost daily use of it. Thirteen cases were successful. Two patients failed to respond at all.

Males he found quite as susceptible as females. The suggestion will, in every case, quiet the nervous system, and prevent or remove the tired feeling which is so often produced by the operation.

The method of inducing susceptibility to suggestion is very

simple. If the patient has already learned the art of relaxation and repose, the preparation is complete, and they are ready to listen to the suggestion of anæsthesia of the tooth substance.

The principles of the art are well explained in Delsarte's dentalizing process, also in a small volume lately published upon "Power Through Repose." The operator needs himself to understand the art of relaxation and rest. A careful study of the volume referred to will make the matter clear.

This accomplished, he will explain to his patient that it is quite possible to obtain complete relaxation and repose, and that in that condition all disturbances will be better borne and that all pain about the teeth will be removed.

Place your hand on the forehead of the patient and say, " You will now rest down and relax all of your muscles ; you will become a dead weight in the chair ; your limbs, body, arms and head are feeling heavy ; your muscles and nerves are resting ; you are feeling entirely comfortable." Repeat this several times. Then say, " Your tooth is now anæsthetized ; the sensitiveness is gone. The cutting will not hurt you ; you will not dread it ; the sound will not disturb you ; if it hurts at all you will not mind it ; it will not shock you." Then proceed to use the engine or excavator, as the case may be, gently and carefully, avoiding any sudden movement or cut ; feeling all the time a repose yourself, and continually repeating the assurance that the anæsthesia is becoming more and more complete.

In this manner the teeth of a patient can be rendered insensible to the cut of an instrument while wide awake and consciousness not in the least affected.

A patient for whom he tried this lately for the first time, laughed outright and said, while he was still cutting what had been previously a very sensitive tooth, " I know and realize this is all so, but I cannot help laughing and I cannot understand it." This patient is one of exceeding good sense, and very far from believing any unreality.

Anyone who will give earnest attention to the matter and study it thoroughly until he can repose himself, will be able to lead his patients to the same goal.

This method and its results are amply sufficient for all dental purposes, and have the merit of being entirely unobjectionable to even the most radical opponent of hypnotism. Patients themselves can induce this repose, and so in such cases the operator can call for it whenever needed.

There is hardly an operator in the land but has had patients fall asleep in the chair while being operated on, and not one of them thought of being disturbed by it. Yet such cases are especially susceptible to suggestion, and such sleep is the quietness and repose and suggestibility that Dr. F. described in his paper.

Saving Materials.

By L. D. S., Toronto.

When I was a student I thought my tutor awfully mean, because he made me carefully save every scrap of wax, and things I called rubbish. We had a "rubbish drawer," into which all "useless" articles were put. "They'll be wanted sometime," I was told; and it was wonderful how often the prediction came true. The idea of not wasting plaster which was only two dollars a barrel, and of being so petty about bits of vulcanite, etc., seemed to me the height of narrowness and meanness. I often feel grateful, to-day, to my tutor, who is dead and gone, for the lessons he taught me in economy. The principle got so bred in me that I believe I save as much rubber, plaster, wax, etc., as most men use.

I think there never was a time when we have such wasteful students as now. My experience of the average Ontario student is, that he is a very nice young man indeed, but that he rarely consults the interest in this way of his tutor. I have seen the most reckless waste of vulcanite in packing, which showed not merely ignorance but pure indifference. The fact is, students in the office are a nuisance. No money compensates a dentist for the abuse of his tools, carelessness with his lathes, etc., and the direct damage to his work by the boys who think because, perhaps, they have paid you a hundred dollars or so, they have a right to be careless, to come and go as they please, and to waste as much of everything as they use.

Aluminum Plates.

By L. D. S., Toronto.

I have given up vulcanite! Anyone who must have a rubber plate will never get it from me. I have done forever with the nasty, clumsy thing—excepting when I use enough of it to attach teeth to metal plates.

For several years I used cast aluminum plates, and, I confess, I had so many failures I returned to vulcanite; but now I am using aluminum exactly as I would use gold, for partial as well as for upper sets, and I have not only satisfaction myself, but I find my patients coming to me and wanting to get their vulcanite sets renewed for this lightest and pleasantest of all metals for the mouth. With care in striking up the plate I can make it yield to every obstruction. I make holes through it, and I secure perfect attachment.

" How do you do in a case of a single tooth, say a lateral incisor, where the space is so narrow you cannot get strength from a rubber attachment? What do you do in close bites where you cannot put any rubber at all?"

Simply this, I line and solder the tooth, and let a tail of gold plate extend beyond the line of the bite; I punch large holes through the tail, or solder a little loop or two to the end. I then rivet this to the aluminum, and there you are.

How are We to Get Our Fees?

By " Licentiate."

The question of fees, of cash and of credit, must always remain a *bete noir* among us, until enough of us take the bull by the horns and insist upon being treated as business men. I have never been able to explain or to get explained, the reason why we dentists are so constantly imposed upon, much more than medical men. It may be that when people are ill enough to call in a physician, their conscience becomes tender; and as life and death are more associated with medical than dental practice, patients want to keep on the right side of their physician. Moreover, there is a great deal of demeaning advertising among us, and the public, looking at the amount of it done even by respectable men, begin to think that dentistry must be more of a trade than a profession, as they do not see this done by respectable medical men. They then argue, that just as one shoemaker is perhaps as good as another, one dentist is as good for them as another, and they shop around, and they beat us down, and they ask credit.

Now, I believe that we must have dentists for the poor as well as the rich. We must let young beginners and struggling men charge lower fees, if they will, than men who have an old-established practice. I have no opinion at all to express as to a tariff, because I believe it is impracticable in a country like Canada, occupied by a population most of whom are not overburdened with superfluous cash.

But there is one feature upon which we can all agree, if we would. In face of discordance of opinion upon many points, as to whether this man or that man should be on the Board, or in the College, etc., we surely have no one to dissent as to the opinion, that whether our fees are low or high, we should have a business method of getting our money. No matter what each one's qualifications may be—all that aside—how are we to get the money we earn?

Now, while admitting that the question is a difficult one in the present way we manage, I insist that by a change of method it could be made extremely simple. I do not write for the sake of spinning fine theories, but to point out plain facts. The public must have our services: but the public has no more right to demand them without paying for them, and paying sufficient to give us a fair profit, than the dentists have a right to get goods from the depots without paying for them. The dentists do not make the prices the depots charge for goods: and the public should not make the fees the dentists charge for their services. Yet some foolish practitioners tempt the public to believe that they can get whatever they want at their own price. I do not even quarrel about that.

My grievance is, that when all is done and said, we do not get what we earn. I find the credit system in Ontario is becoming as bad as in Quebec. It was only the other day that I learned that two dentists, who had been in partnership only three years, had over $7,000 on their books when they dissolved, and that they had to wipe off perhaps $1,500. I say this is a monstrous iniquity.

Now, why cannot our Provincial associations agree, to take up this question simultaneously at their annual meetings, and resolve that the practice of dentistry in Canada will be conducted more upon a cash basis. Accounts should be rendered as soon as the services are completed, and transient and unknown patients should be made to understand that services are cash. One dentist I know, makes no exception to exacting cash for all artificial work. Others render monthly accounts regularly. Others insist upon monthly or bi-monthly notes, even for $5 accounts. I think their plans are practical and justifiable. Our outlay is not only one of material, but of personal energy and skill. When a family account is rendered, why not enclose a blank note at thirty or sixty days? If the debtor prefers to pay cash, he will. If he cannot, he cannot very decently refuse a note. Then, again, there are people who come to us, whom we cannot directly inform that our terms are —to them—cash. There are dead-beats and others we want to get rid off. Why not have a framed card to hang in front of the chair just before they enter the surgery, with some such information on it as this :

EVERY OPERATION AND ALL ARTIFICIAL WORK

ARE

STRICTLY CASH.

NO CREDIT GIVEN.

PLEASE DO NOT ASK FOR IT, OR EXPECT IT.

Hasty Opinion.

By J. H. SPRINGLE, D.D.S., L.D.S., Montreal.

In looking over contemporary American dental literature, one is struck by the number of antagonistic classifications and peculiar nomenclature given to the different conditions with which we are concerned as dentists. It seems as if every man who has, or who thinks he has, any standing, deems it necessary to announce new and often startling theories and names for the conditions which he meets in his practice. Usually no attempt is made to conclusively prove these assertions, either by accurate experiment or by known scientific facts. The work is gone over too hastily, and as soon as it is announced, half a hundred men, who see flaws in it, immediately point them out and take advantage of the opportunity to air their own ideas, and squelch the unfortunate writer, although they are in turn picked to pieces by everybody else. Our American cousins are, perhaps, apt to look at things in a too superficial manner. Life is too short with them to consider a case in all its bearings ; it is only seen in the light in which it first strikes them. Each individual member of the greatest nation on earth is generally of the opinion that mentally he is quite as good a man as his neighbor, if not a few degrees better. Few are willing to recognize and look up to the really scientific investigators, of whom they have not a few, and, in consequence, these men are perhaps better known in foreign lands than in their own, where the loud voices of their pigmy *confreres* dim their brightness. An instance of this is found in the way Dr. Black's scholarly and truly scientific articles in the *American System of Dentistry*, have been received by the different college staffs. Is it not the case that almost every professor of pathology will give a pet classification of his own, rarely supported by experiment or proof and often consisting of several conflicting theories ? In every second article we see the expressions, "*I* hold" this or that idea, "*my* opinion" is so and so. In a recent number of a prominent dental journal, is a controversy between two gentlemen on the presence of uric acid in the disease known as *pyorrhœa alveolaris*. One of them has proved by a few experiments, to his own satisfaction, that uric acid is present ; the other, on the authority of a lesser number of experiments, states positively that it is not present, or if so, is in unimportant quantities. Now, it is evident that one of these gentlemen is wrong, although both write with the calmness of conviction. Would it not have been better if they had both taken a little more time and trouble about these experiments? Even if they had not announced their important conclusions for a year or so, the world would have wagged on in the same old way. Perhaps if they were to read Mr. Chas. Darwin's manner of supporting one of his theories, they might get a few pointers. He brings a great mass of independent evidence together, all pointing in the one direction, and even then he does not say, " therefore my theory is a fact," but, " is it not very probable that my theory is a correct one ? " This is science, and, also, it is hard work.

Proceedings of Dental Societies.

Royal College of Dental Surgeons of Ontario.

Results of the examination just completed :

FINAL YEAR. Passed—Alton Anderson, C. N. Abbott, J. W. Bell, F. E. Beemer, J. D. Cameron, M. F. Cross, Charles Cobban, Donald Davidson, G. A. Dewar, W. R. Greene, H. A. Galloway, F. G. Hughes, V. H. Lyon, A. A. McKenzie, Chas. Colter, D. Marshall, J. McKnight, A. E. McCordick, G. A. Newton, B. F. Nicholls, G. R. Patterson, R. J. Read, W. A. Scott, E. A. Totten, H. P. Thompson, W. T. Wood, J. R. Mitchell, A. E. Webster, F. L. Wood. Passed in anatomy, materia medica, and practical dentistry—J. C. Bansley, O. A. Marshall, J. F. Ross, R. A. Willmott. To take chemistry again—E. B. Shurtleff, T. S. Fairbairn, Charles Neill. To take physiology again—E. B. Shurtleff, W. A. Sangster. To take surgery again—Chas. Neill, W. A. Sangster. To take anatomy again—T. S. Fairbairn.

JUNIOR YEAR. Passed—D. Black, W. C. Brown, W. J. Bruce, I. P. Cunningham, W. B. Cavanagh, Geo. Emmett, W. S. French, E. W. Falconer, W. T. Griffin, J. L. Leitch, C. B. Little, E. W. Oliver, K. Peaker, H. C. Skinner, N. Schnarr, R. G. McLean, F. H. Walters, A. J. Wyckoff, J. N. Wood. T. Levey will take anatomy and chemistry again. G. F. Baker will take histology, comparative dental anatomy and bacteriology again, and take anatomy, materia medica and metal work in final year. C. P. Sherman will take histology again, and complete technique and take anatomy and materia medica in final year.

FRESHMAN YEAR. Passed—R. M. Armstrong, F. Britton, J. A. Bothwell, J. M. Bell, J. J. Brown, T. E. Ball, Wm. Burnett, S. J. Campbell, L. G. Campbell, J. E. Cummings, S. E. Foster, O. H. Hutchinson, J. E. Johnston, W. W. Kenny, G. H. Kennedy, W. E. Lundy, A. E. Little, J. F. McMillan, L. M. Mabee, J. C. Mathison, H. McQueen, F. S. Mercer, A. L. McLachlan, W. A. McLean,

G. A. Roberts, A, P. Rogers, John Sweet, W. G. Switzer, J. G. Somerville, J. A. Simpson, W. T. Templar, E. S. Washington, W. S. Westlund. D. Baird, prevented from writing by illness, permitted to take a supplemental in all subjects. G. H. Sweet will take histology. T. A. Hart will take anatomy and histology. Louis Cashman will take histology. Ford Butler and J. C. Moore take anatomy again.

University of Toronto, Examination for D.D.S., March, 1894.

The following are the results of the recent examinations in dentistry in the University of Toronto :

FIRST-CLASS HONORS—G. A. Dewar, J. McKnight, W. A. Scott, F. L. Wood, W. T. Wood.

SECOND-CLASS HONORS—C. N. Abbott, D. A. Anderson, J. W. Bell, J. D. Cameron, M. F. Cross, D. Davidson, W. R. Greene, V. H. Lyon, D. Marshall, J. R. Mitchell, G. A. Newton, B. F. Nichols, G. R. Patterson, R. J. Read.

PASS—C. P. Cobban, F. G. Hughes, A. E. McCordick, A. A. McKenzie, G. J. Musgrove, H. P. Thompson, E. A. Totten.

D. Baird completed his examination for D.D.S., by passing in anatomy and in physiology and histology. H. A. Galloway must pass a supplemental examination in medicine and surgery before obtaining his degree. J. F. Ross and R. A. Willmott passed in materia medica and in anatomy, as students in the second year in the Royal College of Dental Surgeons.

Toronto Dental Society.

The regular monthly meeting of the Toronto Dental Society was held on Monday evening, April 9th, in the Society's permanent quarters in the Y. M. C. A., Yonge St. An interesting and profitable paper on " Causes of Failure in Dental Operations," was read by Dr. F. D. Price. The discussion of the subject was taken up by Drs. J. B. Willmott and McLaughlin. The election of officers and standing committees for the coming year resulted as follows :—Hon. President, N. Pearson ; President, Wm. Wonder ; 1st Vice-President, Harold Clark ; 2nd Vice-President, J. F. Adams ; Secretary. E. Forster ; Treasurer, A. J. McDonagh ; Membership and Ethics Committee, McLaughlin, Wood and Mills; Programme Committee, Wonder, Clark and Adams.

Selections.

The Golden Wedding of Sir John and Lady Tomes.

Towards the end of last year, as most of our readers may be aware, it was decided at a representative gathering of the profession, to present to Sir John and Lady Tomes a suitable offering on the occasion of their golden wedding. A committee was appointed, and it was decided to bring the subject under the notice of those connected with the various scientific and other societies connected with dentistry.

A meeting of the subscribers to the presentation fund was subsequently held on February 3, at 40 Leicester Square, the chair on the occasion being occupied by Sir Edwin Saunders. This gathering, after hearing the statements of the Hon. Treasurer and Secretaries, unanimously decided that the most opportune way of celebrating the event would be the foundation of a scholarship for original research in dentistry and its allied branches. It was at the same time decided to prepare an illuminated address enclosed in an album, expressing the honor and esteem in which both Sir John and Lady Tomes were held by all, the names and addresses of the subscribers to the wedding gift to be also inserted in the album, together with the names of the ladies who had contributed to the purchase of a special gift to Lady Tomes in shape of a handsome silver-gilt inkstand.

A representative deputation was appointed to wait upon Sir John and Lady Tomes on the day preceding their golden wedding day, and accordingly on St. Valentine's Day, February 14, the following journeyed to Upwood Gorse, Caterham : Sir Edwin Saunders, Messrs. T. Arnold Rogers, S. J. Hutchinson, G. Brunton, G. A. Ibbetson, J. Smith Turner, F. Canton, Walter Campbell, W. F. Forsyth, J. H. Mummery, A. J. Woodhouse, S. Lee Rymer, J.P., E. Trimmer (Secretary of the Royal College of Surgeons), W. H. Woodruff, W. B. Paterson.

Sir John and Lady Tomes, in the presence of relatives and friends, having cordially received and welcomed the deputation, Mr. Thomas Arnold Rogers addressed the assembly, and said :

As Chairman of the Committee, but who has never taken the chair, nor indeed performed any of the duties of the chairman—unless perhaps occasionally to make himself disagreeable—I beg permission to say a very few words of regret for my inability to fulfil those duties. At the moment of summoning the first meeting, I was overtaken by illness which has incapacitated me from taking any active part. But I have the satisfaction of knowing that the work has been done much better without me than it would have been with me. Mr. Hutchinson immediately came to the rescue, and we all know how thoroughly he has performed his part. And Sir Edwin Saunders very kindly, and at some personal inconvenience presided over the last committee meeting, and I need not say that Sir Edwin is a chairman *par excellence.*

My duty on the present occasion somewhat resembles that of " Wall " in the " Midsummer-Night's Dream." I am, as it were, the medium of communication between the lovers. And I do not think I am wrong, in the remembrance of all that has passed, in considering those whom we are met here to-day to honor, and ourselves, lovers in the truest sense, who have ever been desirous of living the life most conducive to the mutual welfare. But I must not say more, lest the fate of " Wall " in the play befall me.

I therefore beg, Sir John and Lady Tomes, to introduce Sir Edwin Saunders as the representative of those who have united to found the Sir John Tomes triennial prize ; and Mr. Brunton, who, happy man, on this appropriate day of St. Valentine, represents the ladies, Mrs. Brunton having taken the initiative in offering their gift to Lady Tomes. And I will now conclude in the words of " Wall " :

"Thus have I, Wall, my part discharged so,
And being done, thus Wall away doth go."

Mr. Brunton, on behalf of the ladies, presented Lady Tomes with a silver-gilt inkstand, and in a few words expressed their congratulations, and the hope that she might long be spared to make every use of it.

Sir Edwin Saunders : Sir John and Lady Tomes,—This flying visit to the peaceful, sylvan shades of Upwood Gorse, at a season which cannot be regarded as the most favorable for the full appreciation of its beauties, demands a few words of explanation. In the first place, let me assure you that you are not being interviewed, so that we may speak with the unrestrained freedom of social intercourse. We are here, then, to signalize a somewhat rare and interesting event. Golden weddings are not of every-day occurrence, and in these days of revolting daughters, emancipated women, of equality of the sexes—which always means the supremacy of what used to be considered the weaker sex—and of general relaxation of the old social order, such events become more and more precious, and ought not to be passed over without some recognition ; for they furnish the best possible, because practical, answer to the somewhat cynical question, " How to be happy though married." We are here in a dual capacity—first, as old friends who have watched with interest your life pilgrimage ; and, second, as representing, at least *pro hac vice,* the profession with which you, Sir John, have been so long, so closely, and so honorably identified. We all represent some society, association, or other interest connected with that profession, and I may truly say that there is not a man present who "hath not on a wedding garment." And we are here in both capacities to bring all good wishes, all kind thoughts, all pious aspirations—thankfulness that you are both in the enjoyment of so large a measure of health and hopeful anticipations for the future.

It goes without saying that when rumor crystallized into fact, and it became known that a golden wedding would synchronize with St. Valentine's Day, there was but one unanimous feeling that it should not be allowed to pass without recognition. But there was room for some divergence of opinion as to the form and method of such recognition. And when I received a letter on the subject from our old friend, Mr. Thomas Rogers, who is never found wanting when anything gracious or courteous is in question, I confess that my imagination did not rise higher than a paragraph in our journal, and a pyramid of cards, letters and telegrams, variously expressing congratulations and felicitations, accompanied more or less by gifts of flowers and works of art arriving on the day. But it soon became evident that a larger scheme was desired, and would find general acceptance, and when it fell into the capable hands of Mr. Hutchinson its success seemed assured. To this I at once gave my adhesion, stipulating only that my own little offering should not be prejudiced, with the presentation of which my share in the day's proceedings terminates, for I am sure that I shall best consult your wishes and your interests by calling upon Mr. Hutchinson to lay before you a detailed account of the scholarship.

The following verses, composed by Sir Edwin, were read by him :

TO SIR JOHN AND LADY TOMES,

On their Golden Wedding.

Dear friends, to-day the golden crown is yours,
The crown of triumph, not of martyrdom ;
Fifty long years of happy wedded life—
Years of sweet counsel, mutual help and love,
Of life made sweeter by companionship.

Fifty years since, a youth and maiden fair
Asked for a blessing of St. Valentine ;
For him, it meant God's last best gift to man,
For her, an added dignity to native charm.
'Twas wisely done—and now the crown is theirs.

Accept, dear friends, this simple offering
Of songs and praises of your patron saint.

EDWIN SAUNDERS.

Mr. Hutchinson then read the address, which had been beautifully illuminated, and was enclosed in an album of white morocco and gold, as follows :

We, who have recorded our names in this book, tender our

hearty congratulations to you, Sir John and Lady Tomes, upon the attainment of this, the fiftieth anniversary of your wedding day.

This event, though in some sense a private one, seems to afford an opportunity which we gladly seize—for expressing in a manner more personal than would be appropriate to any more public occasion, our recognition of your life-work and mutual devotion.

The singleness of purpose with which this object (nearest to the hearts of all of us) has been pursued—whether it be the scientific, the social, or the political advancement of our professional interests—has called forth this expression of regard and esteem, which, it has been thought, could take no form more in accord with your well-known feelings, than that of a personal gift to your devoted helpmate, and the foundation of a Scholarship or Prize Essay, to be awarded triennially to members of our profession, for original work in any direction of scientific inquiry.

This, it is hoped and believed, will commemorate in rising and future generations, the appreciation by us, your contemporaries, of your life-work in the educational reform of your profession, and inspire in them something of the same spirit of high aspiration and self-denial, which have characterized your long and honorable career. We express our earnest hope that you may both be long spared to enjoy your well-earned rest, in the assurance of the warmest good wishes of your many friends.

Sir John Tomes: Sir Edwin Saunders and Gentlemen,—Words will fail to express in fitting terms our acknowledgment of the kind and generous feelings which have prompted your visit and offers, in commemoration of the fiftieth anniversary of our wedding day, offers of gifts that will hand down the name to generations yet to come, by distinctive rewards to future workers in the cause of dental science. Encouragement, if not a necessity, is a great help to the young while gaining the needful equipments for the battle of life. And approval of the results of the fought-out battle is very grateful to the old, cheering the coming time, whether measured by months or years. For the approval you have so kindly expressed at the present time, and provided for in time to come, we offer our most sincere and heartfelt thanks. I do not stand alone ; I have worked with many workers, whose devotion to professional progress taken in the widest sense of the term, is recorded in the minutes of the Odontological Society and of the British Dental Association. You have selected me from amongst them for the reception of honors, in which they must also take a share. There is one, however, whose name will not be found in any record ; yet she, in willingly waiving her claim to what might have been my hours of leisure, has contributed to the results you have set forth in such flattering terms. No one feels more strongly than Lady Tomes that those who have lived by the practice of a

profession, owe a deep debt to that profession payable only by
personal devotion to its general and special interests. It has not
been our custom to mark the wedding day by even a family
gathering; and until ten days ago, when your proceedings were
made known to me, though we might have departed from the usual
habit by asking a few near relations to dine with us, we had no
thought that the event of to-morrow—our fiftieth anniversary—
would have assumed the importance your proceedings have given
to it. Had I been consulted in the later stage of your generous
actions in our behalf, I could not have devised a more acceptable
form of commemoration; for while the connection of the name
with the triennial prize is a great personal distinction, the award
of the prize for an original paper of ascertained merit is a direct
educational gain to the profession as a whole. The very handsome
ink-stand, and the album inscribed with many names, will be
constant reminders of the very kindly feelings entertained by the
subscribers towards my wife and myself. You wish us still longer
life and further happiness. We, in return, wish you one and all,
long life and health, and the measure of happiness in the future
that has marked our past fifty years of unbroken concord.—*Journal
of the British Dental Association.*

Opening of the National Dental Hospital, London, England.

His Royal Highness the Duke of York, attended by Major-
General Sir Francis de Winton and Captain the Hon. D. Keppel,
performed the ceremony of opening the new premises of the
National Dental Hospital and College, Great Portland Street, of
which institution the Prince is President. The new hospital, which
is the gift of the Dowager Lady Howard de Walden, has cost some
£10,000 to erect. It is a handsome building, with an exterior of
red brick, and comprises a large lecture hall, laboratories, special
demonstration rooms, a stopping room capable of accommodating
seventy-five patients, and other offices, the architect being Mr. A.
E. Thompson, of Leadenhall Buildings. Among those present at
the opening ceremony were the Bishop of London, Lord Strafford,
Vice-President of the Institution, the Dowager Lady Howard de
Walden, Mr. L. G. F. Cavendish Bentinck, Mr. Alban Gibbs, M.P.,
Sir W. Gilbey, Major-General A. Ellis, Mr. J. G. Noel, the Rev. A.
J. Robinson, Mr. S. Lee Rymer, Mr. S. Spokes (Dean of the College), Mr. A. E. Thompson, Sir P. Spokes, Mr. Underwood, Dr.
Coupland, Dr. Littlejohn, and Captain Evans. A guard of honor
was furnished by the Honorable Artillery Company, under the
command of Captain J. Pash, and a large crowd assembled outside
the hospital and heartily cheered His Royal Highness, who was

accompanied by His Highness Prince Edward of Saxe-Weimar and the Duke of Fife, both of whom are members of the committee of management of the hospital. On the arrival of the Prince the guard gave a royal salute, and the band played a few bars of the National Anthem. Lord Strafford, having received the Prince, presented the members of the committee of management to His Royal Highness, who afterwards inspected the new buildings. In the lecture hall, where the opening ceremony took place, a dias covered with crimson cloth was erected, and the commodious apartment was ornamented with palms and flowers. The Prince, who escorted the Dowager Lady Howard de Walden, was warmly cheered on entering the hall. The proceedings were commenced by the Bishop of London offering prayer, after which

The Earl of Strafford rose amid cheers to tender thanks to the Duke of York for allowing his name to be associated with the institution as its president, and for being present to inaugurate the new building. He remarked that though dental surgery had long formed part of the instruction at hospitals, yet previous to 1860 there were no buildings specially adapted for the pursuit of that branch of surgical science. In that year a small building in Great Portland Street was established as the first dental hospital in London. Since then many thousands of people had received benefit from it, but the premises were very narrow and cramped, and, considering that a college of instruction with lecture rooms was highly necessary for the furtherance of the objects of the institution, the management felt that the work was somewhat confined in its operations, and were very anxious for larger and more commodious premises. Those premises, thanks to the noble gift of the Dowager Lady Howard de Walden, they were that day in possession of. They now had every hope that the good work of the hospital might be extended. When he mentioned that no fewer than 27,-902 persons had, during the past year, received relief by the surgical skill of the staff of the hospital, he thought they had a fair augury that this beneficent and useful work would in the future be extended. In conclusion, Lord Strafford expressed a hope that the Duke of York and his illustrious consort might be blessed with many years of health and happiness.

His Royal Highness the Duke of York, who was received with cheers, said :—" Lord Strafford, your Royal Highness, my Lords, Ladies and Gentlemen, it gives me much pleasure to attend here to-day, and to assist in the carrying on of such a useful institution. Of the many hospitals engaged in charitable work for the poorer classes, I feel sure that the National Dental Hospital must afford an amount of relief in the particular kind of cases dealt with here, which some of us are apt to overlook. I am glad to learn from Lord Strafford of the good work done here, and whatever may be the criticism sometimes passed upon the establishments of so-called

" special " hospitals, I feel sure that dental hospitals cannot be open to objection.   One peculiar feature is that the actual treatment of patients is mainly carried out, as a matter of routine, by students. I am informed that after a special preparatory stage, the student is entrusted with the charge of patients, under the supervision of the surgical staff.   At the close of the curriculum, when the student presents himself at the Royal College of Surgeons for examination, he has performed all the operations he may expect to meet with during his professional career.   Thus the patient and the student render mutual aid, for the former has the advantage of receiving the benefit of skilled treatment.   As president of the hospital, it will give me satisfaction to know that the same good results are continued in the future.   I must not omit to refer to the munificent action of the Dowager Lady Howard de Walden.   It is due to her generous interest in the beneficial work carried on by this institution for the last thirty years, that we are able to meet in this handsome building to-day.   I have had an opportunity of seeing the excellent arrangements now brought to completion, and I heartily trust that nothing may interfere with the successful attainment of the ends in view, namely, the alleviation of dental troubles amongst the suffering poor, and the education of a race of future dental surgeons who may do honor to the special branch of surgery to which they will belong.   I have now much pleasure in declaring this new building of the National Dental Hospital open for the useful purpose for which it has been erected."

The Prince then left the hall, and proceeding to the entrance of the new buildings, unveiled two tablets, one of which refers to the gift of the building by the Dowager Lady Howard de Walden, and the other to the visit of His Royal Highness·   The proceedings then terminated.—*The Journal of the British Dental Association.*

Correspondence.

To the Editor of the DOMINION DENTAL JOURNAL :

SIR,—I have a very warm feeling of respect for the editor of the *Dental Practitioner and Advertiser*, of Buffalo ; but I cannot discover what we Canadians have done to rouse his ire on the subject of education.

There are a great many men who get credit for being great men, chiefly upon their own declarations ; and I think if we had more bounce in Canada, or more self-assertion, we would be more respected —by some people.   I do not mean to apply this to your contemporary ; but it is generally the case in the United States, that they overshadow us in a great many respects purely by the magnitude of their assertion. I hope I say this in a spirit of fair play, at the same time of self-defence, which will be understood by fair-minded men. We have so many better things in Canada than they have over the border—I do not mean professionally—and I believe if we bragged more about them, they would get more appreciation. One of these is our system of dental education, which we formulated ourselves, chiefly from the British standard. I agree with your repeatedly expressed opinion, that we should not lower our educational level so as to embrace in our ranks the uneducated bell-boy and office-sweep, but that we should raise it, so as to induce the highest university man to join us. The former drag us down to their trade level : the latter lift us up to their professional standard.

Twenty-six years ago I was one of a number of young men—yourself among them, I remember very well—who went to the United States to enter a dental college. I remember the result of our exploration and observation was to satisfy us that our time and money would be wasted, that the medical lectures which we had taken in Toronto and Montreal for two years were superior to what was being given in the Dental College, and the practical anatomy so much more thorough, that we felt we had nothing in that line better there, excepting some valuable instruction on operative dentistry, which we got subsequently much better from the late Dr. Atkinson. I remember the occasion when two of the colleges were publicly cut off from recognition by the Quebec Dental Board for repeated violations of their terms of graduation, and if it is necessary for your purpose, I can supply you with the way in which degrees were conferred upon some men who to-day set themselves up as of superior clay to their fellows. It would be easy, vulgarly speaking, to shut their mouths. Some of these men who sneer at those who did not graduate in a dental school should rise and give us their own personal history, how many days or weeks, when and where they attended college before graduating ; or where, when and how they got other degrees they flourish.

In Canada we have for a long time exacted a preliminary entrance examination. Before the valuable organization of the National Association of Dental Faculties, when its colleges were asking attendance of only eight or ten months to graduate, we were exacting forty-eight months ? The United States " year " was a sessional " year." Ours was a calendar year. We never had, and I believe never will have, anything to learn from our neighbors as to the matriculate standard, as to the courses on anatomy, physiology, chemistry, practical anatomy. But I freely acknowledge that we always had, and I believe always will have, much to learn from the greater population, on the operative and mechanical branches, which in a country having so many more millions of

people than Canada, are necessarily more advanced and practised·
In defending our own system, the DOMINION JOURNAL is defending
our own self-respect ; but we do not respect one whit the less, as
you have fairly shown, the great advances, both in theory and practice and education, made by our good professional brethren in the
United States.   Yours,

Toronto.   L.D.S.

Editorial.

Admission to Study Dentistry.

There still exists a wide difference of opinion between the dental
educationalists of England and the United States, as to the standard of education required from candidates for entrance to study.
It would seem to be inferred, from many contributions in the
journals, that, for reasons unknown or not declared, our American
cousins, with a population of 60,000,000, with richly-endowed universities, a superior system of common-school education, a marvellous supply of literary and scientific institutions, magazines and
papers, are not prepared to raise the matriculation to the standard
required in Britain and in Canada.   The editor of the *International
Journal*. in the March issue, remarks, " It is questionable whether
the profession are ready to advance this beyond what is regarded
as a good English education, and we are not sure that it would be
advisable at the same present time, but it is an additional reform
that must come. We can have no sympathy with the methods
adopted in England and on the Continent in this respect, and do
not believe that the high standard there required can ever be
adopted in this country, as far as dentistry is concerned.   In order
to meet its demands, a young man's best years are sacrificed to
the attainment of information which, while in itself of great value,
is utterly useless in a practical profession such as ours must ever
remain.   The change, if any be made, must be made to a slightly
higher standard."
Why should not the ranks of dentistry be drawn from the higher
educated class of the community ? Why not from the universities
in preference to the common schools ? It may be argued that some
of the best men in our profession had a very limited education. It
may also be stated, as a fact, that some of them had no education
at all.   But it will not be pretended that a low standard of education is a *sine qua non* of professional aptitude, or that a classical
and mathematical education is a bar to success.   If the preliminary
examination at present demanded, would have shut out some of
those who have honored our ranks for many years, could it not be

argued that it is shutting out many to-day who might honor our ranks in years to come? Educationalists are not philanthropists. They should have no sentimental considerations. It is surely time, with all the educational advantages possessed, to demand a higher standard from young men who have to enter at once upon such studies as Anatomy, Physiology, Chemistry, Materia Medica, etc., ignorant of the very elements of the languages from which most of the terms used in these sciences are derived. Such education is but a caricature and a travesty, and will explain much of the peculiar " scientific" discussions for which dentistry, more than any other profession, is distinguished. If educationalists mean to make dentistry nothing better than "practical," it will be in order for medical men to repossess the ground of scientific study and training, while dentistry proper descends again to the ranks of tooth carpentering. But if it is to be classed among the liberal and learned professions, as it certainly is in England and on the Continent, in Canada and Australia, it must at least aspire to exalt its standard of admission, so as to exclude those whose limited education hinders them from fully comprehending and assimilating scientific studies. It need be no barrier to an ignoramus, if the ignoramus determines to prepare himself for entrance. If he is incapable of such preparation, he is unfit to be better than an exclusive mechanic. Dentistry has long ago escaped from its purely mechanical probation, and it is time the reproach was removed that we are " fractionally qualified beings" whose science is mostly smatter.

Sixteen years ago Dr. Charles W. Elliott, President of Harvard University, delivered an address in Boston before the American Academy of Dental Science. We have frequently stated that we might quote eminent authorities in the United States to prove the weakness of American dental education, and it will perhaps suggest good grounds for advancement, by contrasting the situation to-day with what it was when Prof. Elliott spoke: "It is well known," he said, " that thousands of rude, ignorant men have entered the profession, attracted by its apparent profitableness and debarred by no law, no established usage, and by no intelligent discrimination of the public against uneducated practitioners." . . . " As the future of a profession—whatever may be its present—is largely determined by the nature of the education which the youth who enter it receive, it is the condition of dental schools which should first engage the attention of those who wish to place dentistry on a level with the learned professions. All the evils which threaten the profession would gradually but surely disappear if dental schools could be made independent, strict and thorough, and public opinion could be so enlightened as to make the calling inaccessible or profitless to uneducated men." . . . " The first fact which strikes one, at the outset of an enquiry into

the methods and practices of dental schools, is that most of them
do not demand, as a qualification for admission, any preliminary
education whatever. No matter how ignorant and untrained a
man may be, most dental schools are open to him. Until very
recently all the medical and law schools in the United States were
in the same ignominious condition. Among American professional schools, the theological schools alone, and not all of them,
have escaped this degradation. It would be difficult to exaggerate
the effect upon the estimation in which the profession of medicine
and dentistry are held, of the fact that, until within two years,
these professions have been accessible to men who could barely
read and write, and have actually been entered by thousands of
persons who never received, at school or college, the early training
which, in the great majority of cases, is an essential preliminary to
a life of refinement and cultivation."

It may not conduce to the numerical strength of college attendance that such advancement should be made, but there are not
only far too many dental colleges, and too many students in most
of them, but the educational standard of the large majority is not
what it should be. It is very exceptional to find a student who
has graduated in Arts disgracing dentistry by quack methods of
advertising. It is very common to find a large proportion of the
illiterate " Doctors of Dental Surgery " at the head of every unprofessional dodge, as they are, as a rule, at the tail-end of any ethical
or progressive reform. A high standard of matriculation would be
the surest, even if it would be a slow antidote. The facilities for
higher education in the United States are more democratic than in
England.

Speaking of the preliminary examination in Arts required of all
candidates for registration in England, Prof. Elliott adds : " There
is no need of argument to prove that such conditions of entrance
as these will, in the course of twenty years, greatly improve the
quality of the mass of the profession in England, and it is the mass,
and not the few persons of exceptional gifts, that educational regulations are always intended to affect. If American dentistry, as a
profession, is to maintain its rank in the world, it must be defended
by similar requisitions against the incursion of inadequate men."

Prof. Elliott Again.

Our friend, the editor of the *Independent Practitioner and Advertiser*, thought we were rather hard on " American Dentistry," in
our criticism of the colleges in their past career. The remarks
above by Prof. Elliott are very *apropos* to the position we took,
especially with reference to the lack of proper matriculation.
Speaking of the schools of the period, Prof. Elliott denounced the

shortness of the term and the period of study—two years of four months each "year." "Many dental schools accept five years of practice as a dentist, instead of one year of study of dentistry, thus still further reducing the already small amount of intellectual training required for the degree. If a man can bring evidence that he has practised dentistry five years—no matter how ignorantly—he can obtain the degree of one of these schools by attending a single winter session. Is not the public right in regarding the American dental diploma as small of general culture? Is it always good evidence even of thorough acquaintance with dentistry?"

The Doctor touched upon the relations between the degree of doctor of medicine and doctor of dental surgery, and said: "Many eminent dentists have regretted the institution of a special dental degree, and have maintained that every dentist should be a doctor of medicine. Let it be granted at once, as a fact beyond dispute, that the full training of a physician and surgeon would be useful to a dentist. He who should follow the three years' course for the doctorate in medicine, and should then give eighteen months or two years to the peculiar studies of dentistry, would be a much better trained man than he who has given but three years in all to professional study."

The editor of the *International*, referring to the time of which Prof. Elliott spoke, says, in the March number, "The status of dental education at that period was about as bad as it possibly could be. The large majority of the schools were acting under a nominal two years, with courses of from four to five months. The so-called rule of "five years' practice," admitting students to the senior year who could present evidence of having had five years' practical experience, was in full force in the large majority of colleges. The results that had followed the adoption of this rule had become a professional scandal, as it was a notorious fact that a very large proportion thus admitted never had had the practice required."

It is certainly gratifying at this late day to have this unsolicited testimony to the "scandalous" breach of the "requirements for graduation," which provoked the Dental Board of Quebec, twenty years ago, to cut off from the list of recognized colleges two offenders. The storm of defiance and the threats of litigation against the public action of the Board evaporated like smoke in face of the proofs of gross violation, such as the editor of the *International* points out.

It is our conviction that, twenty years hence, the best minds among our cousins over the border will be as much ashamed of the present low standard of matriculation as they are of the past fraudulent "five years' practice."

Dental Education Again.

"ALAS! ALAS!!

The sad, sad condition of American dental schools, especially those of twenty years ago, still rests with overwhelming weight upon the mind of our good brother of the DOMINION DENTAL JOURNAL. He really cannot rest because of what once existed here. We, upon this side the line, have much to cheer us in the fact that a school that will probably furnish us a model for all time has been started in the Province of Quebec, and we regard with as much of complacency as possible the prospect that the superior advantages offered will induce a migration of students to Montreal, and leave us as bare as a plucked fowl.

"Upon both sides of the great lakes it is a singular fact that the would-be instructors of experienced teachers, the men who alone seem capable of properly conducting an educational establishment, are those who are non-graduates themselves. The only men who know all about the schools are those who have never attended them. Singular, is it not, that those who have had college training, and who perhaps have had years of experience in teaching, are the very ones who know nothing about it? Or perhaps it is the corrupting influence of a teacher's life, which so debases them that they necessarily become dishonest, sordid, and possessed by an insane desire to ruin their chosen profession."—*Dental Practitioner and Advertiser.*

The above is the latest contribution of our facetious contemporary to the polite literature of dental journalism. He has abandoned the herring which he trailed across the scent in discussion, and confines himself to the "sad, sad condition of American dental schools" twenty years ago. We have no apology to make for holding opinions on that score, so much more authoritatively expressed by the President of Harvard University, by most of the leading educationalists, and especially by the editor of the *Practitioner* himself.

En passant, the editor knows perfectly well that the college opened in Quebec Province never offered inducements to students, that it has not issued a calendar, and has been barely mentioned, and never advertised, in this or any other journal. Our worthy friend can continue to crow as the champion collegiate rooster, with never a fear of losing to Quebec the smallest feather.

The assumption that nobody knows anything about dental education unless he has graduated in a dental college is puerile and illogical. It might as fitly be argued, that nobody knows anything about the English language or arithmetic, unless he is a graduate of a seminary. If we follow our worthy editor from premises to conclusion, it will appear that the hundreds of graduates who were ignorant of English, and who passed only one session before graduation twenty years ago, are better educators, and must have a better knowledge of the best methods of dental education, than educated men who have passed two or more sessions in medical universities, who have studied the dental education of two continents from an impartial standpoint, who have been earnest students of dental literature and science, and who, as examiners on Dental Boards, had frequent opportunities to detect most thoroughly the deficiencies of the curriculum of the past system. In arguing with our contemporary, it is sufficient, in order to refute his statements in one place, to quote them in another. The case he defends on page 111 of the last issue of the *Dental Practitioner and Advertiser*, he demolishes on page 101. While assuming that the schools of twenty years ago were better than we declared them to be, he says "the curriculum was so narrow, and the term so short, students believed that the objects gained were not sufficient to warrant them entering a college." That is the whole sum and substance of our argument, which some months ago he so severely denounced. He further admits that "the curriculum is not yet what it should be. Three years may be a sufficient time, provided the whole of it is spent in the prosecution of the proper studies. When the winter term is but five months, it may become a mere incident in other labors. Farmers' sons, and those who are engaged in other avocations, can go to college during the winter, very much as in the country the boys and girls attend school during the same months—because there is little else to do. The five-months' term, as Prof. Truman cogently remarks, really means about three and a half, for the first two weeks are spent in organizing the classes, two more are taken out for holidays, while the examinations and closing exercises occupy perhaps three more, so that the time actually spent in study may be made ridiculously inadequate!!"

The worthy editor, further to exemplify his consistency, proceeds to remark : "When the term is short, and confined to the winter months, a poor class of students is encouraged to commence study. They are ambitious to do something besides hoe corn, and they earn sufficient during the rest of the year to keep them during a short term in college, and hence they commence a dental course without the proper and needful preparation. They have not sufficient of education to qualify them for a professional life. Their pecuniary circumstances are such that they cannot pursue their studies between terms, and hence what is gained during their four or five months' work in the winter, is lost when their attention is turned to other matters in the spring. . . . Every honest and competent educator knows that it is quite impossible properly to cover all the studies that should be included in the curriculum, even in three terms of seven months each. . . . As for a five-months' term, it is too often but a travesty upon study."

And any amount more of the same argument. It is quite evident that our worthy friend is ashamed of dental education to-day, and that he will, after all, come around to accept the three and four full years of twelve months each year, prevalent for the last twenty years in the Provinces of Canada he sneers at. There could hardly be greater fun for anyone who has nothing else to do, than pulling to pieces the meshes of such sophistry, and contradicting the positive statements of to-day by the positive statements of yesterday. *Quantum sufficit.*

Graduates and Non-Graduates.

It would seem as if some leading educators imagined, that mere graduation in a dental college in one session of four months, without matriculation, without knowing the language in which the lectures were delivered, without any previous experience or practice, was sufficient to elevate one above the average practitioner, who had built up a successful practice by dint of conscientious study and app ication, and immeasureably greater advantages than any school was able at that time to supply. The travesty of education which put thousands of D.D.Ss. into our ranks, can only find defenders to-day among polemical curiosities, who must play to the galleries, and who are in the habit of hitting heads wherever they pop up, for the mere sake of a sort of pugnacious popularity.

How did most of the leading practitioners who began practice twenty-five or thirty years ago obtain the degree of D.D.S.? How much, if any, time did they put in at college? As a correspondent says, " Some of these men who sneer at those who did not graduate in a dental school, should rise and give us their own personal history : how many days or weeks, when and where they attended college before graduating ; and where, when and how they got other degrees they flourish."

We know men who graduated in one short session who did not know an English letter from a cuneiform inscription—who did not even pass an oral examination through an interpreter. We know men to have stepped out of the stable as hostlers and graduated as doctors of dental surgery in one session. Any quack—we emphasize the " quack "—who chose to declare that he had had five years' practice previous to entrance was exempted from one of the two sessions. The whole system was rotten at the core, and it would be much more honorable to acknowledge it than hypocritically writing twaddle in its defence, in any shape whatever.

It may interest some people to know that when the profession was first organized in Canada the intention—which would have carried in the Legislature at that time—to give dentists the title of

D.D.S. instead of L.D.S., was successfully opposed by the leading reformers of the time. The opportunities to obtain American degrees on the same terms as they were received by our worthy friends, were certainly not wanting to Canadians, and in many cases they were secured. But, to assume that the degree of M.D.S., granted by State Boards twenty-five years ago, in consideration of being in actual practice several years, and after such examination as to literary knowledge as Boards at that remote period thought necessary ; to assume that the degree of D.D.S., granted about the same time in one session, to gentlemen who curiously continued their practice with an occasional run down to Philadelphia to attend the College in session ; to assume that other degrees, conferred after a somewhat desultory course of study, not one of them under conditions which were even tolerated in Canadian education since dentistry or medicine were organized as professions ; to assume that such a travesty of education qualifies the possessors of these degrees to swagger in insolent superiority over men *who could have had them on the same terms*, but who despised them, is an assumption of huge proportions, something akin to the resolution of the other "superior" people in the Western States, who " Resolved that the elect shall inherit the earth. We are the elect."

To sum up, the possession of the degree of D.D.S., obtained twenty-five or thirty years ago, is no proof whatever of superior training, as the training was most deficient. We do not believe it inspired one man to become a better dentist than he would have been if he had never seen the inside of a college. It did no more for him than an honorary degree. The man himself deserved whatever praise was due to his skill or talents. To-day, under the *ægis* of the National Association of Dental Faculties, the D.D.S. is a degree to be respected. We do not think that this journal merits the abuse it has received from the editor of the *Dental Practitioner and Advertiser,* for alluding to facts in connection with the education of the past, in which Canadian dentists, who have contributed their proportion to American colleges in recent years, are as much interested as our facetious and friendly contemporary. The object honest men should have in going to a dental school is to get knowledge, not a bit of parchment.

Head-rests.

Several times we have editorially drawn attention to the uncomfortable head-rests of our modern dental chairs ; but we· perhaps overlooked a dangerous condition of the necessary parts of a dental chair, which ought to be guarded against. A few weeks ago a physician mentioned to us the fact, that he had several patients who had contracted ringworm by contact with a dentist's chair. A curious coincidence occurred in the cases of two other patients of the same dentist, both of whom had ringworm, evidently from the same cause. We were permitted to examine the head-rest. It was never covered with a napkin ; it was greasy and dirty from use and old age. The dentist was perfectly innocent of any danger from its use in this condition, and seemed to be grateful for the suggestion to use napkins.

It is a very simple matter to have a good stock of clean, white napkins for the purpose, and to change them for every patient. Skin diseases have been contracted in barber's chairs, and the dentist's chair is quite as dangerous in this respect.

The Dental Society of the State of New York will hold its twenty-sixth annual meeting at Albany, May 9th and 10th.

The Connecticut State Dental Society will hold a union meeting in connection with the Connecticut Valley Society, at Hartford, third Tuesday in May.

The Illinois State Dental Society, at Springfield, Ill., second Tuesday in May.

Maine Dental Society, third Tuesday in July, at Rockland.

Michigan State Dental Society, June 7th, at Ann Arbor.

American Dental Association, first Tuesday in August, at Old Point Comfort, Va.

Southern Dental Association, July 31st, at Old Point Comfort, Va.

DOMINION
DENTAL JOURNAL.

| VOL. VI. | TORONTO, JUNE, 1894. | No. 6. |

Original Communications.

Dental Dots.

By D. V. BEACOCK, Brockville, Ont.

Don't leave the cover off your vulcanizer when not in use.

Don't mix plaster to pour into a flask or impression cup, and when partially full mix a little salt or potassium with the remainder in the bowl, to make it set; this will spoil all. Put it in just before commencing to pour.

Don't refuse to take a good dental journal. That community is to be more than pitied, whose dentist is too mean to read or subscribe for one or more dental journals.

Don't be too eager to take out six-year molars for children; you may live to regret it. Save all you can, except when common sense combined with dental knowledge otherwise dictates.

Don't use any copper amalgam in any of the teeth near the front of the mouth, no matter how small the cavity. If the patient is young it is sure to stain the tooth. I have seen several beautiful bicuspids ruined or otherwise disfigured for life with it.

Don't forget that kindness shown to children may, when they grow up, bring you many dollars.

2

Don't yield to the whim of every crank of a patient that may come along, by doing just whatever they may suggest, because they tell you that some other dentist does. Have an individuality of your own ; be sure you are right, then stand by your convictions.

Don't refuse to give a hint in the dental journal whenever you happen to have such a thing. Freely have ye received, now freely give.

Don't lower your prices, because some one tells you that Mr. So-and-so will do the same work for so much ; it often happens that they are not telling the exact truth, but trying to beat you down —in other words, shopping.

Don't be in too great a hurry to find fault with some filling you may happen to find in the mouth not very well put in. It may be that the patient will calmly listen till you are through, then look you in the face, and say, "Why, sir, you put that filling in yourself!"

Don't make a funnel of your throat, to pour nauseous drugs and patent nostrums into your already over-jaded stomach, should you unfortunately be the victim of dyspepsia, hepatic or nephritic troubles, with their usual accompaniments, insomnia and neurasthenia, or any of the numerous diseases that dentists are so liable to. It would be much wiser to take a vacation, plenty of fresh-air exercise, using carefully prepared and easily digested food, with a judicious use of dumb-bells and the Indian clubs. These latter will materially assist the metabolism and blood formation by accelerating the cell changes, and this too without the injurious effects of benumbing drugs, such as so-called tonics, nervines, sedatives and drastic purgatives, which too often paralyze instead of strengthen the very organs they are supposed to aid. In fact, try and lead a life more in harmony with nature's law, and less vexing to both body and mind.

A Convenient Method of Making an Articulating Plate.

By R. E. SPARKS, D.D.S., Kingston, Ont.

After making the impression, take a little moulding compound, which has been softening while the impression has been taken, put it in a partial impression tray, and take a second impression. Cool and remove from tray. You are now prepared to proceed as in any ordinary case.

Combination Metal and Cement Fillings.

By B.

It can hardly be denied but that the metals we use in filling teeth, are neither compatible with the tooth structure, nor as perfectly adapted to the marginal edges as the average cement preparations. If the ordinary cements were perfectly insoluble they would oust gold and amalgam from the market. We are so accustomed to extolling the various forms of metal fillings, that we perhaps overlook their disadvantages, and, in some cases, their positive injuriousness. If we could insert gold as easily as amalgam, several of the greatest objections to it would be removed. Any filling that demands great pressure, that requires hammering, etc., for condensation, that is difficult to use in inaccessible cavities, that exacts great strain and exhaustion of nervous force on the part of both patient and operator, that must necessarily be for the not-over-full-purse a costly material, has objections which we would, if we could, remove. Amalgam is no substitute under every circumstance for gold ; and in itself considered, being a conductor of heat, shares in one of the objections to gold.

For several years past I have consistently practised, except in small cavities, a suggestion made before I was born, but which, like many other good ideas, is lost to the memory of some, and perhaps ignored in the practice of others. It is simply the use of any of the best cement fillings, such as made by White, Justi, Sibley, Johnson and Lund, as the base or bulk, with gold or amalgam as a cover.

Now this seems a very simple, old story, but at a dental meeting which some of your readers may remember, I challenged twenty dentists present to insert this combination filling in dead teeth in plaster-of-Paris settings ; and simple as it seemed, only seven of them did it, under those favorable conditions, in a way to make them reliable had the operations been done in the mouth ! The faults perpetrated were as follows : margins left thin or untrimmed, overhanging edges of enamel, improper trimming of the bone cement from the margins, starting the metal filling too soon in cases where gold was used as the covering ; any one of these would cause inevitable failure in the mouth.

Briefly let me say, that I take care to have no possibility of these contingencies. In frequent cases where gold is used, I insert loose pellets into the bone cement before it hardens, instead of subsequently drilling retaining points or cutting grooves. I then use the hot air syringe rapidly, and it is easy to lay loose mats, or attach ribbons to these pellets. Whether I am to use gold or amalgam, in all cavities over the average size, I insert fully three-fourths of bone cement. It is better than metal in contact with the dentine, because it is a non-conductor, because it is more compatible with the tooth-structure, because it is easier upon the patient. When it is covered by secure gold or amalgam, it is better than an all-metal filling. If it was no more insoluble in the mouth than it is out of it, who would use metal as a filling?

In frail cavities, I am in the habit of imbedding in the cement a platinum or gold screw-post ; sometimes bent at an angle so as to sustain the force of mastication, and building gold or amalgam on this strengthener. In dead teeth I have, for experiment, imbedded ordinary safety-pin wire into the pulp-cavity, bent from one canal to the other, sometimes soldering a cross piece on top, which seemed to secure the attachment of fillings, and even of a crown.

How to get Clean Joints.

By CHAS. SUTTON, Coaticook, Que.

I have often read statements in the journals that the way to get clean joints is to grind closely, or to insert plaster, cement, etc., between the joints. Yet in spite of instructions, joints do come out with those reproachful dark lines which offend the eye. I do not pretend that I have made an original discovery, but I worked out the matter for myself, and I never have a dark joint, and this is the way I avoid it :

1. I never let wax get between the joints in preparing the set for the flask. I never melt the wax before or behind, where the blocks meet.

2. One of the last things I do when the case is waxed up, is to remove each block, one at a time, rub the joints on a piece of fine and clean sandpaper and replace them, taking care never to melt the wax where the blocks meet.

3. I then flask the set as usual, and when opening it, I avoid heating it so much that the wax will melt and run into the clean joints. I then *pick out* all the wax possible, especially in the vicinity where the blocks meet.

4. Now comes the secret. If you have not melted the wax into the joints before flasking, or when heating it to separate the flask, you have now perfectly clean joints. But you have to pour hot water into the case to melt out wax you cannot pick out, and when you do that, you just run the melted wax into those joints, and

even if you boil for an hour, and pour gallons of boiling water into the case, you can never cleanse them of foreign matter which not even boiling water will remove.

Now after you have picked out all the wax possible, just run into the joints thin plaster of Paris, and wait till it hardens. *Then* you may pour on your boiling water to remove the vestige of the wax ; but neither the wax nor the water can get between the joints, and neither can the rubber. It is not the rubber that dirties the joints. It is the wax, and the foreign matter in the wax which you run into them when you think you are running it out.

Translations.

(From Foreign Dental Journals, etc., etc.)

By CARL E. KLOTZ, St. Catharines.

NITROUS OXIDE WITH A SMALL PERCENTAGE OF OXYGEN ADDED.—In a splendid work on anæsthetics and their administration Dr. Hewitt says : "Generally the admixture of oxygen with nitrous oxide for anæsthetic purposes is not permissible, and the narcosis obtained by the nitrous oxide alone is in most cases sufficient." By experiment and observation in the last few years it has been found that, in a number of cases, better results have been obtained by adding a small percentage of oxygen to the nitrous oxide. Many operators will look with disfavor on this practice. I will therefore give you a table of comparisons between the two methods, the one giving results and effects under anæsthesia with pure nitrous oxide, and the other with the mixture :

Pure Nitrous Oxide.	*Nitrous Oxide mixed with a small percentage of Oxygen.*
1. Requires a simple apparatus and little practice and experience.	1. By using the mixture you require a complicated apparatus, and a great deal of practice in using it.
2. Patient quickly under the influence.	2. Patient not so quickly under the influence.
3. Face becomes pale and slightly bluish in color.	3. Face undergoes very little or no change of color.
4. Respiration labored and irregular, mostly snoring and stertorous.	4. Respiration quiet and regular, slight snoring sometimes, but never stertorous.

5. Generally twitching of the muscles.

5. No twitching of the muscles noticeable.

6. Pulse frequently faster, but when fully under the influence of the gas it gets slower.

6. Pulse always normal.

7. Under complete narcosis generally dilatation of the pupils.

7. Only slight dilatation of the pupils.

8. Dysphagia and swelling of the tongue and upper air passages.

8. Only slight swelling.

9. Average time to put patient under the influence of the gas is about 51 seconds.

9. Average time required is about 110 seconds.

10. Average time of anæsthesia after mouthpiece is taken from the mouth, 30 seconds.

10. Average time of anæsthesia is 44 seconds.

11. Average quantity required for anæsthesia is about 6 gallons.

11. Average quantity required from 8 to 10 gallons.

12. Bad after-effects (headache, dizziness, nausea or vomiting) are seldom experienced.

12. Bad after-effects are a little more frequent.

13. Exciting and sometimes horrible dreams are experienced by the patient.

13. Dreams are seldom excitable, and very often of a pleasant nature.

It will be seen by the above table that the symptoms of asphyxia, through the addition of oxygen to the nitrous oxide during inhalation, have been thwarted ; its use as an anæsthetic is consequently in many cases less dangerous.

The combination of oxygen and nitrous oxide appears to be principally applicable in the following cases :

1. To narcotize children, in whom you expect a disturbing twitching of the muscles when giving nitrous oxide alone.

2. For anemic and weakly patients, who, like children, frequently have a tendency to contraction of the muscles, and remain but a very short time under the influence of pure nitrous oxide.

3. For all persons who show a remarkable susceptibility for nitrous oxide *per se*. Such patients are frequently difficult to manage, as the anæsthetic effect is of a very short duration.

4. For such patients who have had unpleasant sensations during the inhalation of nitrous oxide.

5. For aged persons.

6. For patients whose tonsils are unusually large.

7. For patients with heart or lung troubles.

—Correspondenz Blatt für Zahuärzte.

Proceedings of Dental Societies.

Dental Association of the Province of Quebec.

The regular meeting for examination of students and other business was held in May. The full Board was present.

The following alterations have been made in the By-laws of the above Board:

By-law 5, Section 1, upon the required course of lectures in the Medical Faculty of McGill or Laval has been expunged, and it now reads after the word attendance on 3rd line, "of two full courses of six months each in the Medical Faculty of any University in this Province."

Section 3 has been expunged, and now reads, "The Primary will comprise Anatomy, Physiology, Chemistry and Metallurgy."

Section 7, Par. 2, the words "except when passed as Primary Examination in McGill or Laval" have been expunged.

Section 15 has been expunged.

Attention is directed to the following resolution passed by the above Board:—

"Any student not complying with the By-laws of this Board by not attending two full courses of six months each, in the Medical Faculty of any University in this Province, the Secretary is hereby ordered to notify him that unless he complies with the same his indenture will be cancelled."

The following gentlemen passed the matriculation examination: Charles Cooper, F. Kent, Maurice Sullivan, D. Bennick.

Primary Examination.—Anatomy. Examiner, Dr. E. Casgrain, Passed: W. Brown, E. Dubeau, C Morrison, A. Gravelle, J. Shaw, J. Adams, James Boyne, John Delisle, J. Roy, H. Kerr, James Panneton, W. Allen, M. Mercier. Chemistry. Examiner, Dr. Hyndman. Passed: E. Dubeau, W. Brown, H. C. McConnell, J. M. Shaw, C. Morrison, E. J. Adams, J. Roy, J. Boyne. Metallurgy. Examiner, Dr. Hyndman. Passed: H. Kerr, H. C. McConnell, J. Boyne, W. Brown, H. Fortin, E. Dubeau, S. Gaudreau, W. Allen, C. Morrison, P. Vosburg, J. Shaw, J. Riendeau, E. Barnes. Physiology. Examiner, Dr. Venner. Passed: E. Barnes, E. Adams, J. Boyne, F. W. Brown, G. Oliver, E. Dubeau, H. Kerr, H. C. McConnell, W. Allen, J. Shaw, C. F. Morrison.

Final Examination.—Passed: J. Gardner, A. Dumont, G. Oliver.

Legislation.

Assembly Bill No. 121, Province of Quebec.

An Act to amend the law respecting dentists.

[Sanctioned, January, 1894.

Her Majesty, by and with the advice and consent of the Legislature of Quebec, enacts as follows:

1. Article 4055 of the Revised Statutes, as replaced by the act 52 Victoria, chapter 40, and amended by the act 55-56 Victoria, chapter 32, section 1, is further amended by adding after the word, "admission," in the fifth line of paragraph 9, the words, "to the study of."

2. Article 4058 of the said Revised Statutes, as enacted by the said act 52 Victoria, chapter 40, and replaced by the act 55-56 Victoria, chapter 32, section 3, is amended :

(*a*) By replacing the first paragraph by the following :

"**4058.** Any person desiring to study dentistry in this Province must previously have passed the examination prescribed by the Board of Examiners of the Dental Association of this Province ; but all graduates in arts or medicine from any Canadian or English University shall be admitted to study dentistry without such examination.

The said Board shall appoint the necessary examiners and indicate the subjects on which candidates for study shall be examined :

(*b*) By adding at the end of the said article, the following paragraph :

" 5. Every student who changes patron must have his indentures transferred to his new patron by his old patron. Such transfer shall be made before a notary and be afterwards registered by the secretary of the Board of Examiners. This transfer is valid only from the date of the registration of such transfer, and confers upon the student all the privileges granted by law to the study of dentistry. Any period of time elapsed between the day on which the student has left his former patron and the day on which the transfer has been registered shall not count in the term of study of such student."

3. Article 4061 of the said Statutes as replaced by 52 Victoria, chapter 40, is amended by replacing the first paragraph by the following:

"**4061.** The examination for admission to study shall be held twice in each year, on the first Wednesday of April and the first

Wednesday of October, and for admission to practise on the first Wednesday of April of each year. Nevertheless, supplementary examinations for admission to practise may be held on the first Wednesday of October in each year, in accordance with the by-laws of the said association now in force."

4. Article 4065 of the said Statutes, as replaced by the said act 52 Victoria, chapter 40, and amended by the act 55-56 Victoria, chapter 32, section 6, is further amended as follows :

(*a*) By striking out from the first paragraph the following words: " for remuneration, or in the hope of being remunerated, rewarded or paid for his services, directly or indirectly."

(*b*) By striking out from the second paragraph the words : " by exacting payment, reward or remuneration for his services as a dentist, by the sale of drugs or medicines, or by barter, exchange or otherwise.

5. Article 4066 of the said Statutes, as enacted by the act 52 Victoria, chapter 40, is repealed.

6. Article 4981 of the said Statutes, as replaced by the act 52 Victoria, chapter 40, is amended by adding after the word, " Quebec," in the fifth line, the following words, " under penalty of the fine enacted by article 4065 of the said Statutes, as repealed by the said act, which shall be recoverable in the manner indicated by the said article 4067."

7. Article 4058 of the said Statutes, as replaced by the act 52 Victoria, chapter 40, and by the act 55-56 Victoria, chapter 32, is amended by replacing the word, " four," in the third line of the paragraph by the word, " three."

8. This act shall apply to students now under indenture.

Selections.

Mr. Tomes' Inaugural Address.

The following extracts from the Presidential address of Mr. Tomes, at the annual meeting of the British Dental Association, in Newcastle, will be read with interest :

" It seems to me that I cannot better employ the short time which I propose to occupy, than by a short review of the conditions of a dentist's life—of that which conduces to his success or failure, and of the manner in which these conditions react upon the man himself ; and in the fulfilment of this task I hope that I shall not be thought to play the part of a too candid friend.

" As a united body—and of this union this Association is the visible sign—we are very young ; counted in the years of a man's life we have not attained to our majority, and what are twenty-one years in the history of a profession? and of youth no one can expect more than promise. And if we venture to think that we show some promise, I also fear that we have many of the faults of youth—faults possessed by youth, however well endowed, faults that pertain to young corporations, and to young nations no less than to individuals. But though there may be excuse for our faults, that is not the less reason that we should try to recognize them, and, so far as may be, correct them. It is in my mind that we expect too much, that we hope to go too fast, and that we are inclined to clamor for a degree of consideration which can only be accorded in the fulness of time, if ever. This consideration may take many forms ; it may be more social recognition, it may be a higher scientific status, or it may be the confidence of the Legislature in entrusting us with more power to work out our ideas. But whatever form it is to take, it, in the very nature of things, can only be of slow growth, and by clamoring for it before it is accorded, we run the risk that is incurred by the pushing youth, of being snubbed for our pains.

"This aspect of things is not confined to our own speciality, it has seldom been better expressed than in the words of Dr. Mitchell Banks, so well known here in the north, and I will read you an extract from his address given last year before the Medical Society of London. Speaking of various medical organizations, he said: 'To become a gigantic mutual admiration body is a mistake. There can be nothing worse for us than to be ignorant of our weak places, and the man who, like the late Dr. Milner Fothergill, points them out to us, is certain to be a thousand times more alive to the real dignity of our profession than the vulgar persons who boast so much about it and add so little to it. By mere virtue of our profession we do not rank socially with other professions—we have to make our social position for ourselves. So much the more reason why our whole profession, down to its youngest graduate, should be men of such good general culture that their company should be welcomed not merely by the rich (for of these I make but little account), but by all of those whose well-trained minds, whose liberal ideas, and whose refined manners, constitute the true society of our country.'

"So I shall not say much of the great strides that have been made, in the education gone through, in the standard of our professional examinations (our students have to pass the same preliminary examination in general education as the general medical students), nor of the progress which legislation has rendered possible in the hindering of irregular forms of practice—this has all been said before, *usque ad nauseam;* but will pass at once to point out the conditions which it appears to me are called for to make the successful practitioner. It goes without saying that he must have fully availed himself of his opportunities of study, for which there is now no lack of opportunity, and it would lead me too far afield to discuss the details of that training of hand and brain, but I should like to say a few words on the matter of a training beyond the ordinary routine of dental education ; for there is a danger lest, led away by the pride of manipulative dexterity, we underrate directions of study which, to the thoughtless, seem to have little practical outcome.

" We have all of us made acquaintance with the self-styled practical man in all grades of society, from the artisan who poisons us with sewer gas, to the politician whose horizon is bounded by the limits of his personal observation, and that none too accurate. Let us quote to you the words of one of the clearest thinkers of our day, Professor Huxley, who thus delivered himself upon the proper scope of education: ' I often wish that this phrase, applied science, had never been invented, for it suggests that there is a sort of scientific knowledge of direct practical use, which can be studied apart from another sort of scientific knowledge, which is of no practical utility, and which is termed pure science. But there is no greater fallacy than this. What people call applied science is nothing but the application of pure science to particular classes of problems. It consists of deductions from those general principles, established by reasoning and observation, which constitute pure science. No one can safely make these deductions until he has a firm grasp of the principles, and he can obtain that grasp only by personal experience of the operations of observation and of reasoning on which they are founded. Almost all the processes employed in the arts and the manufactures fall within the range either of physics or of chemistry. In order to improve them, one must thoroughly understand them ; and no one has a chance of really understanding them unless he has obtained that mastery of principles and that habit of dealing with facts which is given by long-continued and well-directed purely scientific training in the laboratory.'

" I will not weaken these pregnant words by comment, save only to say that every word which I have quoted is applicable to the training of the dentist, but that as yet we are far behind such an ideal as is there propounded. That scientific habit of mind by which we observe correctly and draw conclusions legitimately is essential, but it is fortunately one which can, to a great extent at all events, be cultivated. But do not suppose that I would allow this wider mental culture to at all take the place of that patient acquisition of manipulative, and I may say, empirical skill. To once more quote Professor Huxley: ' Indeed, I am so narrow-minded myself, that if I had to choose between two physicians, one who did not know whether a whale is a fish or not, and could not tell gentian from ginger, but did understand the application of

the institutes of medicine to his art, while the other, like Talley-
rand's doctor, " knew a little of everything, even a little physic,"
with all my love for breadth of culture, I should assuredly consult
the latter.'

" But in real life we are not called upon to make this choice ; the
man who is greedy of learning in his own special line is rarely—I
may say, never—content to be ill-informed outside it. But supposing our young aspirant to start fully equipped with such knowledge as the schools can give him, his success is not yet fully
assured, and there are certain qualities, like all qualities capable of
improvement by cultivation, which will serve him in good stead.
He must have nerve ; not perhaps the nerve of the surgeon in
whose hands lie the issues of life and death, but a certain steadiness
of nerve which will enable him in the face of his special difficulties
to be fully master of all the skill which he possesses, and this will
go far towards securing the confidence of his patients. He must
be painstaking, for it is in attention to *minutiæ* that, just as in
modern surgery, the difference between success and failure lies ;
he must be patient, too, in dealing with all the little obstacles
which crop up. And he must have tact and a quick judgment of
the idiosyncrasies of his patient, which he must be both quick to
appreciate, and, within proper limits, to bend to. For the very
nature of our work precludes the possibility of the patient being
able to judge even of results, except by the test of time, far less
of what is best to be done for him, so that the dentist has ample
opportunity for the exercise of all his discretion in knowing when
to give way to his patient, and when to fight out his little battle in
the patient's own interest. And it is very desirable that he should
cultivate a thoroughly kind and friendly feeling towards those who
honor him with their confidence—I say cultivate, because I believe
that such a habit of mind is strengthened by use, and that it is just
as easy to entertain a friendly feeling towards those to whom we are
able to render service, as it lies deep down in imperfect human nature
to dislike those whom we have in any way injured. He must have a
good physique ; his work is hour after hour exhausting in a degree
that no one who has not tried it can appreciate. With busy practice
comes another difficulty, and that is to avoid being hurried, and to
keep for each patient time enough to do him justice. There is no
temptation for the busy dentist to spend one moment more than is
absolutely necessary over his work ; on the contrary, there is a
very strong temptation in the other direction, as it becomes very
difficult to satisfy all those who wish to be seen, and who do not
realize that dental operations take so long that it is rarely possible
for the dentist, as it sometimes may be for the medical man, to
squeeze in another patient when his appointment book is full. So
that a good deal of moral firmness is needed every day to keep
the dentist out of this pitfall. And he has all the more need of

these qualities in that his patient can never know the extent of the difficulties of his work—difficulties that are great enough, though the work be small—and will often be inclined to rate as high, or higher, the practitioner who attempts nothing difficult, but pilots their teeth towards a gradual and painless euthanasia, as he who renders far more real service, but in attempting much more now and again fails in something that the other would never have attempted.

"It may be said that these qualities which I have sketched would have led to success in any calling ; so I believe they would, and I fancy it is generally true that the man who scores a real success in any calling would have done so in a good many others had his career been a different one.

"One more word before I leave this matter of professional success. By success I do not mean merely pecuniary success. I do not call it real success unless a man stands in the opinion of his own professional brethren at least as high, or higher, than he does with the public. It is, unfortunately, the case that in all branches of the medical profession, and very especially in ours, the ear of the public is sometimes to be caught by self-assertion, and the many hydra-headed forms of quackery. It is sometimes asked why, when the manufacturer or the dealer advertises his goods without exciting the smallest adverse comment, should it be considered disgraceful for a barrister, a stock-broker, or a medical man to advertise himself. The difference is not far to seek, though it is often overlooked. The one advertises an article which he wishes to make known to the public, and it is greatly to their convenience that he should do so ; the one extols a thing, the other extols a man—himself. And there is this further difference—the thing may be new, all that is said about it may be true, but this can hardly be the case with the personal advertisement. For all knowledge that is of importance in a professional sense is very soon public property, for each to make use of as his abilities serve ; but it would hardly have the effect he desires were the advertiser to say : ' I am even as other men are ; ' he must brag in some form, or it would be no good, and when he brags he can hardly be truthful.

"Let us turn from this disagreeable subject to a consideration of the reaction upon the man himself of success in practice. Wealth he can hardly attain—the limits of time preclude it; and the great income of a surgeon or physician in the front rank is impossible. But ease and comfort and moderate savings are within the reach of a large number. He will have but little leisure ; the large expenditure of time upon his operations in order to do them properly not merely sets a limit upon the amount that he can do, but the number of hours during which a man can do such work without undue exhaustion being soon reached, he has none too much energy for other things. One day's work very closely resembles the next, and the next, and though I would not be understood to say that there is not more of variety, and more scope for the exercise of sound judgment than any outsider might suppose, nevertheless, it is all exercised upon a strictly limited class of subjects, and so has its special mental dangers. The dentist in large practice may be compared to a man who daily journeys along a deep lane, shut in with hedgerows on either side. In such a lane there will be much for him who has eyes to see it, more, perhaps, than in a lifetime he can possibly exhaust, if he observes its geology, its fauna and flora, and the phenomena of human life and its ways that unfold themselves there ; but for all that, our wayfarer will never understand even his little world if he never looks outside it. I came across a passage in one of Stevenson's novels the other day which illustrates what I mean : 'The dull man is made, not by the nature, but by the degree of his immersion in a single business.' And all the more if that be sedentary, uneventful, and ingloriously safe. More than one-half of him will then remain unexercised and undeveloped ; the rest will be distended and deformed by over-nutrition, over-cerebration, and the heat of rooms.' And, inasmuch as it is easy to see the mote in our brother's eye, I often fancy that I can trace the cramping and narrowing effect of our necessarily limited horizons, which prevents our even seeing what is really well within their limits. There are countless problems lying before us ; the etiology of the diseases we have to treat, problems of heredity laid out before us—a rich and varied field for observation, yet how many cultivate it, even making due allowance for the fatigues of our routine work. By all means, then, let the dentist who would keep his mind fresh cultivate a hobby. A hobby is more restful than idleness, and is a joy forever, if it be well chosen. I recollect being struck with the sadness of the end of the life of one of the greatest physicians of recent days, who had no hobbies. He broke down in health, so that he could not practise, and then time hung heavy, even on the hands of a bright intellect, because, with failing health and declining years, it was too late to take up a fresh pursuit. And, as a contrast, the end of the life of a great surgeon, who, when he retired from practice, eagerly turned to the pursuit of art, which he had cultivated with a great measure of success throughout a long and busy life. And I think I can trace the same cramping effect in our relations to outside matters.

" Important to the well-being of the individual are his teeth ; yet man is not wholly a complex organism constructed for the purpose of carrying about thirty-two (or fewer) teeth. Useful as I hope we are, we are only a small section of a great community, and while we hope that any legislation which we may be able at any future time to influence, will be upon the lines on which we have sought to improve the position of our profession, we must always remember that it is only because the advancement of our profession is, broadly speaking, for the public weal, that what has been effected in the past was possible, and that which may be effected in the future can come into the sphere of possibility only upon the same grounds of a general public utility."—*Journal of the British Dental Association.*

How Best to Read and Study and Write Dental Literature.*

By C. N. JOHNSON, L.D.S., D.D.S., Chicago, Ill.

MR. PRESIDENT AND GENTLEMEN,—The phrase "dental literature" in the title given the essayist by your committee probably relates more particularly to the periodical literature of the profession than to books, and it is to this phase of the subject that, with your permission, the writer will chiefly devote himself. Most of the dental literature of the present day is made up of matter appearing either originally or finally in dental journals, for there is very little that is published in books but what has, in one form or another, found utterance in periodicals. It may, therefore, be realized what an important place in the general literature of the profession our journalistic literature is destined to fill, and he who keeps well abreast with his dental journals and watches closely the book reviews contained therein, so that he may avail himself of any special book on a subject of interest to him, need not fear of missing much that is of permanent value.

The division of the subject into three parts, to read, to study and to write, very justly implies that there is a distinction between reading and studying, and yet for the purposes of the present paper it may be well to consider the two in the same connection. At the outset it must be assumed—with the possible risk of taking too much for granted—that all are agreed as to the necessity of a familiarity with our periodical literature in order for a dentist to keep himself fully alive to the best interests of his patrons. The question for our present consideration is, how best may this familiarity be maintained?

To gain a comprehensive idea of what is going on in the profession, a dentist should subscribe for five or six journals at least. No one journal can supply the demands of a progressive man, for each journal has its distinguishing characteristics, and therefore represents a different line of thought from the others.

*Read before the joint meeting of the Iowa and Nebraska State Dental Societies, May, 1894.

In reading and studying dental literature to the best advantage it is necessary to plan some system whereby the work may be pursued in a regular and consecutive manner.   The average sub-scriber to our journals probably falls far short of gaining the greatest possible benefit from his literature on account of aimless methods of reading.   To subscribe for a journal and then leave it lying around the office to be picked up in a hap-hazard sort of way whenever chance suggests a spare moment, is to waste, for the most part, the money paid for subscriptions.   Such desultory reading as this leaves no lasting impression on the mind, and results at best in a confused idea of what is going on in dentistry. No one method of reading can be laid down as a guide for all subscribers to follow.   Individual circumstances and conditions operate to render necessary a separate plan for almost every reader. Each one should study out that plan which, to him, seems the most convenient and profitable, and this method when once arranged, should be rigidly adhered to until a better one presents itself   This may at first require some discipline, and usually den-tists are not good disciplinarians (especially when it comes to disciplining themselves), but in the end it will be found that even discipline itself becomes a habit, and if the method pursued be the one best suited to the requirements of the individual, it will soon seem easy to follow.

While, as has been said, no one method can be advanced as suitable for all, yet a few general suggestions may prove of interest. Supposing the subscriber be a young man just starting in practice, the advice is to read carefully every article appearing in the jour-nals.   This may at first thought appear like a waste of time, but there are many arguments to favor its observance.   The beginner often has considerable time not taken by appointments, and that time may be more profitably spent in making himself familiar with the literature of the profession than in any other manner. No young dentist of a receptive nature can read an article treating on any line of practice without carrying the influence of that article to the operating chair or laboratory.   In the early days of practice it may be well to keep the journals at the office for at least the first month of their appearance, where they may be per-used at will during any spare time.   It is far better to keep the mind fully engaged with topics relating to practice than to read light literature during office hours, or to sit brooding over lack of practice.   After the journal has served its purpose at the office, it should be taken to the home and placed in regular order in the library.   During the process of reading the journal, careful note should be taken of those articles which will justify a second read-ing and subsequent study.   To keep a list of these, it is well to have an indexed title book in which to record the title of the article, with the name and date of the journal.   This title book, or something to fill its place, should be made a prominent feature in reading and studying dental literature. By its use, the reader may keep year after year a list of those articles to which he may wish to refer at any time, and if he subsequently drifts into a specialty, and becomes interested in any one line of work, he will find in his book on the one page a list of those articles bearing on his specialty, with the date of publication and the name of the journal containing them. Without a title book of this kind, it is necessary to look over the entire index of every journal in the library in order to examine the literature of any one subject. This indexed title book should be in the hands of every reader of dental literature, young or old. Every dentist can select such a one as seems best adapted to his needs. Probably a small one that can be slipped into the pocket, and thus readily carried between the office and the residence, will be the most convenient to the majority, but an extensive reader could so enlarge the scope of the work as to result in a complete index of the periodical literature of the profession. Such a record kept for several years would eventually prove a most valuable work of reference and save the reader a great amount of time.

In addition to the reading done during his office hours, the young practitioner should religiously set aside certain evenings in the week for professional reading and study. At these times he can pursue a certain line of thought without fear of being disturbed, as he often must be in his office, and the concentration of mind possible in the quiet hours of the evening impresses the subject matter upon him to a degree not approached under other circumstances. While reading, whether at the office or the house, careful note should be made of every word whose meaning is not well understood, and the dictionary should be appealed to in every instance, so that the reader becomes familiar with the technical terms used by writers upon dental subjects. As practice increases, and the time is more fully occupied in the office, it becomes necessary to do less and less reading during the day, and eventually the time comes when all reading at the office must be abandoned, and the journals carried home for perusal. This need not necessarily result in extending the number of evenings to be employed in this work, for by this time the practitioner is presumably in a position to discriminate somewhat in his reading. It has just been stated that the recent graduate should read carefully every article appearing in his journals, to the end that he may keep himself occupied and gain a familiarity with the various writers and their theories, but as this familiarity is gained it will impress the discerning and experienced reader that there is much appearing in our periodicals that does not call for verbatim examination on the part of the advanced practitioner. He will soon learn to select those articles which merit his careful attention, and to dismiss the

3

others with a hasty glance. It will become more necessary each year to exercise good judgment in this respect, so that time—which grows more valuable as age advances—is not wasted on indifferent literature. By careful discrimination and the constant use of the title book, a practitioner may keep himself in touch with the current literature of his profession and still have time for his social and domestic duties, and also for writing dental literature himself.

The time has now arrived when the practitioner should begin to pay back in part the debt he owes the profession by adding something from year to year to its literature. No man should be a drone in the dental hive any more than in the great hive of humanity, and just so soon as his experience justifies it, he should begin to cultivate the habit of writing out the results of his observations gained in practice and by reading, and incorporate them into papers for dental societies or original communications to dental journals.

This brings us to the consideration of the third part of our title —how best to write dental literature. This must be acknowledged a difficult subject to treat in a manner to make it interesting, or of practical value to the average member of a dental society. The suggestions attempted in the present paper are intended to apply for the most part to beginners, and some of the hints given may appear so simple and so patent as not to be worthy of a place in an essay to be read before such a meeting as this. Extenuation is pleaded on the ground that experience has shown how deficient the majority of writers on dental topics prove themselves in many of these minor details.

The first requirement for a paper on any topic, no matter what the age of the author, is for him to have something to say. There should be a distinct idea in his mind that he has a matter of some import to tell the profession. It need not necessarily be—in fact, in the very nature of things it seldom can be—anything strictly original. But it must be something with which he is personally impressed—something which he feels needs more emphasis than has yet been given it. It is possible for some valuable line of practice to be advocated in our periodical literature and remain in print for months, and even years, without the profession generally adopting it or giving it the attention it merits. This is often due to the fact that it has been indifferently presented to the profession by its originator. The man who takes up a subject of this kind and by the very earnestness of his conviction forces the profession to give it due consideration, is often of more practical benefit than the man whose genius originated the idea. If all practitioners cannot be original investigators they can at least be thinkers, and no man should allow himself to be a thinker for any length of time without giving the profession the benefit of his thoughts. In a calling like dentistry he should not be a thinker "for revenue only." The specious plea made by some of our inventive genii that they are able to think out a problem for themselves but are unable to describe the process on paper, so that the profession may get the benefit of it, should not long obtain in this age. Too much literature of all kinds is appearing every day to leave a man long in ignorance of proper modes of expression, and even if a first, or second, or third attempt fails in a clear statement of his idea, this should not discourage him from repeated effort till he gains his point. It would probably surprise the literary novice to be told how many times the MS. of some of our ablest authors of general literature is rewritten. The fact that an article reads smoothly is no indication that it was written easily—the fact is usually to the contrary. Persistent effort of this kind will prove beneficial to the writer in more ways than one. No man can write out an idea without having that idea made clearer in his mind—he cannot describe a method or an appliance without forcing the details more firmly into his brain, on account of having given concise and accurate expression to them. In no department of our work is the saying "practice makes perfect" more true than in this.

After being assured that he has something of interest to tell the profession, the next point for the practitioner to consider is the proper method of saying it. Here we approach a subject upon which it is difficult to give definite instruction. No man can tell another how to write within the limits of one short paper, and in truth it is not altogether clear just how far one individual can impart this knowledge to another, if given the amplest opportunity. The most that can be done is to offer suggestions and point out defects.

In writing a paper, the first thing to do after having the subject well in hand is to arrange the matter in a systematic manner, so that the line of thought will be carried in the mind of the reader in a logical sequence from title to colophon. In order to do this it will sometimes be necessary to make notes, consisting of a series of headings, before any writing is done on the paper proper. For this purpose it is well to have always at hand a slip of paper for some time before the essay is started, while the general idea of the subject-matter is taking form in the mind, so that any heading may be jotted down as it occurs. Often an idea will suggest itself while working at the chair, or in the laboratory, or riding in the street car, or lying in bed vainly dallying with the sometimes fickle god, Morpheus. If the idea is not caught and trapped on the instant, it is quite likely to slip away never to return, or perhaps to return too late. Armed with adequate notes, the writer may properly arrange the headings in orderly sequence, and when this is done it is safe to say that half the labor of writing that paper is accomplished.

If the paper is started without a properly arranged list of headings, it is often the case that ideas occur to the author as the paper progresses, and in order to get them into their proper places, he must insert them in the subject-matter at some point previous to where he is writing—in doing which he usually destroys that rhythmic harmony that should ring throughout the paper from beginning to end.

The preparation of MS. for the printer is a subject which might appear of such minor importance that its consideration would seem uncalled for in a paper like this, and yet it is a matter which in the aggregate causes no end of worry, and—must it be admitted?—considerable justifiable profanity on the part of editors of dental journals. The first copy of a paper is usually disfigured by frequent interlinings, erasures and corrections of various kinds; and no man of any conscience will read a paper before a society in that condition, much less turn it in to the editor for publication. It is well when the first draft is completed to put away the paper in a pigeonhole and leave it for as long a time as convenient, until the author grows unfamiliar with its phraseology. It should then be read aloud to see how it sounds, and it will usually be found that defects present themselves, which in the first flush of composition had been overlooked. When the paper has been carefully corrected, it should be copied in a clear, plain hand, or, what is preferable, with a typewriter. Typewritten copy is manifestly so much better than the writing of the average professional man, that some societies specify that papers presented for publication must be typewritten. No paper should be read before a society or offered for publication without careful attention to a certain point which is quite frequently entirely ignored by authors. This relates to the title of the paper, the name of the author, his place of residence, etc. Too often are papers handed to the editor without the slightest indication, so far as the MS. is concerned, as to what they are about, or by whom they were written, or where they were read ; and the sublime complacency of the authors is epitomized in the remark recently made by one of them, " What are editors for, anyhow ? " It may here be modestly intimated that editors are not for the purpose of divining hidden mysteries such as are sometimes presented for their solution, and the sooner writers recognize this, the better it will be for the author's peace of mind and the editor's prospect of heaven. When the typewritten copy is made, it should contain first the title of the paper, then the name of the society before which it is to be read, with date of meeting, the name of the author, with his degrees, and the town and State where he resides.

The question of punctuation is sometimes a matter of importance, but no rules can be given that will benefit the average writer except probably the one rule of common sense. A word of admonition, however, may be deemed admissible for those writers who fall into the abominable habit of punctuating everything with a dash. The dash is a valuable adjunct in the process of punctuation when properly applied, but it can scarcely be advocated for exclusive use in lieu of commas, semicolons, colons and periods. Some of the MSS. that come to an editor call to mind the remark of a lady writer who on being asked her authority for using so many dashes said, "Oh, when I'm in any doubt as to punctuation I throw in a dash." Some of our writers according to this would appear to be in doubt most of the time, and if their MS. was given to the printer as it leaves their hands the proof would make it appear as if more than half of the author's mind was in a blank. A safer precept than the lady's would be—when in doubt do not use anything.

Moderation is also suggested in the use of italics. These innocent little letters have their legitimate place in our literature, but too often they are dragged out to bolster up an argument which contains little strength outside of the emphasis given it by the conspicuous type. It is sometimes as if the author were aiming occasional blows at the reader to compel his attention to the various points he was attempting to make, in the evident conviction that without this method of typical gesticulation the points would be overlooked.

Offensive mannerisms of speech such as too frequently mar the pages of our journals should be avoided. These are mostly matters of habit and few men realize how badly they have this habit till they conduct a critical examination of their own work. An instance of this kind occurs in a recent issue of one of our most pretentious monthlies where on a single page no less than five sentences are started with the word "Now." This word seemed to be the evil genius of that writer for in a short article of a little more than three pages he made it do duty in this respect ten different times. This in face of the fact that in every instance the sentence would have been strengthened by its omission. It was not used in the sense of stating time but simply as a disagreeable excrescence which jarred on the reader at every turn. In giving full sway to this one mannerism the author made an article sound ridiculous which in other respects was a worthy one. A good way to cure one's self of this habit is to read aloud the MS., as has before been advised, previous to having it typewritten, but in case the habit has become so far a second nature that the author is unable to detect his own mannerism he would do well to hand it to some friend for revision. When his defect is once pointed out he should avoid it in his future writing.

A final word of advice directed more particularly to our young writers must conclude what is already too long a paper. The usual tendency with amateur authors, especially if they chance to be favored with a prolific vocabulary, is to indulge in too much fine writing—in other words to give their work a hifalutin style which shoots wide of the mark in an essay on any professional topic. High-flown, stilted phraseology is being more and more tabooed in the general literature of the world. It is frowned upon by the purely literary individual everywhere, is being less and less indulged in by the newspaper man of the day, and even the novelist himself—that literary Bohemian whose main stock in trade it has oft-times proved itself to be—is now forced to use it, if use it at all, in the face of ridicule and caricature. How far then should it be removed from a place in the literature of a profession like dentistry. Study simplicity of style, plainness of speech, aptness of phrase and brevity of expression. Think out the thing that you want to tell—think it out clearly in your own mind so that the idea is indelibly engraven there before you attempt to put it on paper. When you begin to write keep the idea firmly fixed as your text and write strictly to that text. Go at once to the heart of your subject, say what you have to say about it in the most concise and direct manner, and when you are through—stop.—*Dental Review.*

American Dentistry in London.*

By Frank M. Wilkinson, D.M.D., Boston.

The object of this short paper is to throw light upon a subject of which comparatively little is known in America, and doubtless much chagrin has been experienced by the profession at large on account of the action of the General Medical Council in London in regard to the two dental schools recently disqualified for registration in Great Britain.

Yet when the facts have been clearly set before the profession, it will not be so surprising that such action was taken, but rather that it was so long delayed. American dentistry in England is advertised most extensively and traded upon by those who practise, or pretend to practise it, simply because of the general admission in England of the superiority of it as compared with that practised by other nationalities. The easy credulity of the English public in this matter leads them to be duped by that which is called American, although those who practise under this title are not of that nationality or schooling. The consequence is, that the grossest maltreatment, to speak plainly, is perpetuated, both in supposed-to-be swell private practices as well as in the advertising "limited" companies, who carry on a trade in dentistry rather than a respectable practice. It is well known by the English dentists that this

---

* Read before Harvard Odontological Society, January 25, 1894.

is a great wrong, not only to them, but to the people who are the victims of this avariciousness; they unscrupulously charge the exorbitant fee because it is "American dentistry," while the truth of the matter is, dentists of ability in the States are not guilty of performing operations such as are classed here as American. As a result, the standard of American dentistry in London is anything but what we could wish, and, as seen by most English dentists, is far from being a credit to those who should be representatives of the profession, capable of upholding its high reputation and standard abroad. Why is this? naturally may be asked. The answer is not very hard to find, when it is known that there are several companies in London, with branches throughout England, who claim to be, and advertise as, Americans, and it is certain that many whom they employ are young men from the States. Every dentist who carries on a respectable practice will most emphatically condemn their methods. Some of the work done is not worthy of any American ; yet fee enough is charged to command the best obtainable service from the hands of our experts. Their charges are excessive for what is really bad.

With this state of affairs going on for years, it is not surprising that our standard should be looked upon as no improvement upon that of the English. In private practices, there are many at present who for years worked for these firms, and finally established themselves when their time expired for which they were "bound out," for no one can secure a position who will not sign a contract that binds out of London for so many miles and for so many years. Some of these men go on with the same kind of work, and coin money. Even in the aristocratic West End (which one might think would be free from such) they are to be found. Some who never attended college put "Dr." on their door-plate, and "Doctor of Dental Surgery" appears, in so many words, on advertising cards, in defiance of the law restricting them from practising in Great Britain. There are men who charge five hundred dollars (and it has been paid) for a full denture, gold base and rubber attachment, while if a tooth be a trifle off color, it is cut off and a crown put on at large expense. Many of these charlatans place large fillings over putrescent pulps, while the best is being paid for and supposed to be received. There are many working in this way, against whom the more learned and skilful have to compete, the latter in modest and professional manner, while the former class are obtrusive and gain the patronage of the wealthy and nobility, for the reason that, being Americans, better services are supposed necessarily to follow. What wonder that the standard is not being elevated ! But some there are who are faithful and conscientious, and the English dentist is fair enough to acknowledge a good production from the land of the Stars and Stripes.

Graduates of American schools have practically no opportunity of securing good situations in England at the present time. A law has recently been passed by the General Medical Council forbidding dentists, under penalty of having their names removed from the register, to employ unregistered assistants. The only opening for the graduate is to take the examination for the degree of " L.D.S." (Ireland), " sine curriculo," in Dublin. Three Harvard men have passed successfully, and are now registered. Let those who go to practise in London adhere to the principles they have been taught before leaving this country, and there will be a change for the better.

Let all diplomas be disqualified (as the British diplomas are) when graduates are involved with firms of the aforesaid description, and the day will not be far distant when a different state of affairs will be presented, and firms which bring discredit upon the fair name of American dentistry will have little excuse for their existence.—*International Dental Journal.*

The Advantages of Association.

In proposing the toast of the British Dental Association at the annual dinner, in Newcastle, the President, Mr. C. S. Tomes, made the following admirable remarks as to the advantages of association : " For instance, one comes in contact with a number of people whom you are very glad to know, and whom otherwise you would not have known. They are professional in so far as union gives us a degree of influence that we should not otherwise attain. Another thing is that amongst 800 people (and we are somewhat more than 800) there must be at all times differences of opinion. We cannot all think alike, and it is not desirable that we should. These differences of opinion, if we do not meet, if we do not shake one another by the hand, may come to something more than differences of opinion—they may come to differences of action, and that would be very much to be deplored. The first thing that people who meet together in a proper spirit have to do is to sink their little differences and their own individual opinions. I do not mean to say that a man should be invertebrate, that he should have no opinions of his own, or that if he holds an opinion very strongly, and considers it to be a point of vital importance, he should not stick to it with all the power that he has ; but one may differ on points that are non-essential and non-vital, and when we do so we should differ in a pleasant, good-humored, and a good-natured way ; thresh out our differences, come to an agreement if we can, give way if we can, and go in, generally speaking, for what is comprised under the term of good-fellowship. In this, like every other Association with so many members, there have been differences of opinion. There has been a certain amount of friction as to some points ; some people have thought the action taken has been wrong ; some people have even done so wrongly themselves as to segregate themselves from the general body, because the actions of the general body were not precisely and exactly what they liked. But at this meeting, I myself and—what is of more importance—others have noticed that some of our differences are becoming smoothed over. I won't say are becoming smoothed over, but have become smoothed over, and the difference is now quite a thing of the past. In commending to you this toast, I can do no more than say that this is an essentially auspicious occasion for drinking our own health, because I think that some of our difficulties, and some of the differences of opinion that have troubled us for a considerable length of time, have within these last two days disappeared."

Editorial.

"The Only One."

Mr. Charles Tomes, in his inaugural address, which will be found upon another page, makes some apt remarks upon ' the self-styled practical man" in dentistry. While recognizing the importance, and in one sense the pre-eminence of manipulative skill, it is clear that without knowledge of the scientific principles the purely "practical man" is an empirical "surgeon" dentist.

Many of our readers have no doubt frequently been amused with the absurd claims put forth by some of these purely practical men. Any editor can testify to the fact, that it is by no means uncommon to receive as original discoveries, ideas which are perhaps a century old. In every city there are some practitioners who have learned what they know entirely outside of colleges, journals or books, and who have the temerity to tell their patients the most absurd yarns as to their practice. Recently a very well-educated party told us that a certain dentist claimed to be the only one in his city who filled the roots of teeth ; the only one who made the "proper bridge-work" (which, by the way, was made entirely by a mechanical assistant) ; the only one who made contour gold fillings ; the only one who treated abscessed teeth ; the only one who was "not a mere theorist."

At the same time, when the naked truth was told, he was the only one who had never had any other training than what he received with an obscure third-class dentist; the only one who had never listened to a medical or dental lecture, the only one, in short, who is mean enough to make capital for himself by deliberate falsehood and impertinent assumption, and just as long as the public will swallow the statements of these advertising liars, "the only one" will always get public support, even if he gets professional contempt.

Personal.

Our *confrere* and fellow-countryman, formerly of Quebec city, Dr. W. R. Patton, of Cologne, Germany, writes us that he expects to pay Canada a visit this summer. His old friends will be delighted to see him.

We regret very much to announce the death of Dr. L. W Dowlin, of Sherbrooke, Que., which occurred last month. The Doctor was one of the first to welcome the organization of the profession in Quebec Province, and always took an active interest in its progress. He served as a member of the Board of Examiners for several years, and won the esteem and respect not only of his confreres, but of the public generally.

One by one the fathers of dentistry are disappearing from the scene of life, but never from memory. Not long ago it was the venerable and loved Dr. Allport. To-day it is Dr. W. H. Eames, of St. Louis, Mo., one of the founders of the *Missouri Dental Journal*, and for many years its editor, and later, editor of its successor, the *Archives of Dentistry*. In college work, journalism, in the societies, as a teacher and ever a student, as a President of Association of Dental College Faculties, and whenever he could say a good word or do a kind deed, he was prominent.

DOMINION
DENTAL JOURNAL.

VOL. VI. TORONTO, JULY, 1894. No. 7.

Original Communications.

A Profitable Way to Dispose of Solder Scrap.

By R. E. SPARKS, M.D., D.D.S., Kingston, Ont.

Dealers cannot allow more than about two-thirds as much for solder scrap as they charge for—say 18k. solder. In crown and bridge work, solder scrap may be made as valuable as new solder. Clean all old backings and bits of plate having solder upon them, by dropping them into a bath of dilute sulphuric acid and boiling for a few minutes, or leave in the bath over night. Wash them in clean water. Hammer each piece quite thin and cut into small pieces, and put into a bottle or box for use. They answer every purpose where cusps are to be filled, or any place where bulk of solder is required. To use them, first flow some new solder upon the piece, then add the scrap. The application of heat will flow the solder contained in the scrap and fuse the whole mass together. Should the surface be rough, on account of the insufficiency of solder contained in the scrap, to cover the bits of plate contained in the same, add more solder.

CONVENIENT NERVE CANAL PLUGGERS.—An assortment of canal pluggers may be made by taking spent nerve brooches and removing any remaining barbs by running a fine file over them while they are held flat upon the bench. They are made smooth by rubbing them a few times with fine sandpaper. The point can be snipped off to any desired size. They can be handled with a nerve brooch carrier.

2

A Convenient Dental Instrument.—A jeweller's pin vise, or wire holder, is a tool having a round wooden handle and a clutch, controlled by a clutch screw at one end. It may be purchased for twenty-five cents, and makes a very convenient dental instrument. It is a nerve brooch carrier, canal plugger (made of spent nerve brooches) carrier. By clutching the two ends of a loop of wire, makes a splendid dentimetre. It will hold post wire while a post is being shaped and sized. It also does excellent service as a needle clutch.

Dental Hints.

By G. F. BELDEN, D.D.S., Seaforth, Ont.

A broken gold filling, where foundation is solid, can be made perfectly good by applying rubber dam, drying gold thoroughly with hot air syringe and commencing with Hubbard's No. 4 leaf gold folded twice, using deeply-serrated points. In this way I have built up as much as two-thirds of a central incisor and have yet to hear of one fracture, although some are of three years' standing.

The use of aluminum in connection with a newly-made amalgam filling will give off salts of aluminum, which, if watched closely, will be found forming and piling up very quickly. I first found this out by filling cusps of set crowns to make them stronger, then tested it in the mouth and found the same thing occur. It will do so, no matter how dry it is made, but will not do it with an old filling

Partial impressions can be taken in plaster, no matter how bad the case may be, either lower or upper, by building up impression cups with wax and fitting them pefectly to the mouth. If there are any dove-tailed spaces between the teeth, place in piece of wax, trim evenly with edges of same. Take impression as usual, removing before plaster sets too firmly. Then slide wax out sideways from between the teeth, place in position in impression, run mould as usual; when hard, separate and trim teeth, and you have a perfect reproduction of the mouth—one you can rely on at all times. Use a little more care to avoid air bubbles than when teeth are absent.

You will hear from me again in some future issue on Pyorrhœa Alveolaris, the treatment of which I have been comparatively successful with.

Proceedings of Dental Societies.

Ontario Dental Society and Eastern Ontario Dental Society.

The sixth annual meeting will be held at City Hall Buildings, Kingston, 25th, 26th and 27th inst. We have just time to give the programme, which has just this moment reached us (12th July):

"Modern Dentistry," C. A. Mountain, Ottawa ; "Calcification of Dental Pulps," R. Rose, Peterborough ; Paper, D. V. Beacock, Brockville ; "Disagreeable Odors in Operating Rooms," Stanley Burns, Smith's Falls ; "Treatment of Pulpless Teeth and Alveolar Abscesses," R. E. Sparks, Kingston ; Paper, A. Stackhouse, Kingston ; Retiring President's Address ; A Contribution to Dental Pathology, W. Geo. Beers, Montreal.

CLINIC.—"How to take a correct Bite," W. M. Brownlee, Mount Forest ; Contribution, Paper on Clinic, C. N. Johnson, Chicago ; Contribution, Papers and Clinics from Members of the Profession.

EXHIBITS.—S. B. Chandler; Detroit Dental Manufacturing Company ; S. S. White Company.

Certificate rates will be granted by the G. T. R. and C. P. R. Co's.

Royal College of Dental Surgeons of Ontario.

The following is a digest of the proceedings of the Board of Directors, held in Toronto, March 27 :

After the appointment of professors and demonstrators, fixing the curriculum, salaries of the teachers, etc., the report of the Executive Committee was presented, four meetings of which were held ; report of Committee on Building and Fitting. The following report of the Secretary followed :

To the Directors of the R. C. D. S.:

GENTLEMEN,—1. The business of the College transacted by the Secretary during the past year has been mainly of the usual routine character. The volume of correspondence is yearly increasing at a somewhat rapid rate. Enquiries as to course of study and conditions of graduation have been more numerous than in previous years, many such enquiries coming from the United States. To most enquiries I have been able to make reply. A few are out of the ordinary course, and I have informed the correspondents that they would be referred to the Board. These will be presented to you in due course.

2. As directed at the last meeting, an official letter was written by the President and myself to the National Association of Dental Faculties, tendering, for reasons given, the resignation of the R. C. D. S. from membership in the Association. After the meeting of the Association in Chicago, in August last, I received a communication from the Secretary saying that the resignation had not been accepted, and asking us to send a representative to the next meeting of the Association at Fortress Monroe, in August, 1894. The correspondence will be laid before you for action.

3. During the year I have been advised of four prosecutions against violators of the provisions of the Dental Act. The first was brought by Dr. H. F. Kinsman, against one Shrieve, an itinerant vendor of patent medicines, who was extracting teeth, ostensibly free of charge. The prosecution was successful and a fine inflicted, which was paid over to me as Secretary of the College.

As the prosecution was not understood to have been authorized by the representative of the district, the payment of $40 has not been made to Dr. Kinsman. It will be for the Board to determine whether this should be done.

The second case was Pratt vs. Patterson, of Lucknow, at the instigation of Dr. Guaemar, of Kincardine. A fine was imposed and the defendant gave notice of appeal. The case was then taken in charge by Dr. Stirton, representative of the district, and by advice of the Executive Committee, he retained counsel and prepared to defend the appeal. At the last moment the defendant paid the fine, which was remitted to me, and withdrew the appeal. The $40 allowed by resolution of the Board for each conviction secured by direction of the district representative, has been paid to Mr. Pratt.

The account of Mr. Guthrie, Q.C., counsel in the case, will be presented to you.

The third case was Dowd vs. Beam, near Welland. The defendant pleaded guilty, but subsequently his attorney, in looking over the papers, advised him to apply to have the conviction quashed, on the ground of defective information. By direction of our President, our solicitor looked into the matter, and was so doubtful of success that he would not advise the College to defend. The conviction was quashed.

The fourth case was McCoy vs. Ellis, on Manitoulin Island. Two charges were laid, on both of which he pleaded guilty, and was fined $40 or ten days in gaol for each offence, the sentences to run concurrently. The defendant elected to go to gaol. The prosecutor, who was not authorized by the district representative, sends a bill for $80. Wrote him that it would be laid before the Board. From these cases, it is quite clear that it will not be wise for the Board to incur any liability for prosecutions which are not authorized directly by its members.

4. At the last meeting of the Board, the possibility of holding a combined examination with the University of Toronto, was the subject of some conversation. I then informed the Board that I had secured the passing of a resolution by the Senate, asking its Committee on Examinations to report on the practicability and expediency of holding a combined examination with the R.C.D.S.

The Committee did not immediately report, and the time passed when it could have been carried out last year.

On looking into the matter, I found that the regulations of the College and the University respecting examinations were so nearly identical, that all that was necessary to secure a combined examination was to have a common Board of Examiners.

The President of the University being favorable, the attention of the Committee on Examinations was called to the request of the Senate, and a report was presented and adopted by the Senate approving the practicability and expediency of a combined examination.

As our examiners had been appointed for the purpose of trying the experiment, the Senate appointed the same parties as their Examiners except in the case of Practical Dentistry, our examiner appearing on the Announcement of Trinity University, as one of its Examiners in the Department of Dentistry. The Superintendent of our Infirmary was appointed University Examiner in Practical Dentistry.

Our examination has been held precisely as provided by by-law, and so far as I can learn has been quite satisfactory to the students.

The arrangement with the University was that each should pay its own Examiners, and that the other expenses should be equitably divided. They found the room and attendance, and we paid the stationery, printing, expressage and one-half the wages of the watchers. The financial saving to us is about $35.

So far as I can learn, the examination has been quite satisfactory to the University, every member of this year's Final Class who is writing for D.D.S., having written for the Degree at Toronto University.

If the Board approves of the combined examination, as I sincerely hope it will, it will be necessary to appoint the examiners for next year in conference with the University Committee on Examinations.

5. Applications for examinations have been received from 40 freshmen, 22 juniors and 38 seniors, including five who failed last year, one who was starred at the supplemental examination in October, 1893, and one who claimed to be entitled to examination as being in practice when the Dental At was passed, and whose application was accepted by the Executive Committee.

6. Of the members of the Senior Class, four were attending

lectures, although their pupilage was not completed, intending to graduate at an American College next winter, and pass the examination for L.D.S. in March, 1895.

In the American Colleges, as under our new regulations, Anatomy and Materia Medica are final in the second year. These four men applied to me to be allowed to write off their final Anatomy and Materia Medica with the juniors, who were completing these subjects this year. On communicating with the President, he replied that he saw no reason why they should not do so. They have, therefore, paid the examination fee of $10 and written on these two subjects, and ask you to accept their examination.

7. The tabulated reports of the examiners in the several subjects will be laid before you for action.

8. A supplemental examination was held in October, 1893, as directed by the Board. The tabulated report of the examiners and the action of the Executive Committee thereon will be presented to you.

9. During the year 60 Matriculants have been registered. Of these, 31 presented Departmental Certificates; 8 Matriculants in Medical Faculty, Trinity University; 8 Medical Faculty, McGill University; 7 Medical Faculty, Western University; 1 Medical Faculty, Queen's University; 2 in Faculty of Arts, Toronto University; 1 Arts, Trinity; 1 Arts, Queen's, and 1 Arts, Acadia University, N.S.

All of which is respectfully submitted.

J. B. WILLMOTT, *Secretary R.C.D.S.*
Toronto, March 27th, 1894.

———

NATIONAL ASSOCIATION OF DENTAL FACULTIES.

The Secretary presented the following correspondence (see paragraph No. 2 of his report).

TORONTO, ONT., July 20th, 1893.

To the National Association of Dental Faculties:

GENTLEMEN,—At the meeting of your Association held August, 1892, at Niagara Falls, almost at the commencement of the sessions, an exceedingly unfriendly attack was made upon the Royal College of Dental Surgeons of Ontario, a member of the Association.

The attack was renewed day by day throughout the entire meeting.

During the sessions a notice of motion was given, having for its object the exclusion of the Royal College of Dental Surgeons from membership, by an amendment to the Constitution of the Association.

The result of the discussion, as shown by the series of votes taken, manifested clearly that but a comparatively small minority shared the unfriendly feeling, nevertheless the incident was very unpleasant to a majority of the members, as well as to the representative of the college attacked. As there is no good ground for supposing that the manifested antagonism, based apparently on a misapprehension of the Dental Law of the Province of Ontario, or on ignorance of its provisions, will be withdrawn, and as it is probable the attack will be renewed on the discussion of the proposed amendment to the Constitution, the Directors of the Royal College of Dental Surgeons have deemed it to be due to their friends in the Association that they should not continue to be a disturbing element, and that it is also due to their own self-respect that they should not remain in an association where an influential minority had so plainly intimated that they were not welcome.

We are directed, therefore, to tender, and do hereby tender, the resignation of the Royal College of Dental Surgeons of Ontario from membership in the National Association of Dental Faculties, and ask for honorable dismissal.

By order and in behalf of the Directors of the Royal College of Dental Surgeons of Ontario.

(Signed)   R. J. HUSBAND, *President.*
J. B. WILLMOTT, *Secretary.*

INDIANAPOLIS, IND., August 23, 1893.

Prof. J. B. Willmott:

DEAR SIR,—The communication from the Royal College of Dental Surgeons of Ontario, to the National Association of Dental Faculties, withdrawing from membership in the said body, was reported duly by the Executive Committee on 11th inst. at Chicago. The letter of withdrawal was received with many and sincere expressions of regret, and on motion was laid upon the table for one year, and the Secretary instructed to inform you of the action of the Association and request that the Royal College send a delegate to the next annual meeting of the National Association of Dental Faculties, which will probably be held at Old Point Comfort.

It affords me pleasure to inform you also that my proposed amendment to Sec. VII. of the Constitution failed to pass, and that, personally, I hope the Royal College may continue to honor itself by sending you as its accredited representative. I have the honor to subscribe myself,

JUNIUS E. CRAVENS,
Secretary N.A.D. Faculties.

24 Marion Block.

The Board were unanimously of opinion that it was desirable to retain our membership in the Association if it could be done without sacrifice of self-respect, and in view of the friendly action of the Association, at the meeting in August, 1893, at Chicago, and the courteous letter ot the Secretary, it was

Moved by Dr. Smith, seconded by Dr. Wood, that Prof. J. B. Willmott be, and is hereby, accredited as the representative of the R. C. D. S. at the meeting of the National Association of Dental Faculties to be held at Old Point Comfort, Va., in August, 1894. Carried.

COLLECTION OF ANNUAL FEE.

On motion, the Executive Committee were directed to take such action as might be thought necessary for the collection of any annual fees which may remain unpaid after the election for members of the Board in December, 1894.

Legislation.

Newfoundland.—The Chain Complete!

An Act to regulate the Practice of Dentistry and Dental Surgery.

[*Passed 24th May, 1893.*

Whereas it is desirable to regulate the Practice of Dentistry in the Colony of Newfoundland :

Be it enacted by the Governor, the Legislative Council and House of Assembly, in Legislative Session convened, as follows·:

1. This Act may be cited as " The Newfoundland Dental Act."

2. No person shall *practice* the profession of dentistry or dental surgery in any place in the Colony of Newfoundland in which there shall be residing and practising a physician or surgeon or dental surgeon, without having first received a certificate as hereinafter provided, entitling him to practice dentistry or dental surgery.

3. A certificate shall be issued by the Colonial Secretary upon production to him by an applicant for such certificate of diploma of graduation by him in dental surgery from the faculty of any Canadian Dental College or the faculty of any Canadian University having a special dental department, or from any such institution duly authorized by the laws of Great Britian or any of her dependencies, or from any Dental College in the United States of America, recognized by the National Board of Dental Examiners of the said United States of America, or from any recognized dental institution of any foreign country which required, at the time of issue of such diploma or license, attendance at a regular course of lectures, and an apprenticeship of not less than two years ; and such certificate shall be issued also, as aforesaid, to any person, established in actual practice in the Colony of Newfoundland at the time of the passing of this Act. It shall be the duty of the persons claiming to be entitled to the certificate required by this section, to produce to the said Colonial Secretary evidence satisfactory to him of his being entitled thereto.

4. Notwithstanding anything herein contained such certificate, as aforesaid, may be issued to any dental student who, at the time of the passing of this Act, was actually apprenticed to any surgeon dentist in this Colony, and who shall actually, at the time of applying for such certificate, have served an apprenticeship of at least five years, and who shall also produced a certificate to the Colonial Secretary from such surgeon dentist, testifying to that effect : Provided always, that nothing herein contained shall be construed to require physicians, surgeons or others to take out such certificate for the purpose of qualifying them to extract teeth.

5. Before any such certificate is granted, the applicant shall pay the Colonial Secretary the sum of five dollars.

6. After three months from the passing of this Act, any person not holding a certificate issued by the said Colonial Secretary, as aforesaid, who shall *practice* dentistry or dental surgery, except extracting teeth, in any place in the Colony of Newfoundland in which there shall be residing and practising a physician, surgeon or dental surgeon, shall be guilty of an infraction of this Act, and shall be liable, upon summary conviction before any Stipendiary Magistrate or Justice of the Peace, to a fine of not less than five dollars, nor more than twenty-five dollars, besides costs of suit, to be levied by distress of the defendant's goods and chattels or, in default thereof, to be imprisoned for a period not exceeding one month.

7. No person, who has not received the certificate required by this Act, shall recover in any court of law any fees of money for any professional services, or operation performed by him, nor for any materials provided by him in the practice of dentistry or dental surgery.

8. Nothing in this Act shall be construed to prevent surgeons or physicians from temporarily filling teeth or otherwise attending to them for the prevention or cure of toothache.

Selections.

Discussion on the "Retention of Artificial Debentures in Edentulous Lower Jaws."

(At last General Medical Council, London, Eng.)

Mr. David Hepburn opened the discussion. Having remarked upon the advantage of occasionally displacing a paper by a discussion on some practical subject, he stated that in introducing the subject for which he had made himself responsible, he intended to confine himself to a consideration of those cases, which present themselves happily only from time to time, which gives much uneasiness to the patient and specially tax the ingenuity of the practitioner, cases which for want of a more elegant term he would call "slipping lowers." The difficulty, then, upon which they wished to throw light was that which revealed itself when a patient, probably advanced in years, seeks the aid of a dental practitioner with a view to being supplied with artificial teeth, all the natural ones being lost and not even the roots remaining. A denture is adapted, but as the early days of trial progress it is found that it has a tendency to slip forward, in consequence of which the mucous membrane becomes irritated, and more or less ulceration and pain is set up. These symptoms are relieved by "easing," as it is called, but only temporary relief results ; shortly fresh spots of ulceration appear, and the operation of "easing" has to be repeated. What were the conditions leading to such a result ? It would be well to recall some of the simple anatomical facts connected with the lower jaw which had a direct bearing on the subject. The inferior maxillary bone varies much at different periods of life. It consists of a curved horizontal portion and two perpendicular portions (the rami), which join the posterior portion of the body on either side. At birth the rami join the body at an oblique angle, as maturity advances, and up to middle life, the obliquity diminishes until the junction is rectangular, in extreme old age, or second childhood ; obliquity is resumed, simulating the condition as presented at birth. It was this obliquity in a more exaggerated form which rendered the jaw intolerant of the artificial denture. Comparing the normal outline of the jaw in middle life with that typical of old age, he would draw attention to the position of the mental foramen, noticing it first from its external aspect. It would be observed to be midway between the superior surface of the alveolus and the base of the jaw in the first case ; in the second, the alveolus having disappeared, it opened close to the superior surface of the body of the jaw, at which point its nerves and vessels spread out directly to the mucous membrane. Viewing laterally the internal surface of the inferior maxilla, the mylohyoid ridge would be seen to be directly midway between the superior surface of the alveolus and the base of the jaw. Again, a further point to be noticed on this aspect of the jaw was the group of genial tubercles situated on the inner side of the symphisis; when extreme absorption had taken place they often assumed an indefinite mass and form with their tendinous attachments, on which no denture can rest. An inclined plane is created laterally, and from this eminence a denture will often slip downward and forward. In addition to these immediate aspects of the body of the jaw itself there were conditions of mobility different from, or rather an exaggeration of, those which the joint is capable of performing during the period when the teeth are existent. As most bony prominences become modified with advancing years so it is with this one. Further, all these senile changes were frequently associated with alterations in the spinal column, resulting in a fixed downward and forward position being imparted to the head, causing the jaw to rest most naturally in a state of protrusion. By reason of this the space posteriorly is reduced to a minimum, therefore when the artificial teeth are present there is a tendency for the denture to be tilted and displaced. Affecting also lower dentures, they had the musclar force of the tongue. The points he had endeavored to emphasize might exist temporarily or permanently. With regard to treatment, provided that careful impressions of the part had been obtained, and the most natural antagonism ascertained, the question presented itself as to whether or not spiral springs should be employed. He would suggest that they should be dispensed with, as, by reason of the configuration of the lower jaw, they will tend to displace, rather than retain, the denture. At the same time he thought there existed certain classes of cases which needed the employment of springs where the retention of the denture by suction was impossible. When necessity arises for the fitting of springs certain points must be adhered to : in view of the limited space they must be brought well forward ; further, it should be provided that when the jaw opens the lower swivel will be on a vertical line with the upper swivel; in this position they should be " blocked ;" *i.e.*, stops should be inserted in proximity to the swivel heads. By this means the direct thrust of the spring will be maintained. Deeply cut chambers will sometimes suffice to procure the same result. The consideration of the adjustment of springs would afford a theme in itself for discussion. Dental surgeons will receive eagerly any suggestion which would retain lower dentures in their place, and by the kindness of Mr. Lennox, of Cambridge, he (Mr. Hepburn) was able to show the contrivance which was fully described by Mr. Lennox at the Exeter meeting. The most heroic treatment was that suggested by Mr. Dall, of Glasgow, who created sockets in the lower jaw by drilling, into which he inserted posts, by means of which the denture is retained. Another method was that of weighting lower dentures to ensure stability, the principle, Mr. Hepburn thought, of the greatest service where the muscles were strong, but he had had a case where the muscular resistance was so great that the denture was like "a storm-tossed vessel in an angry sea." With regard to the relief of pain by lining the denture with gutta-percha, the mucous membrane became absolutely tolerant of it, but there was the disadvantage of impurity after prolonged use. The metal moulds required some ingenuity in their treatment. The perishable nature of the base, and the impossibility of paring it away without destroying its surface should laceration occur, detracted from its advantages, and all things considered, vulcanite seemed the best. In conclusion, he would give his own experience in a few words. He believed that the difficulties could only be overcome by personal adjustment of the denture to the mouth itself through repeated trials, consequently, during the initial stages of "fitting," frequent visits at short intervals on the part of the patient were of the utmost importance. Having examined the patient, and formed a prognosis of the difficulties to be dealt with, impressions should be taken, preferably in plaster of Paris. When these were cast, and trial plates prepared, the approximate articulation should be taken, with the head bent slightly forward. The bite having been taken, the upper denture might be made and the lower one set up in wax, keeping the lower front teeth well within the upper teeth as to position and height ; if springs were used they should be temporarily adjusted. Almost· invariably the articulation, notwithstanding the precautions, would be found at fault—the lower would slip forward. He would then cover the crowns of the teeth with a moulding of pink wax while the wax was soft ; taking the dentures out of the mouth, the two should then be united according to the indications thus obtained ; the bite might then be finally adjusted. In doing this the teeth should again be set well back, and no prominent cusps be allowed to interfere with the free movement of the jaws. In the upper denture additional canines in the place of first bicuspids would allow of freer movement without tilting.

Mr. Lawrence Read said, with regard to the remarks of Mr. Hepburn as to the lining of the lower pieces, this was a matter in which he had taken some interest, and had devoted a good deal of time to some six or seven years ago ; the difficulty of finishing the rubber he had now quite overcome ; it was a very simple matter when once one knew how to deal with it. His method was to take a large piece of steel wire, about a quarter of an inch thick, with a rounded end, make it red hot, and run it over any rough surface that it was desired to polish. If it was then treated with a little chloroform on wool, a beautiful polished surface was left, just as if it had been baked in a metal mould. It took no time to do, and every edge could be finished off as nicely as could be desired. He had had some lowers with the soft rubber linings, which had been worn for seven years, and were still quite perfect in every way. It was not at all necessary to make them on metal moulds, and they could be finished off, if a little rough, just as readily as a piece of hard vulcanite could be polished.

Mr. S. A. Coxon (Wisbech) demonstrated, by means of diagrams on the blackboard, the plan he adopted in order to get the swivels for springs exactly opposite one another. His method was to take a small strip of No. 7 gold, fold another piece over it, pressing it tightly, thus forming a bolt which could be drawn either forward or backward, and permitted of the springs being put in absolutely true. Another advantage was that the swivel could be attached without getting twisted.

Mr. F. J. Bennett, commenting on the model shown and explained by Mr. Hepburn as being in an oblique position an inclined plane being formed, thought that the condition would bear another interpretation. As it stood, undoubtedly there was an inclined plane, but he (Mr. Bennett) doubted whether in nature they ever got that condition of the mouth if left to itself. If artificial teeth were placed in the mouth it might be so, but without them there was no longer an inclined plane, the lower and upper jaws became parallel. He thought that these facts should teach them to make the bite as shallow as possible; in that way the inclined plane would be reduced to a minimum. Mr. Bennett then criticised at some length the anatomical accuracy of the diagrams by which Mr. Hepburn's opening was illustrated.

Mr. G. Brunton said there was a point which he had been expecting to hear mentioned, namely, that where springs were worn they not unfrequently twisted round, in consequence of which the upper denture is twisted in one direction and the lower in another. He might say that he personally very seldom used spiral springs, but he had seen such cases, and it occurred to him that the reason of the twisting was that the two spiral springs were both coiled in the same direction; he thought that if they were coiled in opposite directions the difficulty would be overcome.

The President remarked that he had himself seen cases similar to those alluded to by Mr. Brunton. They were usually cases where the denture had been worn for many years, and he was inclined to attribute the twisting to the absorption of the alveolus at the sides, leaving the plate nearly impinging on the palate in the middle. He had never seen the twisting in freshly-made plates.

Mr. W. A. Vice narrated an instance which had come under his notice only the previous week, and which supported the view just expressed by the President. The denture had been worn for a long time ; the lower arch was absorbed very much, until the lower piece would not fit at all. The lady dated the movement round to the left side from the time of her having a new spring on the right, and Mr. Vice thought that she was probably correct ; there certainly was some difference in the strength of the springs, the old one on the left being much weaker than the new one on the opposite side.

Mr. S. J. Hutchinson said that Mr. Hepburn had spoken of the loose membrane which was sometimes the cause of trouble in fixing a lower denture. His usual plan was to snip off the membrane with a pair of scissors, allowing the wound to cicatrize, and in this way the difficulty was overcome most satisfactorily.

Mr. H. Baldwin narrated particulars of a case in his own practice, presenting some very interesting features. It was an instance in which an artificial denture, fitted to an edentulous mouth, hurt the patient, not because it slipped forward, but because it moved about so much. But little remained of the lower alveolar process. The attachments of genio hyoglossus and mylohyoid muscles stood up from the general level of the lower jaw. It was an interesting point, Mr. Baldwin thought, that these muscles were preserved when there had been the greatest possible removal of the rest of the alveolar process. To make the plate more comfortable, vellum rubber was tried as a lining, but it had to be given up, as the patient, a man aged sixty, found it induced a tendency to champ his jaws together. The greatest success in treating this case was ultimately obtained by setting up the teeth on a Bonwill articulator, paying great attention to the practical hints upon which Dr. Bonwill laid stress, that was to say, taking care to have the line of articulation of the two rows of back teeth bending decidedly upwards, and further, providing that in all possible movements of the lower jaw the lower denture would strike the upper one at *three points* at once. Considerable care and trouble was necessary in order that this requirement should be fulfilled, but it could be done.

Mr. W. A. Maggs thought that perhaps Mr. Hepburn laid too much stress upon the mandible ; personally he had always regarded the articulation as responsible for the forward movement. The fact that the *eminentia articularis* in aged skulls was so much diminished would tend, of course, to the free movement of the mandible. No doubt the articulation became very lax, and if it were possible to examine a sufficient number of skulls, a considerable difference in the neck of the condyle, and probably in the condyle itself, would be found. He thought that the cases just mentioned by Mr. Baldwin were probably aggravated by the continuous wearing of the denture. While it was difficult to do without the teeth, yet they knew that continuous pressure produced absorption, and he thought that if the denture were not so constantly worn, the tendency to wasting of the jaw would be diminished.

Mr. J. H. Badcock said that in cases where one had great difficulty in making a lower remain in its place, a model taken in the ordinary gutta-percha or stent would show a ridge all round; if, however, a model of the same jaw were taken in plaster of Paris they would find no ridge ; for this reason he strongly advocated plaster of Paris in preference to gutta-percha for taking impressions in such cases. If the model were taken so as to rest only on the floor of the mouth, and not at all upon the bulging sides, there would be very little difficulty, and there would also be much less trouble *afterwards* in easing the case away where necessary. With regard to smoothing the vellum rubber with a hot iron, he thought the whole secret of success lay in having the iron hot enough.

Mr. R. H. Woodhouse did not think that the discussion ought to pass without an allusion to the extreme importance of preserving the natural teeth. They knew that the alveolus was so subservient to the presence of the natural teeth that the retention of even a single tooth, if prolonged, might save all the trouble that had been described that evening.

Mr. W. Hern desired to touch upon a point with regard to the muscular attachments referred to in the mylohoid ridge. He thought it would be found a considerable advantage if the denture were left a little low. He agreed with Mr. Badcock as to the superiority of plaster models. There was a little point about the tray for taking impressions ; if the tray was a little deep one got the frænum of the tongue thrust down, giving a false impression. With regard to the turning of the dentures in opposite directions, as referred to by Mr. Brunton, he (Mr. Hern) thought that it was due to the thrust of the swivel being inaccurate ; so long as the denture fitted well the plates were correct and retained their adaptation, but when the mouth began to change and the fitting was not quite so correct, then the upper and lower dentures turned round as the consequence of the thrust of the swivel being wrong. It seemed to him that the excellent device brought forward by Mr. Coxon would correct this.

Mr. Coxon had omitted to mention that if one got a slight soreness of the mouth it could be relieved by shifting one of the bolts a little. His contrivance also afforded an opportunity to the patient of seeing if he could do without springs.

Mr. Betts stated that he found it very useful to ask a patient to protrude the tongue ; by this means, in conjunction with a shallow tray, the floor of the mouth was raised and one got a much more satisfactory impression.

Mr. Storer Bennett, after the exceedingly interesting and able manner in which Mr. Hepburn had introduced the subject, wished only to touch upon an anatomical point, to which allusion had been made in the opening. In going through the museum, certain variations in the height to which the *eminentia articularis* was raised would be observed. He gathered that Mr. Hepburn was of opinion that a good deal of the forward movement of the lower jaw in old people was due to the fact that the *eminentia articularis* in them was much lower than in people of middle life. This view should not go forth on the authority of the Society without a reservation. He (Mr. Bennett) thought that the protrusion was probably due more to the fact of the ligaments yielding and the jaw becoming exceedingly lax in old age, than to any absorption and flattening of the *eminentia articularis* itself.—*Dental Record (London, Eng.)*

Gum Lancing in Difficult Primary Dentition.*

By Dr. E. C. Kirk, D.D.S.

I should feel myself constrained to offer you an apology for bringing to your notice such an antiquated topic, were it not that, old as it is, the vexed question of its legitimacy is still in dispute, and the procedure has not gained general acceptance among medical and dental practitioners. It is not my purpose to enter into any historical *resumé* of the views entertained by various writers of greater or less prominence, who have recorded their opinions from the times of Hippocrates and Galen to the present time; but in this paper to call your attention to the main differences in the two principal schools of thought on this subject, and urge upon you the necessity of investigating it for yourselves, not from the point of view of the medical practitioner, but from the background of the special training and culture which you possess as dentists. I think we may safely dismiss from consideration the views and theories of earlier medical writers upon this subject, and confine ourselves wholly to an investigation of the more recent, for in a certain and more or less difinite degree the former are included in the latter—at least, so much of the former as has been considered valuable. The question of gum lancing in difficult primary dentition has been the subject of much animated discussion during the past eighteen months. Especially since the publication of a book by Dr. Forchheimer, of Cincinnati, Ohio, on "Disease of the Mouth in Children" (non-surgical), in May, 1892, in which work the author took most positive ground against the operation as a therapeutic measure for the relief of diseases inci-

*An address before the Woman's Dental Association of the United States.

dent to the teething period. His conclusions respecting the operation were tersely stated as follows:

1. It is useless—(a) as far as giving relief to symptoms; (b) as far as facilitating or hastening teething.

2. It is useful only as blood-letting, and ought not to be used as such.

3. It is harmful—(a) in producing local trouble; (b) in producing general disturbances on account of hæmorrhage; (c) in having established a method which is too general to do specific good, and too specific for general use.

4. It is to be used only as a surgical procedure to give relief to surgical accidents.

I have quoted these conclusions at length, because they fairly represent the opinions, and are the arguments generally put forward by that class of medical practitioners who do not know anything about the operation from practical experience, and still less from an intelligent understanding of the *rationale* of the procedure.

A critical review of Forchheimer's book appeared in the *Dental Cosmos* for June, '92, pointing out some of the fallacies that were apparent in his conclusions, and advocating the operation of gum lancing on rational grounds, from the standpoint of accepted knowledge of the anatomy, physiology, and nervous relationships of the tissues and organs involved. The subject was further discussed by numerous authors and editors in medical and dental periodicals, and finally Dr. Magitot presented it in a communication to the French Academy of Medicine. In his paper the author took the ground that inasmuch as dentition was a purely physiological process, there could be no such things as "accidents of dentition," or, as we express it in this country, diseases incident to or dependent upon dentition. His argument to sustain his position was, like that of Forchheimer, based solely upon analytical reasoning from premises which could not be accepted by anyone conversant with the clinical aspects of the subject.

As a sequel to this discussion of the French Academy, M. Poinsot, one of the participants, has elaborated the subject in an interesting volume recently published, entitled, "Accidents of the First Dentition."

It will be seen, then, that the class of practitioners who are antagonistic to the operation of gum lancing are those who, like Forchheimer, object to it because they do not understand why it should be done, nor how to do it—mistaking gum scarification for gum lancing,—and those who, like Magitot, oppose the operation as a therapeutic measure because dentition is a physiological process; *ergo*, there can be no diseases due to or caused by it; hence lancing the gums for the relief of any disorders intercurrent with dentition is irrational and unnecessary. During the past twenty years it has been my lot to have been somewhat closely related

3

to medical as well as dental work, and to have had rather frequent opportunities to observe cases of difficult dentition, and the effect of an intelligent use of the gum lancet as a therapeutic measure for the relief of disorders incident thereto ; hence my faith in the efficacy of the operation is the outgrowth of personal experience as well as observation, and if I shall seem to advocate it somewhat dogmatically, it is because I am convinced that the facts sustain my belief.

The argument of Magitot and his followers, it seems to me, is easily demolished after an investigation of his major premise, viz.: that dentition is a purely physiological process. The answer to this is simply that dentition, while it is generally a physiological process, is not always so, and like all physiological processes, if interrupted or interfered with, may become pathological in its expression. We have only to call to mind the many accidents and fatal pathological phenomena which may attend parturition to find sufficient proof of the utter fallacy of Magitot's proposition.

The proruption of a tooth is a complex process, and includes a number of factors which, when they proceed harmoniously, produce no untoward results, and the teething process in its physiological expression is unattended with disturbances to the health status of the infant. A perfectly normal process of dentition rarely occurs. There is generally a condition of nervous excitation attendant upon the teething period, which in many cases is so slight as to express itself only as a somewhat increased nervous irritability in the child, productive of wakefulness, etc. Or the nervous irritation may be so increased in degree as to cause the most alarming and even fatal consequences. The period of teething is generally made manifest by this increased nervous irritability, and an increased flow of saliva from the mouth. The gums may be more or less congested over the presenting teeth, the positions of which are usually clearly discernible by reason of the gum being elevated and made tense by the erupting tooth crown beneath. The tumefaction or congestion of the overlying gum may be entirely absent, even in cases where the most profound manifestations are present, due wholly to the peripheral nervous irritation caused by the advancing tooth. It is this class of cases where the local manifestations are but slight, and the general disturbance is profound, that has been the cause of the controversy which has been waged around the question of gum lancing. Those who hold to the belief of Forchheimer deny that any relief of general systemic disturbances can follow the operation in such cases. Where they have to deal with a case presenting a congested condition of the gum tissues, they admit that the operation may be useful by letting blood, but no further. The explanation of this belief is not far to seek. It is due to the fact that they understand the operation of gum lancing to mean a superficial scarification of the gum tissue, to empty the congested vessels of the parts and so reduce the local hyperæmia.

I have taken some pains to investigate the matter when opportunity has offered, and I have never found an operator who objected to gum lancing who did not have exactly this conception of the operation. This is gum scarification, and not gum lancing. Gum lancing is a totally different procedure, undertaken not for the relief of congestion of the gum, but for the purpose of freeing the tooth from restraint by the unyielding gum which covers it, causing backward pressure of the undeveloped tooth root upon the formative dentinal papilla at its base ; the irritation of this latter is the cause of the nervous disturbances which it is the purpose of the operation to relieve. The conditions which demand relief by gum lancing are so graphically told by the late Dr. J. W. White, in the *American System of Dentistry*, that I cannot do better than quote from him :

"The direct pressure of the advancing tooth upon the fibrous integuments is not the only nor the principal factor in the disturbance of equilibrium in pathological dentition. The most serious complications are, it is reasonable to suppose, caused by the resistance of the gums, and consequent pressure upon the nervous and vascular supply of the pulp, giving rise to severe and unremitting pain—a true toothache, comparable only to that exquisite torture which is experienced in after life from an exposed and irritated pulp. The condition, when a tooth is thus situated, is not unlike that which is found in whitlow, vascular and sensitive tissues bound down by unyielding coverings. If such a perversion of this physiological process is possible, there can be no question as to the extent of the mischief which may result—an irritability of the general system which finds expression in loss of appetite, sleeplessness, nausea, thirst, fever, diarrhœa or constipation, convulsions, paralysis, and other serious lesions, many of which, as strabismus or epilepsy, remain throughout life."

If, then, morbid symptoms, coincident with the teething period, manifest themselves, and their history and character point to a dental origin, the operation of dividing the gum over the presenting tooth should be so performed that the crown shall be completely freed from its imprisonment by the overlying tissues. It is frequently necessary to include in the operation not only the teeth immediately presenting, but those next in order of eruption in each jaw. If the operation has been properly done, it should be followed almost immediately by marked improvement in the general condition of the infant, and instant relief to the nervous distress.

The technique of the operation is quite simple. The child should be placed on a pillow lengthwise, supported on the lap of the nurse or assistant, seated on a chair facing the operator, and with the back toward the source of light, which should come preferably from a north window. The operator seats himself in front of the nurse, with the end of the pillow supporting the child's head in his lap. He then has command of the territory of operation, and can, by holding the child's head, guard against any sudden movement. The hands and body of the child are to be firmly held by the assistant. The best form of lancet for the operation is a small curved bistury, such as is sold at the depots for the purpose, but with the needle-like point ground off to a small but keen, rounded edge. The lancet is to be passed through the overlying tissue until it is felt to come into contact with the enamel surface, and the tissue divided a sufficient distance to allow the tooth to erupt without resistance.

For the incisors, a single linear cut along the incisive edge is sufficient ; for the cuspids and molars, a crucial incision is required. The operation is not excessively painful, and the pain is reduced to a minimum when a properly sharpened knife is used dextrously. Little hemorrhage follows, but if persistent, some slight styptic, such as powdered alum or phènal sodique, may be used.

Nearly all medical writers agree that the teething period is one fraught with danger. Statistics show that the percentage of infant mortality is markedly higher during teething. A long series of infantile disorders occur most frequently during that period, and while recognizing this coincidence we find many otherwise intelligent practitioners ignoring the possibility of a casual relationship between these diseases of infancy and the teething process, and, consequently, condemning the operation of gum lancing, not only as useless, but dangerous.

A recent published work on "Diseases and Injuries of the Teeth," by Messrs. Morton Smale and J. E. Coyler, of London, contains the following suggestive statement : " Many healthy children pass through this period without any untoward symptoms, but many succumb, as may be gathered from the tables of mortality, teething being the cause of over 4.8 per cent. of deaths in children under 12 months, and 7.8 per cent. between the ages of 1 and 3 years." These same authors, however, notwithstanding this statement, are inclined to regard gum lancing as not useful save as a blood-letting measure. I have been unable so far to find any reported case of fatal result from gum lancing, nor have I knowledge of any untoward result occasioned by it when correctly performed. It is quite true that no precise scientific demonstration by the microscope or by post-mortem examination has been made to settle the question of the exact rationale of the procedure pro or con. The conditions are such that it perhaps never can be made, but this same objection might be as potently urged against many other well-established therapeutic measures in constant legitimate use.

The value of gum lancing in difficult dentition is established almost solely on clinical evidence, though it is difficult to understand why the perfectly plausible hypothesis of the rationale of its action should be rejected by its opponents as imperfect, when that

set up by them in rebuttal is so manifestly illogical and inconsistent. Clinical evidence depends for its value upon the character
and relationships of the phenomena observed, and the frequency
with which certain related phenomena repeat themselves under
similar conditions. If, for instance, infantile convulsions occurring
coincidently with difficult or delayed eruption of the teeth are found
to be relieved by a judicious use of the gum lancet, and a favorable
result is obtained invariably in a number of cases so treated, we
should be justified in assuming the casual relation between difficult
dentition and infantile convulsions within certain limits, and be
justified iu the use of the lancet as a therapeutic measure for their
relief. This relationship has been repeatedly observed. I have in
several instances seen teething children, where convulsive seizures
had supervened until the child was almost comatose, relieved at
once and veritably snatched from the jaws of death by freely
dividing the gum over the retarded teeth.

But convulsive seizures are not the only pathological result of
delayed dentition. The irritation caused by the advancing tooth
is but slight at first, and extends over a considerable period of
time. The impress upon the nervous system of the child may be
comparatively slight, so that its expression may not be manifested
in the explosive outbursts of the nervous system which we know
as convulsions. The nervous stress is more commonly manifested
in loss of appetite, impairment of the digestive function, and
nausea. Impairment of the digestive function, due to interference
with the innervation of the stomach, whereby the food ingested
becomes itself a source of irritation through the establishment of
fermentative processes throughout its mass, leads to and is account-
able for the train of intestinal disorders, infantile diarrhœas, intestinal catarrhs, etc., which so often accompany the teething process,
and constitute the *bete noir* of mothers in rearing their children
through the much dreaded second summer. Where the digestive
sequelæ of pathological dentition have established themselves, the
lancet cannot be expected to effect a cure unaided. Its use should
be followed by appropriate constitutional treatment.

. The close relationship of difficult dentition aud capillary bronchitis in infants has frequently been noted by medical writers and
practitioners, but the idea of pathological dentition as a predisposing, not to say exciting, cause seems to have been overlooked until
recently, notwithstanding the fact that in very many of the fatal
cases of croupous pneumonia in young children there has been a
definite history of difficult dentition immediately antecedent to the
pulmonary attack. Recent observations lead me to suspect that in
these cases the antecedent condition of difficult or pathological
dentition has been the cause which induced the subsequent attack
of capillary bronchitis.

In this connection it may be well to call to your attention the investigations recently published by Dr. Emil Schreier, of Vienna, with respect to the nature of the infecting organism in apical pericementitis. This observer found in all the cases of apical inflammation about the roots of teeth which he examined, twenty or more in all, the diplococcus pneumoniæ, invariably present as the exciter of the inflammatory process. This is in line with Miller's investigations, which showed that the diplococcus pneumoniæ was a constant inhabitant of the mouth. As a further link in this particular chain of evidence, Dr. C. N. Pierce recently recounted to me two cases of incipient croupous pneumonia which occurred at different times in a family who were patients of his. In each instance the child was suffering from difficult eruption of the teeth, and in each case croupous pneumonia was set up as a sequel. In both cases Dr. Pierce performed gum lancing, and in both cases there was subsidence of all the distressing symptoms in a few hours, with rapid and complete recovery. To any one who has investigated this subject, especially from the clinical standpoint, there can be no doubt as to the great utility of the operation in relieving in many cases the most alarming symptoms. It is simply and easily performed, and there are no weighty objections which can be urged against it, so that is a matter of continued wonder that there can be found in the ranks of medical practitioners those who still strongly oppose it.

It may be asked of what interest can the question be to the dentist, who is seldom, if ever, called upon to operate in these cases. To this I would answer, prepare yourselves by an intelligent understanding of the operation, and its correct relationships, and you will be consulted with respect to these matters when it is known that you are competent to give judgment upon them. Or if the knowledge has no usefulness outside of your immediate family, it may still afford you the opportunity to save the life of some one dear to you, as I verily believe it has upon more than one occasion in my own family circle.—*Dental Practitioner and Advertiser.*

Death Under Nitrous Oxide Gas.*

By JOHN ADAMS, F.R.C.S. Eng.

The patient came to the dentist on Monday, February 21st, about 1.30 p.m., and had an hour previously partaken of a light lunch. After waiting half an hour, he was shown into the operating room on the first floor. He seemed in good health, and wished to have a second right upper molar extracted whilst under gas.

* A Paper read before the Society of Anæsthetists on March 15th, 1894.

There was nothing tight about the neck, nor was there anything in his appearance to lead one to think he was not a fit subject for the anæsthetic. He had a small receding jaw, and a short, thick neck, but no abnormal swelling of any kind which prevented his closing his mouth, as reported in *The Lancet* of the above date. An ordinary prop, attached to a strong fishing-line, was placed between the upper and lower central incisors. After taking three or four inspirations of nitrous oxide gas he took off the face-piece and said he felt nervous, but at his own request I proceeded to go on with the administration. His respiration was shallow. but regular, and after taking about two-thirds of the ordinary quantity of gas, the tooth was extracted quickly and without any difficulty ; the respirations at once became irregular and the patient became more cyanosed, his muscles rigid, and after three or four respirations, he ceased to breathe, but no danger appeared imminent. Breathing not continuing, the prop was at once removed, the patient taken from the chair on to the floor, and artificial respiration commenced within thirty seconds after the extraction. The tongue was pulled forward. The heart was beating regularly but not strongly, the body remained rigid, and there was no inspiratory effort. About two minutes after the tooth was extracted, two or three expirations took place, showing there was no considerable obstruction in the larynx. Nitrate of amyl was applied to the nose and mouth ; but as no inspirations took place, it could not have affected the patient. A subcutaneous injection of ether was given over the præcordial region, as the action of the heart now became feeble. These measures failing, tracheotomy was performed within three minutes of the time the gas was discontinued to be administered ; the position of the patient was awkward for the operation, and the extremely receding lower jaw, with a short, thick neck, made it somewhat difficult to perform, but as everything was at hand and ready assistance given, I fortunately made an entrance through the upper rings of the trachea without loss of time. The tracheal wound was kept open, and on resuming artificial respiration, a quantity of mucus (about an ounce) was forced out, nearly clear and only slightly blood-stained. Although one could hear air passing in and out of the opening in the trachea, there was no voluntary effort of breathing from first to last. The patient now became still more cyanosed, and the heart could no longer be heard beating. Artificial respiration was continued for twenty minutes longer, although there was little hope of its being of use. Micturition took place after the commencement of taking the nitrous oxide, a symptom which I have not infrequently noticed when cyanosis becomes well marked, and also in children. I will recapitulate shortly the methods adopted to restore respiration : (1) artificial respiration within half a minute after the patient ceased to breathe ; (2) nitrate of amyl within one minute after respiration ceased ; (3) subcutaneous injection of ether within two minutes after the patient had ceased to breathe, and (4) tracheotomy within three minutes after the patient had ceased to breathe.

The necropsy was performed by Dr. Norman Moore, at the request of the coroner, twenty-five hours after death, in the presence of the medical attendant of the deceased and myself. Dr. Moore has kindly looked over and corrected the description of the morbid appearances. The body was well nourished and muscular, of a man about twenty-six years of age. The face, neck and back were all deeply cyanosed ; there was a mark of a recent tracheotomy wound. On removing the skull cap, which was unusually thick, venous engorgement was visible on the surface of the cerebral hemispheres ; nothing abnormal was noticed in the cerebral substance. On opening the chest, the veins were noticed everywhere full of dark fluid blood. All the internal organs were healthy. The pericardium contained the normal amount of fluid. The heart was normal and the valves competent. All the cavities of the heart were empty, except a small quantity of fluid blood in the right ventricle. No clots were present. The lungs were engorged with dark fluid blood, and were nearly airless. On opening the bronchi, the mucous membrane was dark in color and engorged, and a quantity of thick mucus was found in all the larger bronchi. The trachea was also engorged, but contained less mucus. The upper three rings were divided. The larynx, tonsils and tongue were removed together for examination. The larynx showed no swelling, and very little engorgement, and contained no appreciable quantity of mucus ; no foreign body or abnormal substance was found. The tonsils showed old enlargement, but did not meet in the middle line. The stomach contained a small quantity of undigested food, with a good deal of ropy mucus. The œsophagus was normal. The liver, kidneys and spleen were all dark in color, showing venous engorgement, but without any signs of disease. The bladder was empty.—*Dental Record, London.*

Editorial.

Newfoundland.—The Chain Complete.

When we announced some time ago that the chain of dental legislation in the Dominion was complete, we felt a professional and political yearning that our oldest island, Newfoundland, could come in with the family as a full partner in the professional advancement. It will not be long, we trust, before it will complete the chain of British Confederation on this continent, and give us then a Dominion of 3,616,583 square miles. In the meantime, our readers will be delighted to hear from Dr. T. L. Hallett, of St. John, Nfld., that the dentists of the little island empire, have secured an Act of Incorporation, which we publish on another page. This really completes the chain from the Atlantic to the Pacific.

Personal.

[We should feel obliged if our readers would send us matter for this department. A few lines on a postal card would frequently be sufficient.—ED.]

Dr. E. B. Ibbotson, major of the Royal Scots, Montreal, has been appointed to the command of the Bisley Team, which sailed for England on the 23rd of last month.

Dr. H. Ievers, of Quebec, is having great success with his " Frank-incense and Balsam," for temporary use in carious teeth. It is a most convenient and comforting little addition to the domestic remedies for emergencies.

In reply to several inquiries, we are glad to repeat that Dr Haskell's Post-graduate School of Prosthetic Dentistry is flourishing as of yore at 211 Wabash Avenue, Chicago. We have had several letters, thanking us for advising applicants to attend the school.

Dr. G. Lenox Curtis, our clever oral surgeon, of New York, stole away for a few days from his patients to tempt the trout in our Laurentian lakes, and had good luck. Dr. C. H. Wells, of Huntingdon, Que., accompanied him. They are both members of " The Trotters," founded by Dr. Young, of Concord, N.H.

It is a curious coincidence that when " The Trotters," after the Vermont State Dental Society meeting, were in session, enjoying the songs and stories, and the relaxation of spirit which wearied dentists know so well to appreciate, one of the members suggested that the ancient rite should be introduced at the American Dental Association, and that the first Great-Grand-Big Knight of the O.S.C. should be the jolly editor of the *Dental Practitioner and Advertiser*. As a man of weight, and one who knows how to tell a good story and enjoy a hearty laugh—well, our memory goes back to old times in Toronto when he made it lively enough May the spirit of good fellowship bloom forever in his heart.

Dr. Chas. Barnes, of Syracuse, N.Y., died suddenly on the 3rd of last month. He was born in England in 1837, and came to Syracuse as a boy and became a student of the late Dr. Westcott. He occupied several offices in the State Association and bore a first-class reputation as a scientific and practical dentist. He was, socially, one of the best of companions—an enthusiastic cricketer and base-ball player.

The Royal Arcanum, one of the very best of the Fraternal Beneficiary Orders, has got a good foothold in Canada. It provides the social enjoyment of a grand fraternity ; the financial protection of a powerful life insurance corporation ; sympathy and aid to the member while living, and to his bereaved family a payment of $3,000. It is managed by a brotherhood bound in *self-interest,* and is as safe as the best bank. In the last list of death claims, we observe the names of Dr. C. W. Wardle, dentist, and no less than six physicians. We commend it very strongly, after several years' experience, as one of the few perfectly safe and reliable organizations.

DOMINION
DENTAL JOURNAL.

VOL. VI.   TORONTO, AUGUST, 1894.   No. 8.

Original Communications.

Translations.

(From Foreign Dental Journals, etc., etc.)

By CARL E. KLOTZ, L.D.S., St. Catharines, Ont.

TREATMENT OF TEETH WITH DEVITALIZED PULPS.—Dr. Glesch, of Zomber, Hungary. After the pulp has been devitalized and rubbed down in position, the pulp is removed out of the pulp chamber and partly out of the canals with spoon-shaped excavators. An antiseptic is applied to the cavity. When the cavity is dried he takes a pellet of cotton moistened with distilled water and dips it into powdered borax. The borax, adhering to the cotton, is placed into the pulp chamber and part of it worked into the canals till it touches the nerve stump. The remaining borax is wiped out of the cavity. Being moist, the borax will permeate the remaining nerve fibres left in the canals, which it would not do if applied in a dry state. The borax in the canals is covered with tin-foil, also the pulp chamber is filled with it. The cavity is filled with any desired filling material—gold, amalgam, etc.—*Zahnärztliches Wochenblatt.*

TROFRACOCAIN is an alkaloid similar to cocain, but not near so poisonous, as Dr. Hugenschmidt, of Paris, says. When used as an anæsthetic it is without the disagreeable after effects as very often experienced with cocain.—*Zahntechniche Reform.*

2

BLACKEN your hickory or orange wood wedges with your lead pencil and see if they don't go in between the teeth much nicer. Try it.—*C. E. K.*

A PECULIAR case of blood-poisoning which caused quite a sensation among the dentists of Berlin. Dr. Bernheim, a dentist of Berlin, extracted a tooth for a lady and got his finger into her mouth, whereupon she closed her teeth with a convulsive firmness on his index finger. After a few hours symptoms of blood-poisoning appeared on the doctor's hand and spread so rapidly that even an immediate amputation did not check the spreading. He became delirious and, notwithstanding the efforts of two physicians, Dr. B. died the following day.—*Berlin Journal.*

AMBLYOPIA CAUSED BY DENTAL IRRITATION.—Patient complained of headache, weakness and seeing specks before her eyes, and, a few days later, of a weakening of the sight of the right eye. Her vision was so impaired that she could scarcely count her fingers at a distance of ten inches from the eyes. The cause could not be discerned by an opthalmoscopic examination. She was treated with iodide of potassium for optic neuritis, but her vision became dimmer. A physician suggested to examine her teeth and found five ground-off roots on the right side, upon which a vulcanite plate rested. The roots were extracted, and four days later her vision was better. In less than two months her eyesight was completely restored and remained so, as subsequent examination showed.—*Deutsche Monatsschrift für Zahnheilkunde.*

A CASE IN PRACTICE.—Some time ago I was called to the house of a lady who had been suffering from toothache for some time. When I arrived the lady told me that Dr. ———— had treated her for a length of time but could not relieve her of her pain, and finally told her that she was not susceptible to medicine, and that she would have to consult a specialist. Upon examination I found that the lady had a copper amalgam filling in the first upper molar, and first and second bicuspids badly decayed. I extracted the molar at once and found the roots abscessed, with a large sac on one of them. I expected that this would relieve her of her pain, but the following day she came to my office and complained of having the same pain. I now treated the bicuspids and dismissed her to come again at a certain time. The second following day she came with the same complaint. I removed the dressing from the bicuspids and devitalized the pulps, extracted them, and prepared the canals with an antiseptic dressing, intending to fill them the following day. (This was not done in one sitting ; it took several.) When she came she complained that the pain was worse than ever. Now I was in a dilemma, and did not know what to do. I again examined her teeth very carefully and found every one apparently sound. I happened to remember a case I had many years ago, where all the teeth in a patient's mouth were sound, but that one molar had a peculiar sound different from the rest when tapping it. I extracted this molar and found, after splitting it, that the nerve was dead and the odor from it was anything but pleasant. I now determined to drill into the second molar, and as soon as I reached the pulp chamber with the drill a quantity of pus was discharged and the pain was immediately gone. I treated the canals and in due course of time filled them as well as the canals in both bicuspids, and—quietness reigns supreme. This case shows that in apparently sound and healthy teeth deceased pulps may be present.—*Monatsschrift Deutscher Zahnkünstler.*

MOUTH POULTICE.—Dr. Hugenschmidt recommends as the only practical poultice that can be used in alocolar abscess, a fig boiled in a solution of boric acid and cut in halves, and the cut surfaces sprinkled with powdered boric acid. It will in most cases cause the abscess to discharge into the mouth. Should the abscess be far advanced and threaten to break through the cheek, then apply an ice-compress with the above.—*Journal für Zahnheilkunde.*

Address of Dr. F. Kilmer, as Retiring President of Ontario Dental Society.

Gentlemen of the Ontario Dental Society and of the Eastern Ontario Dental Society :

It is with pleasure I welcome you at this union meeting of these two important societies—important because they embrace in their membership and attendance the most ethical and progressive members of our profession, because a broad, liberal spirit of good-will and brotherly feeling is developed by the social intercourse at these gatherings, and because the kind and generous criticisms of our methods and their practical application in our clinics give a stimulus to intelligent and scientific methods of investigation.

I wish to thank you for your generous response to the call of this union meeting, and I think I can safely assure you that any sacrifice of time or convenience to attend this meeting will be more than amply repaid by the opportunity you will have for the free interchange of thought and of good-will.

There are, no doubt, many careful and conscientious dentists in the Province who are not members of either society, who would, I am sure, be benefited by identifying themselves with us, and the society too would be equally benefited by their presence, and by their discussions on the various subjects presented at our meetings.

There are various motives by which we are induced to attend conventions. Some come to read papers, to take part in, or intelligently listen to the discussions, with the view of being practically benefited by them. Some go to see the sights, to hear the big guns, if there are any on hand and heavily loaded, and to tell their patients when they return home that they have been attending a professional meeting. Some go merely to see the exhibits of the dealers, to see what new things they may have on exhibition, and then to put in what is generally designated "a big time."

The first of these are the life and energy of the associations, and we are hoping each year to see this number materially increase. Unfortunately there are some who never attend a convention for any purpose ; they never read a journal, and are absolutely ignorant of improved and advanced methods. They know not the influence of professional fellowship or fraternal feeling, but seem content to settle down into a groove so deep that their condition could not be better described than one of narrow and dense ignorance of their best possibilities. Time in its onward march will do much to lessen this class. Recent graduates from our college, with the impulses of a high matriculation, an extended term of studentship, and an extra college term, where lectures and demonstrations are faithfully given by a Faculty that in point of ability stand the peers of the Faculty of any dental college on the Continent, will come into our societies, their minds in favor of professional progress, and they cannot to the same extent drop into these grooves of professional narrow-mindedness because of the bias given their minds by a more extended and scientific training. To them we may look for the main hope and strength of our societies.

It is a fact, however, that occasionally a graduate is apparently so constituted that he cannot wait to conscientiously gain the confidence of the public, but resorts to the tricks of the ignorant pretender. He might not care to be called a quack, but such he is, no matter what his college standing may have been, so long as he practises the deceptions of quacks. If these men could be brought under the influences of our societies, they might be restrained from gliding into this bombastic assertion of their special abilities, and the unparalleled advantages of their secret specifics, destroying thereby their self-respect, and only gaining in its place that credulous portion of the public who are found always standing around open-mouthed ready to be duped. Our society would be doing good work to appoint a committee of resident dentists in Toronto, to canvass the graduating class each year and try and induce them to join our association, and subscribe to our code of ethics. If this could be successfully done, I think the conscientious dentist would be less often filled with disgust, by seeing in many papers advertisements claiming exclusive knowledge of some wonderful drug that does every possible and a great many impossible things, from restoring a necrotic pulp to vitality, to developing new teeth in an edentulous jaw like mushrooms springing from a hot-bed, or claiming the special control of some mechanical device that renders their work superior to that of everyone else. Such knowledge and such skill is apt to discourage the more modest dentists, because they will occasionally find that specifics fail, and that special mechanical appliances sometimes require just a little alteration to meet their case in hand. More especially are they likely to be discouraged when they remember that these men of prodigious secrets and marvellous appliances neither distinguished themselves during their college course, nor followed habits of life after entering upon active practice that would indicate either studious or scientific investigation, and then suddenly hear them announce that they have made a great discovery that they possess a secret drug that performs miracles.

Discouraged, indeed, they might well be if these men were the brains of the profession and the skilful manipulators of its many intricate and difficult operations, and appropriately they might exclaim with Dogberry, " Oh! that I had been writ down an ass." But let them take courage, and opposite this superior, secret and exclusive knowledge write QUACK in big capitals, and let them remember that the *materia medica* is the property of every intelligent dentist, and that the physiological, therapeutical, and toxical actions of its various substances are thoroughly investigated and recorded by men who are not so exclusive with the secrets their investigations reveal. One needs but read the best medical and dental journals of to-day to feel assured that the most careful and scientific investigators freely and fully give their investigations to those less qualified by opportunity or ability to investigate for themselves. There you find reliable reports of experiments with all kinds of drugs that are specific in their character. There, too, you become acquainted with the latest theories, and methods of treatment based thereon. Bacterio pathology is fully discussed, and there you learn about psycho-therapeutics or hypnotic suggestion as a sedative and obtundant. There you will even find scientific men, thinking it for the benefit of less informed and more credulous to analyze and put before them the composition of these secret preparations, showing that they are well-known drugs simply clouded in secrecy and palmed off as new discoveries by unscrupulous nostrum vendors. I would advise you to summarily dismiss anyone calling on you in your office with a secret specific, or some improved patent which, for a small consideration (compared to the priceless advantage it will be over your neighbor across the street), he will give you a town or county right for its sole use. How that "sole right" does catch these men who want the earth! I would absolutely refuse to accept any preparation that I did not know its ingrediency and there relative proportions, or for which I was required to enter into a covenant not to divulge its formulæ. When I receive a circular headed something like this: "In daily use by more than all others combined. The only practical, reliable, harmless and effective anæsthetic," and so on to the end of the chapter, even though a three dollar syringe is thrown in with a ten dollar purchase of the shotgun mixtures, it has about the same effect on me as flaunting a red rag before an infuriated bull, and I want to gore somebody, and I would like it to be both the vendor and the unprofessional quack whose testimonials and advertisements flood the country. In this connection I will quote from the *Cosmos*, for May, 1893, as follows: "If we are professional at all, it is entirely inconsistent with the pretension that anyone should secure control of procedures or the use of appliances for his own exclusive benefit, and unworthy of those who are under the moral obligation to fulfil the maxim, 'Freely as ye have received, freely give.' The endeavor to impose upon the profession by dispensing for gain secret formulæ of any of the preparations or materials we use, is a still more reprehensible practice, and the use of such should be excluded from any and every society. To effectually stamp out this evil there appears only one means of action, which is for each practitioner to refuse any preparation the ingrediency and proportion of which are unknown to him." Testimonials might often tempt one to accept these nostrums, but they are too frequently unreliable. They may have been given as the result of a combination of circumstances that would not exist in your relation with your patient. Belief in the potency of the nostrums by the operator, and the soothing charm which springs from unhesitating faith the patient has in the operator and his methods, is a combination that does not always exist. I would, therefore, say, do not be over-ready to give a testimonial until you have had time and opportunity to form a clear judgment. I was waited upon by an agent with an electric appliance for painless extracting, and was shown testimonials, some from men I knew at college, and in whom one had no reason not to place confidence. I was induced to invest; paid a small amount; agreed to pay a certain sum at stated intervals, failing that to forfeit what I had paid as well as the appliance. My experience, like Mr. Taylor's, mentioned in the *Items of Interest* was that no person gave it unqualified approval. "Some spoke of it as Josh

Billings did of tight boots. He said : ' Tight butes is a blessing, inasmuch as they make a man forget all his other troubles.'
So patients have said the electricity is worse than having the tooth
out." Before the first date of payment had come around I notified
the agent to take his appliance away, as it would remain in the
office at his risk. This taught me the value of testimonials, and
but that the agent lacked the physical proportions I would have
given him another bill to have kicked me around the office until
my physical discomfort would have been more in keeping with my
loss of self-respect for being so easily duped by a nicely worded
testimonial.

Leaving these things aside, I believe there is a growing professional spirit among the dentists of Ontario. I believe the spirit of
free interchange of thought and of methods is rapidly growing, and
as a result there is a proportionate decrease in the tendency and
disposition to misrepresent and take advantage of each other.

By cultivating its growth we will increase our respect, and en-
thusiasm for our profession, and command as well more perfect
respect from the public. It will bind us together in earnest effort
for the highest excellence. It will impel us to give our best
service to our patients, and extend the kindest courtesies to our
professional brother, helping us in all circumstances to apply the
golden rule in our relations with each other.

There are many causes for these hopeful signs. Some arise
from the influence of our conventions, and many from the influence
of our DOMINION DENTAL JOURNAL, which, by the way, should
be subscribed for by every dentist in Canada, and last, but not
least, much of this spirit may have come with the changes made in
the management of our College, and in the election of its Board of
Directors. These changes will manifest themselves in our conventions, and we should expect to see our associations improving.
Heretofore the tendency was to have discussions on College affairs
and matters of legislation take a most prominent place. With the
present condition of things we can, and should, give most prominence to subjects of especial interest to the individual dentist in his
private practice. Subjects that heretofore received a good deal of
explanation and repetition for the enlightenment of the profession
will now not be necessary, owing to the general distribution of the
proceedings of the Board of Directors. Each of you have, no
doubt, received a copy of this report, and have, I hope, carefully
read it. It is indicative of progress, and I am satisfied, after seeing
the immense amount of work accomplished during the past two
years, the steps taken by the Board to protect the dentist, as well
as the best interests of the public, and to guard against any legislation that would interfere with the privileges and rights of the
Board, or of the licentiates, you will have the utmost confidence in
the Board to manage their affairs that used, at least every second

year, so much to agitate us, and that the best of our time and energy will now be occupied in the friendly discussion of those topics that touch us in our every-day practice.

The districts into which our province is divided for electing the Board of Directors would be an excellent division for more limited associations, which, if once formed, would create a more professional spirit in the local districts. They would encourage the best methods and the most careful investigations in a greater number than could be reached by the more general association. They would, also, be a means by which the representatives to the Board of Directors would be enabled to gauge the general sentiment of the profession, which would be of material help to them in their official duties. If such societies were in active existence what a resource our general society would have to draw from, and in return how it could extend its influence.

Through the printed transactions and reports in the various journals, and by the stimulus given to those who were present, what an influence the Dental Congress of last August in Chicago will have. It will extend to hundreds of dentists who were not present, helping them to more fully appreciate the dignity of their chosen profession, and elevating them in no small degree in their ethical standing, and what is true of the World's Columbian Dental Congress is true in a more limited sense of every dental convention.

Let us then strive each year to have a convention that will be universally attended that the best good may result therefrom. Such has been our endeavor this year by this union meeting, but in conclusion I wish to say, that it ought to be of paramount importance that there should be one society that would be an aggregation of all that is best in the various local societies that now exist in, or that may be formed in the Province, and that society should be the Ontario Dental Society.

Modern Dentistry.*

By C. A. MARTIN, L.D.S., Ottawa, Ont.

When asked for a title to a solicited contribution I did not then know what I would write about, so I selected "Modern Dentistry," believing it to be a most comprehensive subject, affording great scope. Do not for a moment expect a long dissertation on the many additions and improvements to the dental science during the past twenty years. It should be considered presumptious in me (one of the old practitioners before the introduction of L.D.S.) to

*Paper read at Union Dental Meeting, Kingston, July, 1894.

attempt to advance new ideas, or even lecture to the advanced graduates of modern colleges. Somewhat bewildered, I come in an inquisitive mood to speak on some of the modes of practice of the present. I do not wish to emulate the divers lecturers and writers of the day with sensational descriptions of extraordinary, wonderful discoveries and successful achievements of exceptional character. That gushing period has passed away from me. The hard, practical facts only remain. In the struggle for existence, increasing responsibilities necessitate the elimination of the superfluous and many modern adjuncts. One must adapt himself to his environments, and adopt a line of practice wherein he is most proficient and capable of giving conscientious value to his patients. Few of us become equally proficient in all branches of dentistry. Believing this, and being sufficiently employed otherwise, I have not tried the Land system of porcelain work, a most beautiful process. When properly performed by experts it is capable of embellishing as well as saving conspicuous defective teeth. The mixing of colors to produce imitation of natural shades is a work of art requiring special and continuous attention. I have not inserted teeth on what is called bridge work, believing that two or more roots should not be kept immovable by a rigid fastening which is irremovable. Although I have seen some nice work in that line, apparently giving satisfaction, still I have met some disastrous consequences when disease or mechanical fractures occur. I think all such work should be made so as to be removable at will by the wearer. I have never implanted teeth, having no faith in the system. Some appear to prove satisfactory, but many come to grief, and all are more or less a source of annoyance and trouble. To my mind the system is contrary to nature's laws, and will be tolerated only in exceptional cases. I do not cap exposed, bleeding or congested pulps, feeling safer to extirpate and fill root canals. A few accounts of horrible suffering, sometimes a demand made to have all the teeth removed to get relief, induced me some years past to eschew the practice. I have never tried the electric vibrator! I have still in my possession a forceps with a hole in the handle which was used, about thirty years ago, by my brother and myself for extracting teeth *without pain.* We wore a kid glove and attached a wire to a galvanic battery and let her go. It acted on the same principle as the method employed by French-Canadians to remove or abate pains caused by burns. They dip the painful part three times in boiling water. I tried the freezing appliance for a short season. Its effect was something similar. I have not used any of the numerous local anæsthetics advertised widely and extravagantly—some with highsounding names, extracted from the Latin principally, others from the Greek and Hebrew. These names alone show considerable labor in research, and the numerous testimonials prove the article worthy of trial. But there are so many on the market that it is difficult to select one.   Apart from the cost (which is an item), an old practitioner who has been successful in other ways, cannot afford the time.   I do not use the electric mallet for filling.   It is hard for me to acknowledge that I am growing old—therefore callous in the adoption of modern improvements ; but my patients protested so much for a time against the use of the dental engine that I dread the introduction of more machinery.   My sons may get it !

There are quite a number of dental appliances and medicinal preparations which I did not try, and which have proven useless. By being thus slow in adopting new things I have saved money, and my patients more or less torture.   Most of my patients object to being experimented upon, and many continue to come through confidence in my old system of practice.   I have never used nitrous oxide gas although I know it to be a good thing.   I prefer sending patients who wish teeth extracted by its use to other dentists who employ it.   In the case of patients desiring an anæsthetic, they or I procure a physician who administers.   I only operate. Perhaps my bump of caution is too large, and may prevent me from securing a wider practice, still I continue to make the sacrifice, and distribute that line of practice to the fearless or more confident.   I once tried to make a plate for a cleft palate, but the girl died before the operation was completed.   I have never tried another case since, patients presenting themselves being generally poor.   I have been successful in some cases of complicated irregularities, one of the most successful occupying nearly a year in making and adjusting various appliances according to changes until perfected ; was not fully paid for, the party leaving the limits forgetfully.   In some cases, after expressing a desire to have their child's teeth regulated, and after the trouble of constructing one or more appliances, the indulgent parent gives way to the child's request to be relieved of the troublesome nuisance, and otherwise honorable people grumble at paying for services rendered.   I have improved and made more symmetrical irregularities in adults' teeth by grinding and polishing.   I have still a few patients of fourteen years of age and over who are themselves anxious to have their teeth straightened.   In such cases I generally succeed.   I have never inserted what is called a Richmond crown, or that mode of pivoting teeth with a gold band exposed on the labial surface.   I have seen considerable irritation and inflammation with a strong tendency to permanent recession of the gum's margin, caused by the presence of gold bands pressed into the alveolar process.   I prefer the Martin crown, where a gold band fits around the lingual part, and the mineral crown champered and fitted to root as a continuation of band, and not hammered in, but gently pressed to place.   I inserted, a few days ago, a right lateral incisor, with gold backing, so as to regulate position, on a root slightly out of arch, for a citizen who has firmly fixed on the left central and lateral incisor roots, crowns—the old-fashioned pivot-holed mineral crowns, fastened with platinum pins, which I inserted fourteen years ago. For the same person I am crowning two bicuspid roots with gold. I believe the gold crown to be one of the most successful as well as useful additions to the dental art. For bicuspids and molars they are invaluable in restoring masticating surfaces, and also in being a complete protection and preservative of roots. But the use of them on cuspids and incisors I consider hideous in appearance. While visiting the Art Gallery at the World's Fair, my brother, who resides in Chicago, introduced me to a local dentist, who, in speaking, displayed three! No less! Three gold incisors! The effect was shocking to me! No doubt he used them as an advertisement, and advised his patients to have the same kind inserted. Well, everyone to his taste. Among the English and Canadian people, very few, if any, would approve of or even tolerate them. Accompanying the last circus which visited Ottawa was a man selling tickets. While extolling the wonders of the side show, he exposed to view a gold incisor, highly polished, which glittered in the lamplight, and seemed to make him proud of his adornment. By the way he twisted his mouth to better expose the glittering object, he no doubt imagined that he was causing envy amongst the supposed backward Canadians. It reminded me of a brass door-plate minus the inscription. I think that I can safely state that we Canadian dentists endeavor to so closely imitate symmetrical natural organs as to deceive the eye, not only of the general public, but of intimate acquaintances. I felt a sense of pride when a patient asked an acquaintance who happened to come into my office, the question, " I have just had a tooth put in. Can you tell which it is?" The acquaintance, after closely scrutinizing, pointed to a natural tooth! We can do this conspicuous kind of work, but we do not recommend it, and we would endeavor to dissuade those who might ask for it. From the craze of having half a front tooth built up with gold it has come to this. I begin to think that there is some truth in the report that some Chicago dentist has inserted diamonds and rubies in teeth for ladies!! Modern art employed to imitate savage tastes! I immediately adopted the rubber dam and clamps, and consider them a boon to the profession. I approve of gold lining to vulcanite plates, also the addition of aluminum for strengthening and stiffening, admitting these plates to be made thinner. The gold plate, however, still holds supreme. The various makes of zinc cements are valuable acquisitions. The improved alloys for amalgams have enabled us to successfully save valuable teeth for people of moderate means. I have frequently seen teeth filled with the filings of a silver quarter doing good service after twenty-five years' use. If all teeth were of as good material and the elements of contact were no more injurious, we could hope to attain equal results with the cleaner material now used. There are many new medicines introduced for the treatment of abscess, etc. I have tried some with beneficial results. Others that are undoubtedly good but slow in action, I seldom use. I have discarded creosote completely, as I obtain better success with carbolic acid and oil of cloves. I still use tannic acid, seldom salicylic or iodoform, but I have added sulphuric acid, acid. eugenic, oil of eucalyptus, peroxide of hydrogen, and tincture of iodine generally. It is unnecessary for me to enumerate the several medicines now in use for the treatment of diseased teeth. The fact that different treatment with different medicines proves equally successful is sufficient guarantee that the dental profession of to-day can cause to be retained in the mouth teeth that were invariably condemned and lost twenty-five years ago. The graduates of our college have generally a uniform system of treatment, which is a benefit, for one knows what to do with another's patient in case of need. The future dentist's manipulations and mode of treatment will become more and more identical, and as the teachings at dental colleges assimilate, so will the mode of treatment become general, and as soon as the old fossils drop off—some of them like barnacles clinging to and retarding the ship of progress—I say as soon as these and the ideas they stubbornly cling to have died out, the dental profession may become one universal system ! If no other benefits were derived from dental colleges, this one fact should be sufficient to uphold their existence, and that is, a professional dignity is visibly extending, an ethical code of procedure is gradually developing, such as is taught in our college, and which seems to be strengthened by each graduating class. This result alone would be sufficient to raise each individual dentist in the estimation of the public. More harmony exists now than formerly among dentists in cities and towns, notwithstanding the continued increase in numbers. In Ottawa the Ontario code of ethics is, I believe, well adhered to, perhaps one or two exceptions where a speciality is announced, with professional card. The growing tendency is upward and onward. I believe the coming dentist will become a specialist in certain branches in which he is most proficient. The present large establishments where numbers of dentists are engaged will eventually disappear, as they somewhat mar professional dignity. Judging from advertisements embellished with pictures of the artists, they appear to represent factories instead of professional offices. In conclusion, I repeat that when the dental profession becomes composed entirely of graduates of recognized high grade colleges, they will stand the equal to the medical profession in fact, and will be so recognized by the public.

An Ethical Resume.

By SENEX.

It is surely a matter for profound and sincere congratulation that, notably within the preceding decade, there has been such a steady and visible inclination of the profession of dentistry in Canada to a higher plane of ethical morality, and the consequent elevation of the professional status of our vocation in the eyes of the laity in general.

For some time this good work of advancement has been going on, though, perhaps, it has been more noticeable during the past few years, thanks to the efforts of some noble characters, to the unselfish and undeviating energy of the dental journal, to the influence exercised by the various societies and associations ; and also the result is due in no limited degree to raising the standard of the preliminary education required for admittance to our colleges, from a mere nonentity to the requiring of an examination second to none, not excepting any college or university in America or the mother country.

And still we would be pleased to see the standard again raised, and we think in Ontario, at least, the time is opportune when this might be accomplished with absolute justice and propriety and beneficial results. While excluding from our ranks men of questionable abilities, a high standard of qualification would serve as an attraction to those with intellects expanded by a generous and liberal education—men capable of instituting original researches, and donating from the store-house of a cultured brain, appliances and literature that would advance, instruct and elevate not only the technical departments, but also the clerical equipment of our profession.

These are the sort of students we want at our colleges—these the sort of confreres we would welcome with our outstretched hands, for it is the liberal and intelligent man every time that maintains the honor and dignity of his profession, and has the stability to say "no" when he is tempted for the sake of a few paltry dollars, and at the sacrifice of a great amount of self-respect, to do something he knows is unprofessional, that he publicly renounced when he affixed his name to the code of ethics.

We think, however, the ninety and nine of the practitioners of Canada to-day consider themselves morally amenable to the code, and conscientiously endeavor to fulfil not only the letter but also the spirit ; who try not to see how frequently they can contravene the edicts of the code, or how many dishonest and disreputable acts they can do clandestinely, and still, like the Pharisee, go up to the temple and attend the convention, and be looked upon by their fellows as ethical and honest, and their reward is immediate, for, by respecting themselves, they are respected by the profession, and appreciated in the community in which they reside, and the unfailing concomitant—an ever-increasing practice—is the result.

But we have also tares among the wheat. We have men at this moment practising dentistry, of whom nothing good can be said, whose sole aim and ambition in life is to get money—to get it any way so long as they get it. They offer up everything, their position in society, the friendly intercourse with their brother-practitioners, they lose their professional standing, they are ejected from the associations in short; they suppress all the finer qualities of their natures, and everything is offered a willing sacrifice upon the altar of avarice. These men would fall far short of what Bacon considers the duty of every man deriving his living from the practice of some profession. "Every professional man is a debtor to his profession; from the which as men of course do seek to receive countenance and profit, so ought they of duty to endeavor themselves by way of amends to be a help and an ornament thereunto." While there are quacks in medicine, quacks in law, and quacks in religion, neither can we truthfully claim them any *rara avis* with us. We have men who travel up and down the country in dental cars, that make the natives gaze with staring eyes and gaping mouths, and with an outfit that reminds one of the tail end of a circus caravan that has lost its bearings.

Then we have the individual who has an advertisement in the daily press or local paper, of huge dimensions, with unlimited cuts of forceps, dentures, molars, excavators, and other little attractions the people love to gaze upon, the reading matter calling attention to the fact (or the lie) that there is only one "dentist" in that portion of heaven's footstool, and he is that one. These men are endeavoring to be a help and an ornament to their profession. Assuredly they are an ornament to the doctorate!

But why go on. We might find unlimited examples. It has always been a mighty mystery to us why some men, by their own mean ways and contemptible actions, relegate themselves outside the pale of professional recognition and the hope of ultimate prosperity, for, at best, their success is only shortlived. The public is quick to recognize and to appreciate professional ability and worth, and equally quick to recognize and estimate at their true value assertions of superiority, whether in the possession of a heavenly spirit or of superlative knowledge and skill. Cant, religious or professional, is always distasteful. "I am holier than thou" is said to have provoked Omnipotence. The essential spirit of cant is an assumption of superiority—always offensive, sure to awaken a feeling of sentiment in human nature, to destroy confidence and weaken influence.

My friends, don't be quacks. Quit yourselves like men. Be honest, upright and just, with high aspirations, and conduct your practice in a legitimate manner, and great and permanent will be your reward.

Proceedings of Dental Societies.

Union Meeting of the Ontario Dental Society and the Eastern Ontario Dental Society, Kingston, 25th, 26th, 27th July.

The sixth annual convention of the Ontario Dental Society, held jointly with the Eastern Ontario Dental Society, was held in Kingston. This was the first time since the organization of either society that a joint meeting has been held. A welcoming address was given by Mayor Herald. Those present belonging to the Ontario Association were: Dr. Baird, Uxbridge; W. P. Brownlee, Mount Forest; J. A. Marshall, Belleville; Dr. Klotz, London; R. Meek, Orangeville; Dr. Rose, Peterboro'; Dr. McBride, Campbellford; William Leggo, Ottawa; C. P. Lennox, Toronto; F. Kilmer, St. Catharines; Dr. Brimacombe, Bowmanville.

Dr. Lodge, Ohio, is a guest of the society.

Those present of the Eastern Ontario Dental Association were: Dr. A. Stanley Burns, Smith's Falls, vice-president; George H. Weageant, Cornwall, secretary-treasurer; R. E. Sparks, A. Stackhouse, J. A. Clark, Kingston; C. A. Martin, J. C. Bower, Ottawa.; D. V. Beacock, Brockville; A. A. Smith, Cornwall; G. E. Hanna, Kemptville; A. E. Webster, Arnprior; C. H. Wartman, Napanee; W. A. Leggo, Ottawa; W. N. Cleary, Renfrew; Dr. Howes, Vankleek Hill. The meeting was called in the City Hall at eight o'clock. On suggestion of Dr. Kilmer, President of the Ontario Association, Dr. Martin, Ottawa, was voted to the chair. He felt flattered at being given the chair at the first union meeting, and he felt sure the hopitality shown them by Kingston before would be renewed. The chairman proved himself a very humorous speaker, and kept the members in an uproar.

The Mayor welcomed the societies, by saying that the citizens were pleased to have strangers from the outside visiting the city. Kingston was a city to be proud of, and every visitor should enjoy himself. From the west the cool breeze of the lake was charming, while the ever-new river scenery of the St. Lawrence to the east could not be excelled. Kingston's public institutions were worthy of a few hours' time for visitation. The joint meeting of the societies could not but be profitable to all present. The interchange of ideas was a good thing. He was glad to welcome them professionally. The practice of medicine was so diverse that there was hardly an organ of the human body that was not specialized. Many of the diseases called upon to treat came from the teeth. He hoped all would go away bearing a good opinion of our ancient and historic city.

The chairman said the welcome was well received and understood. Such a warm-hearted welcome was proverbial of Kingston. There was no town where such a warm feeling was shown, due in a large degree to the unanimity of the local dentists. The antagonism existing among the dentists in some places should be done away with. Kingston showed the benefits of unanimity. Two years ago the Eastern Society met in the city, and was glad to return. The time was not far distant when dentistry would not only be recognized by other institutions but by the people at large. If the teeth were kept in good order the doctors would have less trouble in keeping the internal machinery in order. The speaker was glad to notice the advancement that was being made in Kingston. The last time he was here he felt like joining the humane society to go in against the horse cars. Now, he believed, he had taken a nine-mile ride for five cents. No, he paid for the two other fellows, whom the conductor thought were patients for the penitentiary.

Dr. Kilmer thanked his Worship on behalf of the Ontario Dental Society, and the Mayor replied that he was pleased if they were pleased.

Dr. Kilmer, the retiring president of the Ontario Society, was glad to meet gentlemen where a broad and liberal spirit was developed. Any sacrifice of time or expense to attend the meeting would be well spent. Many dentists not belonging to the society could be greatly benefited. Unfortunately some attended the convention for no purpose whatever. To the students the main strength of the society could be looked forward to in the future. A resident committee of dentists should be appointed in Toronto to canvass the graduating class of the Dental College. He dwelt for some time on the wonderful discoveries made by quacks and the worthlessness of their medicines. The World's Chicago Dental Convention was one to be proud of; so should all other conventions.

In the absence of Dr. Brace, Brockville, Dr. Burns read the retiring address of the former for the Eastern Ontario Society. About fifteen years ago the Eastern Ontario Society was organized in Brockville, and he had been a charter member. The society had had its ups and downs. The change made in the Dental Act, whereby the members of the Board could be voted on by mail was a good one, but why the fee was levied he could not understand. He did not think there was any better place than Kingston to hold the convention. The officers elected by the Ontario Dental Society were :— President, Dr. Klotz, St. Catharines ; Vice-President, Dr. Leggo, Ottawa ; Secretary, Dr. Brownlee, Mount Forest ; Treasurer, Dr. Lennox, Toronto ; Auditors, Drs. Brownlee Marshall ; Ethics Committee, Drs. Klotz, Rose, Peterboro' ; Baird, Uxbridge ; Executive Committee, Drs. J. B. Willmott, J. Marshall, H. R. Abbott, F. Kilmer, R. Meek ; New Members, Drs. Meek, Orangeville ; McBride, Campbellford.

THURSDAY MORNING SESSION.

The Convention met at nine o'clock, when Dr. Rose, Peterboro', read a paper on " Calcification of Dental Pulp," followed by a discussion on the subject by Drs. Lennox, Martin, Burns, Kilmer, Marshall and Brownlee. Dr. Beacock, Brockville, read a paper on " Heredity and Environment," and Dr. Martin, Ottawa, on " Modern Dentistry."

THE EXCURSION—A VERY ENJOYABLE TRIP DOWN THE ST. LAWRENCE.

The steamer *Maud,* having on board the members of the Ontario and the Eastern Ontario Dental Associations, left the city about two o'clock. On the outward trip the boat kept to the Canadian channel, winding in and out among the islands in order to give the visitors the best possible opportunity of seeing the magnificent scenery of the river and islands. She passed Gananoque, crossed to Thousand Island Park, and without stopping returned by the American channel.

On the return trip refreshments were served by the ladies, and Misses Orser and Greenwood sang a number of very pretty duets. Prof. McKay contributed a couple of humorous recitations, and Drs. Martin and Lennox contributed to the general amusement by telling several excellent stories. All the city members of the medical profession had been invited, and on their behalf Hon. Senator Sullivan moved, and Dr. Lavell seconded, a vote of thanks to the Eastern Ontario Dental Association, both mover and seconder expressing the pleasure they had experienced in the hospitality of the Society. Principal Grant also extended an unofficial welcome to the visitors, which Mayor Herald made official in a fitting address.

As the boat approached the wharf, at about half-past seven, " Auld Lang Syne " and " God Save the Queen " were sung by the excursionists, thus concluding one of the most enjoyable trips of the season. A large number of ladies and many city medical men accepted the invitation to be present.

At 8.45 o'clock the delegates repaired to the City Hall to finish the day by several hours of work. The chairman, Dr. Martin, remarked they looked happier and more genial, and showed signs of much greater exhilaration when they took their seats to resume the regular business of the convention than they had previously done.

Before settling down to business, Dr. Burns, president of the Ontario Dental Association, rose and requested the chairman to inform the president and members of the Eastern Ontario Dental Society that the Ontario Society had held a special meeting a short time previously, at which it was moved by Dr. Marshall, seconded by Dr. Brimacombe, and unanimously resolved, " That the members of the Ontario Dental Association express their sincere thanks for and appreciation of the great kindness and hospitality extended by the Eastern Ontario Dental Association during their stay in the city of Kingston ; also their due appreciation of the arrangements made by the local committee for an enjoyable trip down the River St. Lawrence and among the Thousand Islands." Dr. Burns asked the chairman to convey to the members of the Eastern Dental Association the thanks of the sister association in accordance with the resolution, and, in a brief but pointed speech, thanked the corporation and citizens of Kingston for the treatment accorded the visiting dentists during their stay. He regretted the meagre attendance, and said that if those who had remained at home could have known that such a warm welcome awaited them they would have attended the convention.

The chairman, Dr. Martin, in conveying to the Eastern Association the thanks of the Ontario Society, heartily approved of all that Dr. Burns had said. He made a very witty address, and paid a high compliment to the Council and people of Kingston. The dentists were always well treated when they came to this city and it should not be forgotten. The dentists to-night could say to the citizens of Kingston what the Mayor said last night to them (the dentists): " If you're pleased so are we."

Other members followed in a similar strain, all expressing the utmost satisfaction with the way in which they had been treated during their stay in the city.

Before he forgot it, the chairman desired to inform those present that the penitentiary and the asylum were both open to inspection by the dentists, and were well worth seeing.

Dr. Stanley Burns, of Smith's Falls, read the first paper, which was entitled " Disagreeable Odors in Operating Rooms."

A very instructive discussion followed the reading of Dr. Burns' paper, in the course of which several of the dentists present gave the meeting the benefit of their experience in the matter. The chairman remarked that he had long ago discarded creosote, and in its stead now uses carbolic acid, a few drops of which, with enough oil of cloves to obliterate the smell, works wonderfully well. Another member said that many dentists have a habit of keeping the old and decayed teeth they have extracted. These give rise to an odor which is not by any means pleasant. Several members expressed their opinions as to the best method of cleaning spittoons—one holding that the most effective method was to use plenty of soap and water. Many hints which will, no doubt, prove of value to those who heard them were given, and several subjects of deep interest in this connection to the profession were discussed.

Dr. R. E. Sparks, of Kingston, read the second paper, which, he informed the audience, had been written by Dr. Abbott, of New York, some time ago. It was entitled "Treatment of Pulpless Teeth and Alveolar Abscesses."

In the treatment of pulpless teeth and alveolar abscesses the writer regarded as invaluable the bi-chloride of mercury and chloride of zinc. The treatment of teeth is unique.

Cleansing and disinfecting the teeth are first necessary. There are many means of doing this—with creosote, carbolic acid, etc. But beyond disinfection the pus-forming membrane must be rendered inert, and to do this bi-chloride of mercury, in the proportion of 1 to 1,000, is most effective. Then the foramen through the root should be closed with a small pledget of cotton ; the root is then to be filled with oxychloride of zinc, containing in the liquid a small percentage of bi-chloride of mercury. The cotton prevents the filling from being forced through the root and irritation is not likely to follow. But should any periostites occur, paint the gum with a mixture of iodine and aconite.

In treating alveolar abscesses, chloride of zinc is one of the most valuable remedies, as it destroys the lining of the sac, and is both astringent and stimulating to the membrane and facilitates a return to normal conditions.

In the discussion which followed the reading of this paper, Drs. Klotz, Marshall, Baird, Rose, Brownlee and Leggo participated. The opinions of these went to show that thorough disinfection is the most effective treatment of such cases as were under consideration.

Dr. Stackhouse addressed the meeting on " Items of Interest to Dentists."

Dr. Brownlee next engaged the attention of the members by demonstrating " How to Take a Perfect Bite," preparatory to fitting artificial teeth.

The Ontario Society will meet next year at Toronto. The Eastern Ontario Association has not yet decided on its place of meeting for next year.

Selections.

Caries of the Alveolus.

As a general rule, dentists have not in the past given as much attention to pathological studies as they should. Our best men have been ambitious to shine as operators, or as mechanics, and have neglected the first and most important of all studies, if we are to be considered in any sense as medical men. Beautiful fillings are too often inserted in teeth that are not in a physiological state, or which are in relation with diseased tissues, and the consequences are sometimes very serious. Many teeth are extracted simply because an otherwise excellent operator is not skilled in diagnosis and treatment. Diseases which, if properly treated at the outset, might be easily cured, are not promptly recognized, and are temporarized with, receiving only topical applications, until the general surgeon must be called in to remedy the effects of the lack of knowledge. Serious tumors have been dallied with until they have invaded tissues which should have been saved from their ravages.

Many of our schools have not given the attention to surgical pathology that is its due. In some, there is no real comprehensive course of lectures upon this subject, the usual diseases of the teeth themselves comprising the instruction in this department, surgery of the jaws and face being entirely relegated to the general practitioner. There is some excuse for this in the fact that our curriculum is already so broad that it is difficult in a term of six months to find time for the other lectures and demonstrations. Yet the dentist certainly should be able to diagnose any diseased condition, even though he should desire to turn it over to a specialist.

But there are some conditions requiring surgical interference that should never be allowed to go out of the dentist's hands. One of these is caries of the alveolus. This is a disease that is far more common than the average dentist is aware of. By it is meant the death and disintegration of the alveolar portions of the bone, cell by cell, and without any serious complications. It differs from necrosis in that there is not usually any formation of pus, or at least but little, no special tumefaction or inflammation of the soft tissues, and no tendency towards a sequestrum. In necrosis there is a stoppage of nutrition throughout a considerable portion of the osseous tissue, while in caries it is a slowly progressing ostisis that breaks down the bone one cell at a time.

Not infrequently, in the filling of cavities in proximate surfaces of the teeth, which extend well up in the cervical region, the alveolus between them is injured by wedges, or matrices, or separators, and this induces an ostitis which results in a caries that causes the loss of the whole of the septum. It is at best but a thin lamina, and hence is specially liable to loss of nutrition through injury. We have known cases in which true necrosis has been the result of such injuries, and a real sequestrum of bone has exfoliated.

Sometimes when there has been violent periostis about a tooth root, the inflammation has spread to the bone and a carious action been set up. In many instances this will continue after extraction. The cavity, perhaps, will not fill up by organization of the plastic exude, the gum will not heal over, and a small cavity will be left. There will be little of inflammation or soreness, and the attention of the patient will not be called to it until the cavity has assumed considerable proportions. If, then, an examination be made with an exploring instrument, the bone will be found bare, and it will be soft and spongy. It will not feel precisely like necrotic bone, but the difference between this and sound tissue can be readily recognized.

A carious condition of the alveolus will sometimes be the result of an anæmic or atonic state. It may be indicative of an inherited syphilitic taint. Of course it will be most often found in those who are in a debilitated state. The dentist should always examine for this when such patients who have been subjected to dental operations fall into his hands. It may be that he will need to scrutinize closely, for sometimes it is not very manifest.

The treatment, of course, is carefully to remove that which is cárious and spongy, apply antiseptics, these to be followed by stimulating applications, like iodide and chloride of zinc, ten to twenty grains to the ounce of water. If the caries is at all extensive, the patient will probably be in atonic condition, and alteratives, with liberal diet and careful hygienic precautions should be prescribed. Proparations af iron may be administered, the hypophosphites are are useful, and tonics generally. If there is reason to suspect any constitutional taint iodide of potassium may be prescribed. or the syrup of iodide of iron, from twenty to forty drops three times per day.

But if the dentist does not desire to attempt general remedies, at least he can and should remove the carious bone by means of bone curettes, or perhaps the engine bur, and give such topical treatment as is needed. Unless he is competent to diagnose the condition and do this much, he can scarcely call himself a surgeon dentist.— *Dental Practitioner and Advertiser.*

Reviews.

A Treatise on Pyorrhœa Alveolaris. By JUNIUS E. CRAVENS, D.D.S, Professor of Operative Dentistry in Indiana Dental College, etc. Mrs. W. M. Herriott, publisher, Dental Depot, Indianapolis, Ind.

This little volume of forty-eight pages, the printing and publishing of which is a decided credit to the lady-publisher, is the condensed result of over twenty years' observation and study of this puzzling part of dental pathology, "a despair to conscientious practitioners and a humiliation to science." Dr. Cravens differs considerably from most authorities as to the etiology of the disease, and offers many interesting suggestions as to treatment. We shall refer to it again.

Editorial.

The Same Old Herring.

Our friend, the editor of the *Dental Practitioner and Advertiser,* is a Master of Evasion. We do not know if he has also got that degree, but at any rate he is entitled to it "*without attendance at college.*" No doubt he enjoys it as a harmless joke. All the same it is not fair play.

We questioned from facts, the worth of dental education in the United States *twenty-five and thirty years ago,* and proved from facts that it was largely a travesty, and that the D.D.S., as then granted, in many cases after a few months' attendance upon lectures without matriculation, to Cubans and others who did not know the language in which the lectures were delivered, was a farce and frequently a fraud. In the same editorial we did justice to the *present* state of education.

Now, our worthy friend started out by editorially accusing us of attacking the American dental education *of to-day;* and by ingeniously omitting the context made it appear, as the devil is said to quote Scripture, that what we thought about the colleges over a quarter of a century ago is just what we think about them to-day!

The fun of the thing is this. We quoted Dr. W. C. Barrett against Dr. W. C. Barrett, and the editor of the *Practitioner* against the editor of the *Practitioner, from the same number of his journal!* We quoted exclusively American journals and American writers on the question of American dental education *in the past,* and we were unable to find one apologist for the state of affairs a quarter of a century ago.

If the editor of the *Practitioner* takes the position, that it is heresy for a Canadian neighbor to discuss in calmness a question so broad as education, which he and other Americans have discussed in heat and fury, he must take a very narrow view of the rights of journalism and the common interests of the profession, and if he cannot find any better argument than evasion, he had better not trail that same old herring across the scent. It is high time it was disinfected or interred.

The Annual Meeting.

The meeting of the Ontario Dental Society and the Eastern Ontario Dental Society in Kingston last month cannot be said to have been a numerical success, owing, no doubt, to the unbusinesslike way in which the " union " was brought about. It was impossible for this JOURNAL to get any information in time, as to when and where the meetings would be held, and the fact that the programme was not received until a few days before the meeting, shows that the members at large have some excuse for their absence. Kingston is such a delightful city in itself, its people are so hospitable, its dentists so united, that we looked forward to one of the very best meetings in the history of the Ontario Society. It is a great pity that the arrangements had not been made earlier, and we trust that the Eastern Ontario will endeavor to unite next year with the Ontario, and hold a regular rouser in Toronto. We owe it to ourselves as professional men. We owe it to ourselves as Canadians. Our neighbors give us many splendid examples in this direction, which should inspire us in our Society and in our journalism. Where are our young men these days?

The Report.

It is not the business of a busy editor, who was prevented by illness from being present, to make up a report of a meeting out of a batch of newspaper cuttings. That is exactly what was sent to us, and nothing more. The facetious newspaper reporter dealt largely in such lively expressions as " jaw smiths," etc., under the delusion that it was very witty. It must certainly tend to raise the dignity of the profession in the county of Frontenac, that leading newspapers could, without correction, be permitted to stigmatize the profession in such vulgar and ignorant language. If we do not educate the press to appreciate the difference between a "jaw smith," a "tooth carpenter" and an educated surgeon-dentist, we must not complain, if its reporting idiots continue to indulge in this cheap and obsolete species of wit.

Important Reductions in Teeth.

It will be learned with pleasure that our dental manufacturers have made important reductions in the price list of teeth. It came into force on the first of last month. The S. S. White Co., H. D. Justi & Son, Johnson & Lund, and, we suppose, other manufacturers (we have not received any other notices) have placed gum sections and gum plate and rubber at 12½ cents each tooth, with reductions in lots of $10 to $300 varying from 12 cents to 9 cents. Plain rubber and plate 12 cents each, running to 8 cents for $300 lots. The various crowns are also reduced in price. We could not get along without our manufacturers and *vice versa* ; and it makes things pleasant, in hard times, when the necessities of professional life, are brought more to the level of the average pocket than has existed for several years.

Not the " Printer's Devil."

One of our friends in Boston kindly writes us, " Did you ever see a 'debenture' that was not artificial?" See July number of DOMINION DENTAL JOURNAL, page 158, also index on cover. .

The fiend who haunts the printer's case is not to blame this time. We were unable to see the proofs of the July number because we were unable to see anything. When the flowers that bloom in the spring bring to an editor the very worst affliction in the way of rose fever, mistakes will occur. For " debenture " read " denture."

Annotations.

DR. BEACOCK'S PAPER.—Dr. Beacock's valuable paper, read in Kingston, will appear in the next issue.

In the last list of death claims of the Royal Arcanum there are the names of Drs. E. A. Whitehead, Luther H. Varney and C. P. Southwell, dentists, and three physicians.

DR. MARTIN'S PAPER.—There is a lot of food for thought and discussion in Dr. Martin's paper. It pricks into bubbles of the past, and what many think are bubbles of the present. It is a paper sure to be much approved and much denied.

DOMINION
DENTAL JOURNAL.

VOL. VI.   TORONTO, SEPTEMBER, 1894.   No. 9.

Original Communications.

Heredity and Environment, Beginning with the Primordial Cell.*

By D. V. BEACOCK, Brockville, Ont.

It has been said, " The child is father to the man," and that if we would comprehend a character, we must trace his birth, his surroundings, the method of his growth, the forces that have shaped him and made him what he is.

The past is fixed; the future lies before us like the block of rough marble before the sculptor. It can be shaped into beautiful designs according to his tastes and fancies, or left untouched with all its beauty and usefulness undeveloped.

The famous inscription of the Oracle of Delphi said, " Man, know thyself." And to do this thoroughly, we have not only to know ourselves but our ancestors as well, and the best way to do this is to begin at the very commencement of life, the primordial cell or germ. We shall then be able to get at the root of health and disease—heredity and environment—the latter two factors having a great deal to do with man's proper development, happiness and misery.

In order that we may properly comprehend the great importance of heredity, it will be necessary to review some of the elementary principles of organic and inorganic nature.

The verdict of modern thought is almost unanimous in asserting that there was a time when the material universe was in a chaotic state—that it was without form; in other words, in a nebulous

---

* I am indebted to Prof. Huxley and Dr. Holmes for many valuable ideas in this paper.

condition, when the plastic material had been created but the magical touch of the Supreme Intelligence had not yet moulded the chaos into wondrous designs that now furnish food for the souls of finite beings. Architecture was then unknown, and without architecture of what use were the materials—the soft clay or the perfect marble? Beauty and utility were yet latent. But ere long the designs and specifications of the Supreme Architect were revealed, and the product of two mighty forces—vital and physical —by the union of mind and matter, produced a living cell. The Great Architect had united the material with the immaterial, the visible with the invisible, and out of the chaos of a dead universe there evolved the greatest mystery of creation—life.

Now, let us take a retrogressive step and look back into the synthesis of living beings. No analytical or synthetical chemistry can give us the origin of life or tell us what it is. The principle that gives the inert mass the power of life is the secret of the Creator, and will never be comprehended by the finite mind of man. What life is, no one knows. It is said to be the result of the activity of the cells. Now, a cell is the lowest form of life, both animal and vegetable, and from these single cells all life is produced.

Let us examine a simple living cell. If we study it carefully we shall find that it is composed of an unresponsive, powerless mass of protoplasm and a vital force. By the union of these two factors it becomes an independent organism, possessing well-marked functions. This is the first step in the wonderful evolution of life.

Protoplasm (from *protos*, first, and *plasma*, mould, or what has been formed) was first so called by Hugo von Mohl as recently as 1846; and the simplest form of life which first emerges from the inorganic to the organic world consists of protoplasm, or, as Huxley calls it, the physical basis of life. It is a colorless semifluid or jelly-like substance, which consists of albuminoid matter. It exists in every living cell, both animal and vegetable. It is just as certain that all individual life, from the most elementary protoplasm up to the highest organism, man, originates in a minute or embryo cell, as it is that oxygen and hydrogen combined in certain proportions make water. Our most delicate means of research throw no light on the purely vital endowments of protoplasm, which not only direct and control its activities, but are transmitted in well-defined characters from parent to offspring. One thing we do know, that there is no life without pre-existing life from which it is derived, and the physical basis through which it acts or is made manifest furnishes no satisfactory explanation as to its real essence and constitution.

It is impossible to procure pure protoplasm for chemical analysis, as it contains many extraneous substances ; and even if this could be done, a chemical analysis of living protoplasm cannot be made.

And it is a well-known fact that there is evidence to show that there is considerable difference in the chemical properties of living and dead protoplasm. For instance, carmine and other coloring matters do not color living protoplasm, while on the other hand they give a brilliant stain to dead protoplasm.

To illustrate : Analytical chemistry is the pulling down of substances ; synthetical chemistry is the building up of a more or less complicated product from its elementary constituents. For instance, if we heat a little sugar to redness in a test tube it leaves a black deposit, which is carbon, while a liquid, which is water, distils over ; and on electrolyzing this fluid we resolve it into hydrogen and oxygen, so that we can thus show that sugar is composed of carbon, hydrogen and oxygen. This pulling down or taking to pieces of sugar (analysis) is an easy matter, but the putting these same elements or pieces together again (the synthesis of sugar) is a very different matter and much more difficult. You may put together carbon, hydrogen and oxygen in due proportions, and shake them all together, or heat them or cool them, and yet you will never get them to combine again so as to make sugar.

The analysis of dead protoplasm, animal or vegetable, is an easy matter, and consists of carbonic acid, water and ammonia. But no chemist has ever succeeded by synthesis, and probably never will succeed in putting these three simple ingredients together again, and thus making protoplasm. Chemical investigation can tell us little or nothing, directly, of the composition of living matter, inasmuch as all such matter must needs die in the analysis. Out of these three simple forms of matter, carbonic acid, water and ammonia, the vegetable world builds up all the protoplasm which keeps the animal world agoing. Withdraw any of these simple elements from the world, and all vital phenomena comes to an end. They are related to the protoplasm of plant life as the protoplasm of the plant is to that of the animal. It will thus be seen that plants are the accumulators of the power which animals distribute and disperse. We must bear in mind that no animal can make protoplasm, but must take it ready-made from some other animal or plant, the animal's highest feat of constructive chemistry being to convert dead protoplasm into that living matter of life which is appropriate to itself. Therefore, in seeking for the origin of protoplasm we have to turn to the vegetable world. The animal can only raise the complex substance of dead protoplasm to the higher power, as one may say of living protoplasm, while the plant can raise the less complex substance, carbonic acid, water and ammonia, to the same stage of *living* protoplasm. The fluid containing carbonic acid, water and ammonia, which offers such a Barmecide feast to the animal, is simply a table richly spread to the multitudes of plants, and, with a due supply of only such materials, many a plant will not only maintain itself in vigor, but grow and multiply until it has increased a million-fold the quantity of protoplasm which it originally possessed, in this way building up the matter of life, to an indefinite extent, from the *common matter* of the universe.

No matter under what guise it takes refuge, whether fungus or oak, worm or man, living protoplasm not only ultimately dies and is resolved into its mineral and lifeless constituents, but it is always dying, and strange as the paradox may sound, could not live *unless* it died.

Notwithstanding all the fundamental resemblances which exist between the powers of protoplasm in plants and animals, they present a striking difference, in the fact that plants can manufacture fresh protoplasm out of minerals and mineral compounds, whereas animals are obliged to procure it ready-made, and hence, in the long-run, depend upon plants for their supply. At the present time we may look upon protoplasm as the basis of physical life in the same sense that some form of it is the essential and active constituent of every living cell or tissue, whether vegetable or animal, and that it is only formed through the physiological activities of living organisms. In the absence of life, protoplasm cannot be formed, and, so far as we can perceive, there are no manifestations of life without it.

Living substance or protoplasm must be looked upon as constantly undergoing changes that vary with the functions required of it. These changes, without attempting to distinguish between them, as chemical, physical, or more strictly speaking, biological, are most conveniently expressed by the general term metabolism, which is both constructive and destructive.

Dr. M. Foster says : " We may picture to ourselves this total change, which we designate by the term metabolism, as consisting, on the one hand, of a downward series of changes (katabolic changes), a stair of many steps, in which more complex bodies are broken down into simpler and simpler waste bodies, and on the other hand, of an upward series of changes (anabolic changes), as also a stair of many steps, by which the dead food, of varying simplicity and complexity, is, with the further assumption of energy, built up into more and more complex bodies. The summit of this stair we call protoplasm."

All work implies waste, and the work of life results, directly or indirectly, in the waste of protoplasm. Every word uttered by a speaker costs him some physical loss, and, in the strictest sense, he burns that his hearers may have light—so much of his body resolved into carbonic acid and urea.* It is one of the funda-

---

* It is said that urea circulates in the blood, and is excreted by the kidneys, and the more mental work the more urea is produced. A fretfulness that produces activity, but no actual results, causes a loss of just so many grains of urea. Therefore, for every footpound of thought you will have a given amount of urea excreted.

mental doctrines of physiology that every part of our organism has its own definite term of vitality, and that there is a continuous succession of the destruction of old cells and the formation of new ones in all tissues, and especially in those in which the most active vital changes are going on, as, for example, in the nervous and muscular tissues. Even the most solid portions of the animal frame, such as the bones, and, to a less extent, the teeth, are undergoing a perpetual, although slower change of this nature, and throughout the body there is a continuous removal of effete or worn-out tissues, and a corresponding deposition of new matter. Every blow we strike, every thought we think, is accompanied by the death and disintegration of a certain amount of muscular or nervous tissue as its necessary condition, and thus every action of our corporeal life, from its beginning to its close, takes place at the expense of the vitality of a certain amount of organized structure. This we term molecular* death. It must be clear to every intelligent mind that this process could not go on forever without the capacity of being repaired.

We therefore have recourse to food to supply the waste. Broadly speaking, the animal body is a machine well adapted for converting potential energy into actual energy. The potential energy is supplied by the food we eat ; this the metabolism of the body converts into kinetic or actual energy of heat and mechanical labor. So we may say that our bodies are delicately constructed heat engines.

Energy, like matter, is indestructible and of two kinds—kinetic, or actual, and potential, or positive energy. Our whole life consists but in the transformation of these two different kinds of energy. We procure food which we eat, the greater part of which, under chemical action of various juices of the digestive organs, is absorbed into our system, which thereby enables us to perform a certain amount of work, mental or physical ; in other words, to transform a certain amount of potential into kinetic or actual energy. *For a certain amount of work* to be done (without waste or injury to the system), a certain amount of food must be absorbed, that is, digested. If the absorption be in excess of the expenditure, then nature stores this energy up in the form of fat ; if the expenditure be in excess of absorption, then nature works upon our bodies and we grow thin. If the absorption equal the expenditure, then we are in a state of what the doctors term physiological equilibrium, in perfect good health.

Energy is expended in building organic substances, or, in other

---

* Speaking of molecules, scientists state that a cubic inch of oxygen, at ordinary temperature and pressure, contains so many molecules, that a number equal to the population of our globe might escape every second, and it would take over six thousand years to empty this small space. Or if a single drop of water could be magnified to the size of the earth, the molecules would be the size of billiard balls.

words, in converting food stuffs of any kind into protoplasm, the summit of the double stair of life, and its potential energy is the transformed or stored energy of the above mentioned constructive process.

Man, like all animals, is born of an egg, or ovum, which was the first germ of our existence, and is a small cell about one-hundredth of an inch in diameter, consisting of a mass of semi-fluid protoplasm enclosed in a membrane, and containing a small speck or nucleus of more *condensed* protoplasm. This nucleated cell is itself the first form into which a mass of simple jelly-like protoplasm is differentiated in the course of its evolution from its original uniform composition. This nucleated cell is the starting point of all higher life, and by splitting up and multiplying repetitions of itself in geometrical progression, provides the cell material out of which all the more complicated structures of living things are built up. At first the egg behaves exactly as any other single-celled organism, as, for instance, that of the ameba, which is considered the simplest form of all organized life. One of the simplest forms of this is nothing but a naked little lump of cell-matter, or plasma, containing a nucleus ; and yet this little speck of jelly moves freely. It shoots out tongues or processes and gradually draws itself up with a sort of wave-like motion ; it eats and grows, and in growing reproduces itself by contracting in the middle and splitting up into independent ameba.

Even if a drop of blood is drawn by pricking one's finger, and carefully viewed with proper precautions and under a sufficiently high microscopic power, there will be seen among the innumerable multitude of little circular discoidal bodies or corpuscles which float in it and give it its color, a comparatively small number of colorless corpuscles, of somewhat larger size and somewhat irregular shape. If this drop of blood be kept at the temperature of the body, they will be seen to exhibit a marvellous activity, changing their forms with the greatest rapidity, drawing in and thrusting out prolongations of their substance, and creeping about as if they were independent organisms. This substance which is so active is simply a mass of protoplasm, and its activity differs in detail, rather than in principle, from that of protoplasm of plant life. The simplest form of life, as it emerges from the inorganic to the organic world, consists of protoplasm. In the earliest state of the human organism, in that in which it has just become distinguishable from the egg in which it arises, it is nothing but an aggregation of corpuscles or cells, and every organ of the body was once no more than such an aggregation. Thus a nucleated mass of protoplasm turns out to be what may be termed the structural unit of the human body, and in its most perfect state it is a multiple of such units variously modified and differentiated. Let us look at this little cell, nestled in a congenial environment. It is alive, it moves, it comes in contact with small particles of inorganic matter ; it shapes itself so as to surround them, and the little particles are absorbed into its organism and they become a part of the living cell. That function of the cell which enables it to absorb the latent forces of the inorganic matter unto itself, we call nutrition. If we watch it still further, we shall see that it increases in size, it grows. But this little cell we have been studying has yet a still brighter future : it has a latent force within that has thus far been unobserved. Growth is the balance of repair over waste, and when through assimilation of food into its substance, this cell reaches a certain size, the force of cohesion is overcome by the release of the energy derived from food, and the cell divides equally at the kernel or nucleus, the soft slimy protoplasm distributes itself around each nucleus as the two part company, to grow and divide again in like manner *ad infinitum*. You here see the function of perpetual existence has been added—the function of self-preservation, by making two living things out of one : the origin of parent and offspring, the beginning of reproduction.

The fundamental principles of life were embraced in these four functions : nutrition, growth, motion and reproduction. The living cell being completed, it has since been allowed to work out its own destiny. It began to unfold the mysterious possibilities that were concealed within its little structure, and the unnumbered ages have witnessed a mighty growth and development—a wonderful evolution of life.

Thus far we have learned four functions of the organic world—nutrition, growth, motion and reproduction. We find by experimentation that if we diminish the nutrition the growth diminishes and the motion lessens. If nutrition ceases, growth and motion both cease and the cell dies ; the two factors that were combined to form the living cell dissolve, and the organism ceases to be. Let us consider the relation these four attributes of organic life bear to one another. Since living organisms can move, grow and reproduce only by means of nutrition, it is evident that they depend upon nutrition for their continued existence. Therefore nutrition is essential to the other three functions, for without it the others would cease to act and the organism would die.

But nutrition and growth cannot be acquired unless the organism exerts itself in selecting food, and subsequently in assimilating it. Thus we learn that without exercise, or the function of motion, the functions of nutrition and growth will cease. Exercise is, therefore, absolutely essential to nutrition and growth. Without the judicious exercise of each function of an organism the other functions will not be normal ; with a little exercise of these functions it may simply continue to exist ; but when they cease to act, the organism must die.

In life, as in death, decompositions are continually going on These decompositions are in kind not different, only during life the products of decomposition are removed and after death they remain in the body and thus poison the individual cells—that is, so alter them that their conditions no longer fulfil the requirements of life.

Scientific authorities everywhere are unanimous on this point: *Omnia vivum ex vivo* (all life comes from life), or, as some put it, *Omne vivum ex ovum* (all life comes from an egg), which is only another way of expressing it, as some animals are viviparous and others oviparous.

The germ, in both animal and plant life, is itself simply a detached portion of the substance of a pre-existing living body. Life, therefore, can be produced from a living ancestor only. And the individual as it develops from the egg cell epitomizes the history of the ancestral forms of its species.

Scientifically it seems impossible man can come from such an extremely minute and apparently insignificant speck as the germ constituting all there is in his beginning. We sometimes wonder at the smallness of the egg of the little humming-bird; but even such a shell full of embryonic germs of human beings would be enough to people a city. Think of it! Man, the lord of creation, yet in his beginning such a mere speck that it takes the most cultured eye to discover it and the best microscope to examine! No wonder science stands appalled and scientists sit by as pigmies. We must remember, too, that infinitesimal as is the human egg, it is *not* the germ; this is merely the mass, a comparatively crude mass. The germ within, as with other eggs, is very much smaller. We speak of the egg as a mere speck. What name shall we use to designate the smallness of this germ? Yet, though so small, it is a complete, living, active, complex organization, a cluster of inspired molecules, wonderfully tenacious, and most mysteriously at work from the first of its impregnated life. Molecule after molecule moves toward the surface of this minute cluster, arranging themselves into three distinct tiers like trained soldiers. The potentiality that resides in this human ameba, that is, the ovum already vivified, lays the foundations of the three embryonal sheets so called, the epiblast, the hypoblast and the mesoblast, the enfoldings of which give us the entire system of primal parts. Every time that you have a reproduction of tissue it has to go through this same process: First, indiscriminate chaos; then completely digested food or peptones; then protoplasmic mass; then the embryonal corpuscles out of which all the tissues arise, as exemplified by all reproduction of structure where there is fracture of the tissues. If they are favorably situated they simply repeat the embryonal condition and series of changes, so that they are indistinguishable from the original material.

Quite as mysterious is the fact that this minute cluster of molecules called a human germ—apparently a mere atom of jelly —not only comprises the beginning of all the vessels, tissues and organs of the matured body, but it brings forth the special characteristics of the parents, holding the potentiality of father and mother wherein heredity is involved, the mental and physical peculiarities, the general bent of disposition, the special traits, tastes, preferences and idiosyncrasies, and often the particular marks, growths, and physical and mental expression. Shakespeare says : " There's a divinity that shapes our ends, rough-hew them how we will." Can anyone doubt it?

Now, since we know that with judicious exercise and normal nutrition there will be normal growth and development, and consequently a normal body, we also know that with normal growth and development and a normal body, it naturally follows that there will be a normal reproduction ; for, if the ancestor is normal, the offspring, which is a part of it, must be normal. But if any function of the organism is varied from the normal, it follows that the others will vary from the normal. If there is abnormal exercise, there will be abnormal nutrition ; there being abnormal exercise and nutrition, there will be abnormal growth and development, and consequently an abnormal body. With all these abnormal conditions there will be abnormal reproduction ; for, if the ancestor is abnormal, the offspring, which is a part of it, must be abnormal, and we call this heredity.

There is a mysterious principle in every living organism that enables it to select from its environment such ingredients as are necessary to produce the different tissues and organs peculiar to its own nature. Thus, if we plant a rose, or a lily, or a grain of corn in the same soil, and give them the same care, each one will select the ingredients from its environment that are essential to its growth and development, and with that subtle chemistry that is everywhere at work in the organic world, will produce its kind. This law holds good in the animal kingdom as well as among plants. If a number of animals of different species are taken in their infancy and subjected as nearly as possible to the same influences, it will be observed that each will develop into a distinct type, differing in almost every respect from the others. The observance of this law convinces us that the principle of each plant or animal, which enables it to preserve the peculiarities of its species, is an inherent principle which is part of its nature, inherited from its ancestors, and by it given to its offspring. Thus we have a universal law which enables each individual to transmit to its offspring certain essentials that are common to all the individuals of its species. Yet there are differences or peculiarities that distinguish each member of a species from all others. Now, how are we to account for these individual differences? This is the province of heredity and environment. It is a well-known fact that no two persons are identical. It is also a self-evident fact that identical causes will produce identical effects, and that unequal causes will produce unequal effects. We know, too, that the latent powers, the latent possibilities that are concealed in each embryonic life, are variable quantities. We also know for a certainty that the influences which surround these individual lives—the environment—for moulding and shaping into a fixed state the plastic, latent, inherited predispositions are never identical. Therefore, in the question with which we have to deal, we have not only two unknown quantities, but two variable unknown quantities that are never the same or alike in two individuals—heredity and environment. Now, since there are no two persons with identical predispositions, what will be the result if we expose them to equal influences? Or the reverse: If we expose a number of persons of unequal predispositions to equal influences, the result must be unequal. If the environment is an uncongenial one, the person with an inheritance most approaching normal will possess the greatest power of resistance, and consequently will be the last to yield to malignant influences. The inverse of this is also true. Suppose, for instance, that all men were born equal, how long would they remain so if exposed to unequal influences? Dr. Weisman says : " We cannot, by excessive feeding, make a giant out of a dwarf, nor convert the brain of a fool into that of a Leibnitz, or a Kant, by means of much thinking." Spencer says : " There is no political alchemy by which you can get golden conduct out of leaden instincts. The inherited differences of individuals are known as individual predispositions. These predispositions render the individual more or less susceptible to external influences.

Heredity is therefore that law of nature whereby parents transmit to their offspring certain variable powers termed predispositions, which render their offspring more or less *susceptible* to their environment. Heredity is the condition within the body, and *environment* consists of the influences that act upon it from *without*. To properly adjust these two factors is the rationale of individual development and organic evolution. To balance some *inward* evil with some purer influence acting from *without*, will enable our environment to *correct* our heredity.

Every-day experience familiarizes us with the facts which are grouped under the name of heredity. *Every one of us bears* upon him obvious marks of his parentage, perhaps of remoter relationships. More particularly, the sum of tendencies to act in a certain way, which we call character, is often to be traced through a long series of progenitors and collaterals. So we may justly say, that this character, this moral and intellectual essence of a man, does veritably pass over from one fleshly tabernacle to another, and does really transmigrate from generation to generation. In the new-born infant the character of the stock lies latent, and the ego is little more than a bundle of potentialities. But very early these become actualities. From childhood to age they manifest themselves in dulness or brightness, weakness or strength, viciousness or uprightness, and with each feature modified by confluence with another character, if by nothing else, the character passes on to its incarnation in new bodies. The Indian philosophers call this character karma.

The mysterious manner in which heredity performs its wonders is not yet known. But Sir James Paget said to his class, " We should not throw away what we do not understand." And Hippocrates, the Grecian physician and philosopher, said, " You will, as a rule, find that the form of the body and disposition of the mind correspond to the nature of the country."

The faculties of every animal depend on two causes : First, heredity, or those that have been evolved from the type and become fixed by succession through a long series of ancestors ; secondly, adaptation, or those which are acquired by education, including *everything* that places the animal in harmony with its environment.

Let us now take a retrospective view of ancestral inheritances. As we do so, you will find a sympathetic chord has been touched in our nature, for a most melancholy vision is presented to us— diseased bodies, dwarfed and deformed ; weak minds, so weak in fact that they cannot see truth, or if perchance they do see it, distort it till it is no longer truth ; souls so black that they feast in darkness on the very dregs of perdition. What a vision to behold ! And do we call these men ? Men who were intended by the Great Creator of the universe to be the crowning piece of His handiwork ! What a fearful manifestation of *penalties* for *broken* laws !

There are three causes that lead to all this depravity and misery, viz., an abnormal inheritance, an abnormal environment, and the improper use or abuse of our functions. If the fountain-head of the stream of life is not pure, we cannot expect the waters below to be pure. If in the laboratory of nature we combine two parts of hydrogen and one of oxygen, we call the resulting compound water ; but, in the chemistry of life, if we combine two parts of immorality, which is moral depravity, one part of insanity, which is mental depravity, and two parts of disease, which is physical depravity, who can tell us what the product will be ? Do we not have this identical problem to deal with in heredity ? Every day of our lives we see this sad debauchery in chemistry, and the experimentation makes the world *shudder* to look at the *fearful results*.

If in the sacred laboratory of wedlock we combine these three ingredients, immorality, insanity, disease, we must remember that the laws of nature are never false. If the resulting compound is not as we would have it, it is because the proper ingredients were not used. We must ever remember that, being in the midst of conflicting influences, it is impossible for man to remain in a state of equilibrium. In the rebellion of influences, the stronger will be victorious, and after each conflict he is either raised one step higher in the scale of life or descends one step lower. By yielding to degrading influences, man's powers are weakened, and he is rendered less able to battle with the lurking foes awaiting him. By yielding to ennobling influences his powers are strengthened, and he is led to still greater conquests.

If we would only make a wise selection of our environment, for, bear in mind, it is the circumstances of the environment from the cradle to the grave that determine our future destiny and a judicious use of our functions, we should always be found in the upward road to perfect development. But if we choose an abnormal environment and aid it by functional inactivity or functional excesses, we shall find, as we are carried downwards in the road to degeneracy, that our only blessing will be ignorance and immorality, poverty and disease. In all nature there are no evils without a remedy, if we but wisely seek it. So it is with evils of heredity. Nature furnishes poisons for the assassin; she also furnishes antidotes for the physician. As we deal with disease so should we deal with crime, as we cannot isolate either from heredity.

Children should be taught by wise mothers and fathers that ignorance of the laws of nature does not necessarily mean innocence in character; it is by *knowledge* that we gain power. A well-known gentleman has said, one who is born with such congenital incapacity that nothing can make a gentleman of him, is entitled, not to our wrath, but to our profoundest sympathy.

Those unfortunate victims who receive moral poisons from their ancestors, and those who receive bodies tainted with impurities, have no moral right whatever to entail upon helpless offspring the bitter fruits of their own ancestral sins. Such homes are the incubators for vice and moral depravity, and it is at their firesides that we find the congenital criminal.

It may appear rather a drastic measure, but there should be a gulf put between congenital criminals and the rest of mankind by means of compulsory celibacy, by isolating them from the world at large or by physiological annihilation,* which will render posterity safe from such contamination. The pure crystal streams of life should not be allowed to be polluted by the streams that flow into them, otherwise the waters of both will become con-

---

* Sexual perverts should not be allowed to procreate, and if the merciful act of asexualization was performed on all habitual criminals, it would not only relieve our gaols of more than half of the inmates but would make them industrious and useful citizens.

taminated. The ideal of a perfect physical nature is perfect health ; the ideal of a perfect mental nature is a normal brain ; the ideal of a perfect moral nature is a perfect conscience, and the ideal of a perfect being is the blending of these three into one symmetrical whole. A sound mind in a sound body should be the desire of all, and if we have lived in accordance with the natural laws of our constitution, the termination of our lives will have a peaceful and happy ending, when, the intellect unimpaired and the other senses uninjured, the same nature which put together the several parts of the machine, takes her own created work to pieces. In many cases the weary pilgrimage of life is brought to a close with little apparent derangement of mental powers ; the final scene may be short and painless, and the phenomena of dying almost imperceptible.

In such an ending the stock of nerve power is exhausted—the marvellous and unseen essence, that hidden mystery that man with all his wonderful powers of reasoning, that physiology with all the aid that science has lent it, and the genius of six thousand years has failed to fathom. In that hour is solved that secret, the mystery of which is only revealed when the book of life is closed forever. Then we may hope, when nature draws the veil over the eye that is glazing on this world, at the same moment she is opening to some unseen but spiritual eye a vista, the confines of which are only wrapped by the everlasting and immeasurable bounds of eternity.

Pope expresses this view of death most pathetically, when he says :

> " Vital spark of heavenly flame !
> Quit, oh quit this mortal frame !
> Trembling, hoping, lingering, flying,
> Oh the pain, the bliss of dying !
> Cease, fond nature, cease thy strife,
> And let me languish into life !

> " Hark ! they whisper ; angels say
> Sister spirit, come away !
> What is this absorbs me quite ?
> Steals my senses, shuts my sight,
> Drowns my spirits, draws my breath ?
> Tell me, my soul, can this be death ?"

"Cheap Jack" and Quackery.

By MARK G. McELHINNEY, D.D.S., Ottawa, Ont.

The profession has a grievance. For a long time there have been heard sounds of complaint. At different times they have assumed various forms, but no one doubts the existence of a widespread and active evil. The Cheap Jack is the evil, he and his tribe. So accustomed have we become to it that we now almost believe it to be a necessary evil. When mankind cannot combat a wrong, he invariably labels it a " necessary evil." The writer has lately come to the conclusion that it is possible to greatly mitigate, if not to altogether eradicate, this evil, and henceforth refuses to believe that it is a necessary one.

There exists in almost every city a class of men calling themselves dentists and doing everything in their power to drag their profession down to the miry level of unskilled labor. They cut prices like rival insolvent dry goods houses, they haggle over prices like fish-wives, and finally accept the recompense of a corporation laborer.

They imagine that the profession has done them an injustice, that their confreres have slighted them, and consequently they endeavor to make it as unpleasant for their fellow-practitioners as possible. They continually have a grievance against the rest of the profession, and in retaliation they forget that it is their own noses that get cut.

There is a peculiar sensitiveness to slights and oversights that marks the *parvenu* and guttersnipe prince the world over, and the class in question possesses it to perfection.

The family that has known pinching poverty and whose immediate ancestors were strangers to refinement and station, often becomes, on accession to wealth, most noticeably disagreeable. Its members are rude to servants, fault-finding as to all services rendered, and open to insult by the most trivial oversight. This is because they are out of their element, and they know it and it irritates them accordingly. The profession of dentistry is rather too good company for some of those in it, and they, being unable to come up to its level, are endeavoring to bring it down to theirs.

Look at any Toronto paper and their trail can be seen all over. Toronto being the largest city within the jurisdiction of our college, it is the most cursed by the evil. According to their own story, there are men who never fail, men who can perform all operations painlessly, men who will guarantee their product for years ; and moreover, they will perform all this and much more for fees that are beyond comprehension for cheapness.

Yet so despicable in their meanness are these same men that they will not reveal these wondrous secrets of success to us their brethren. Being young my experience is limited, but it has not been too short to make the acquaintance of some of the experts of the profession and see some of their best efforts. It is beyond doubt that even these experts do occasionally fail, do even give pain sometimes and cannot conscientiously guarantee any work for even three days. One of the most skilful dentists in America has told me this in almost the same words. And further, these experts cannot afford to give their services for an office boy's wages. Those who advertise infallibility, painlessness, best material and workmanship " at rock-bottom prices," are merely liars seeking to gull the public.

They probably give the best material they can afford and the best workmanship of which they are capable, but neither, in the eyes of an expert, are cheap at half the money. The Cheap John knows how little his services are worth and charges accordingly. He is not to blame for he is the creature of his circumstances, nor can we hope to reform him, for he is without the incentive to self-advancement. He is also morally wanting, for he will appropriate to himself the processes and preparations that some reputable man has spent twenty years in perfecting, and this abominable parasite will next door, perhaps, parade them at half price, thus robbing the reputable man of his well-deserved reward.

Who is to blame for the existence of the charlatan? Who makes dentists? The School of Dentistry. Who founded the School? The College. Who constitutes the College? The profession at large. That means you and it means me and all of us. We, in fact, are to be blamed for our own degradation. Since quacks cannot be cured they must be prevented. Dentistry is one of the protected professions, and apart from the right of any class to protection, dentistry seems likely to be protected for some time.

Let us get what benefit we can from this protection while it lasts, for its days are perhaps numbered. The ultimate downfall of class legislation seems inevitable, then will it be re-introduced in a viler form—mass legislation. Class legislation has abuses, but mass legislation has not one redeeming feature. The profession of dentistry is in Ontario represented by the Royal College with its regulations and examiners. It is within the power of the college to pronounce upon the fitness or unfitness of a candidate. Let them do their duty and quackery will be stopped at the fountain-head. They cannot do that duty unless backed up by the solid sentiment of the profession. At present anyone may become a member of our profession if he can pay certain fees and lie or cheat his way through examinations. It matters not how unsuitable or how immoral, how ill-bred or how useless. The laxity of the procedure in this respect is notorious.

We have cut a rod for our own backs. Our chickens are coming home to roost in the annual output of unsuitable persons. At the opening of the session the school gobbles up everything that can pay, and at the conclusion of the course vomits them forth upon the profession irrespective of all considerations whatever, and the manner of it offends our nostrils greatly.

It is not possible that out of a class of twenty-five or thirty students, picked at random from the schools, workshops and farms of Canada, each one can be a fit and proper person to practise a learned profession. It is probable that at least one-quarter of the number should be sent back.

There have been sessions at the conclusion of which every member graduated. There could be nothing worse for the honor of the profession. The general effect is demoralizing. Subsequent students cultivate carelessness. A reasonable number of "plucks" each session would produce a wholesome respect for the examinations and more careful attention during the term.

There would be fewer "Smart Alecks" and so-called "Dead game sports" in our ranks if the way were made a little more difficult. I am not one to find fault with anyone for having a good time. A cigar and a glass of beer are excusable occasionally, but if there is a kind of man that I detest it is one of those "sporty" students. He drinks to excess and brags eternally about it; swears loud, sings questionable songs likewise, and imagines that the whole female sex is at his feet because he has perchance overcome the scruples of some fifth-rate servant girl or been the favored lover of some wretched prostitute. This language is strong, but it is true and should be driven into unwilling ears with a speaking-trumpet. The members of the profession must be awakened to the necessities of the hour. It were time that the Augean stable of dentistry was purged of its uncleanness.

From the general expression of the joint meeting of the E. O. and the Ontario Dental Societies, some of the members, at least, are fully awake.

Let us carry the conflict into the enemy's country and either gloriously rescue our profession from infamy or perish in the general destruction, lost in the sink of quackery, charlatanism and incapability.

The ethics of a profession are second only to its educational attainments, and should, I believe, be a part of the student's indenture and of the final degree. Whoso will not uphold the dignity of the profession should lose his license. The profession in self-protection should be empowered to seize it and drive the offender forth, with stripes if need be. The five and eight dollar plate man, the painless operator, the discoverer of nature's panacea (who probably does not know the chemical construction of water), and the low brute who insults women, whoever they be, in his chair are the natural and special enemies of every honest dentist, and should be treated accordingly. They do not develop these traits suddenly in after-life. They are the men who, in mistaken charity, the examiners allow to pass. They are the men who should be sent back whence they came.

I have at some length, perhaps, reviewed the evil ; also to some extent hinted at a cure, or at least a means of prevention. The plan of campaign would be this—subject, of course, to additions and corrections by older and wiser heads :

For prevention—A more rigorous adherence to the percentage required to pass candidates, a stricter supervision to prevent cribbing, the doing of metal work for examination by persons other than the candidate, and recognition of the fact that a habitual drunkard and loafer, a man who will steal instruments and material from the college and his fellow-students, and a libertine, are not fit men to practise a respectable profession.

For cure—A general education of the public by the spreading broadcast of the knowledge that good services cannot be got for nothing. The best way to do this would be the issue of brief leaflets bearing the authority of the Association, and explaining in plain terms the exact relations between the dentist and the patient, and the different attitudes of the charlatan and of the reputable dentist toward these relations. There could be no better use for the funds of any association than the printing and distributing of knowledge of this kind ; not only would it lessen the number of dupes, thereby starving out the quack, but it would call the attention of the general public to the matter, which attention could not but bring forth good results.

In this imperfect and disconnected way have I put down a few thoughts that occur and re-occur to me almost daily, trusting that in them may be found something useful and nothing altogether bad, for whatever may be faulty with my expression or my method, I feel that there is nothing wrong with the sentiment that calls for the preservation of the dignity of the dental profession.

To Utilize Old Gold Filling.

By G. V. N. RELYEA, L.D.S., Oswego, N.Y.

Gold fillings that have been doing good service for many years often become loose, either from slight decay or accident. We will suppose such a filling in either the incisors or cuspids, which the patient wants refilled. The party may not be willing or in circum-

3

stances to pay for another gold filling, and to fill with any other material may be out of the question.   If the gold is in a solid condition, and other circumstances favorable, excavate what may be necessary, then mix a little phosphate very thin, line the cavity with it and place the old gold in its former position, gently press and hold it until the phosphate sets, and if kept dry by the rubber dam it will again do service for many years.

It is very perplexing to find that a full upper denture, after being prepared, has, in part, if not wholly, lost its adhesiveness. This I attribute to the expansion of the plaster, or hastily or carelessly removing it from the flask before being sufficiently cooled. To avoid against expansion, embed the plate in two-thirds of plaster *that has gone through the vulcanizer.*   To guard against the latter, *take time.*   To be a thoroughly successful dentist, be a painstaking one.

Proceedings of Dental Societies.

National Association of Dental Faculties.

The eleventh annual session of the National Association of Dental Faculties was held at the Hygeia Hotel, Old Point Comfort, Va., commencing Saturday, August 4, 1894, the president, Dr. H. A. Smith, of Cincinnati, in the chair.

The resignation of Dr. J. E. Cravens as secretary was accepted, and Dr. Louis Ottofy, of Chicago, was made secretary *pro tem.*

The following faculties were represented :

Baltimore College of Dental Surgery—B. Holly Smith.
Boston Dental College—J. A. Follett.
Chicago College of Dental Surgery—T. W. Brophy.
Harvard University, Dental Department—Thomas Fillebrown.
Kansas City Dental College—J. D. Patterson.
Missouri Dental College—A. H. Fuller.
New York College of Dentistry—Frank Abbott.
Ohio College of Dental Surgery—H. A. Smith.
Pennsylvania College of Dental Surgery—C. N. Peirce.
Philadelphia Dental College—S. H. Guilford.
State University of Iowa, Dental Department—W. O. Kulp.
University of Michigan, Dental Department—J. Taft.
University of Pennsylvania, Dental Department—Jas. Truman.
Vanderbilt University, Dental Department—H. W. Morgan.
Louisville College of Dentistry—F. Peabody.

Southern Medical College, Dental Department—C. V. Rosser.
University of Tennessee, Dental Department—J. P. Gray.
University of Maryland, Dental Department—F. J. S. Gorgas.
Royal College of Dental Surgeons of Ontario—J. B. Willmott.
Columbian University, Dental Department—H. C. Thompson.
Northwestern University Dental College—G. H. Cushing.
American College of Dental Surgery—Louis Ottofy.
National University, Dental Department—J. Roland Walton.
College of Dentistry University of Minnesota—T. E. Weeks.

The following schools were admitted to membership during the meeting:
Western Reserve University, Dental Department, Cleveland, O.
—H. L. Ambler.
Western Dental College, Kansas City, Mo.—D. J. McMillen.

With reference to the application of Howard University, Dental Department, the Executive Committee recommended that in consequence of changes in and inadequacy of its dental department the application be rejected. The report was adopted.

The report of the Executive Committee recommending the admission of the University of Buffalo, Dental Department, to membership, was amended by the addition of the following clause, and then adopted: "When the honorary degrees conferred on Messrs. Southwick and Howard are returned to the university and revoked, and official notification of such revocation filed with the secretary of this association."*

The amendment to rule 5 offered by Dr. Hunt last year, making the rule read as follows, was adopted unanimously:
"(5.) STANDING OF UNDERGRADUATES IN MEDICINE.—Undergraduates of reputable medical colleges, who have regularly completed one full scholastic year, having attended at least seventy-five per cent. of a five months' term, and passed a satisfactory examination in the studies of the freshman year, may be admitted to the junior grade in colleges of this association, subject to other rules governing admission to that grade."

The following new applications for membership, with their recommendations, were reported by the Executive Committee:
Dental Department, Cleveland University of Medicine and Surgery, Cleveland, O. Recommended by Drs. J. Taft and J. E. Garretson.
Cincinnati College of Dental Surgery, Cincinnati, O. Recommended by Drs. James Truman, T. W. Brophy, F. J. S. Gorgas, and J. A. Follett.

---

* The Dental Department of the University of Buffalo complied with these condition on August 13, 1894, and is therefore admitted into full membership.—LOÚIS OTTOFY, *Secretary.*

Birmingham Dental College, Birmingham, Ala. Recommended by Drs. H. W. Morgan and C. V. Rosser.

University College of Medicine, Dental Department, Richmond, Va. Recommended by Drs. F. J. S. Gorgas and H. W. Morgan.

Atlanta Dental College, Atlanta, Ga. Recommended by Dr. H. W. Morgan and the faculty of the University of Tennessee, Dental Department.

The amendment to by-law 4, which was offered by Dr. Hunt last year, was laid on the table.

The resolution offered last year by Dr. Sudduth, directing the addition of Latin and physics to the entrance examination, was also laid on the table.

The special committee appointed last year to consider the matter of the vote of censure passed upon the Baltimore College of Dental Surgery reported, through its chairman, Dr. C. N. Peirce, recommending that no further action be taken. The report was adopted.

Dr. Louis Ottofy offered a recommendation, which was adopted, that all colleges, members of this association, shall increase the college course of 1895-96 to not less than six months.

The following resolution from the Executive Committee was adopted:

Resolved,—That any college or colleges making application for membership in the National Association of Dental Faculties shall be required to secure and present to the Executive Committee the approval and indorsement of the board of dental examiners of the State (where such boards exist) in which such colleges are located, before this application can be considered.

The following from the Executive Committee was laid on the table :

Resolved,—That we regard it as inconsistent for any member of a faculty of any college holding membership in this body to at the same time be a member of any State board of dental examiners.

The report of the *ad interim* committee with reference to charges preferred against the University of Maryland, Dental Department, was referred to the Executive Committee, which reported as follows :

" Your Executive Committee respectfully report that they find that the University of Maryland, Dental Department, in the reception of certain students did violate the regulations of this association, through a misapprehension of the rules, as it is interpreted by your committee that the regular sessions of all colleges close with their commencement exercises."

The report was adopted.

Dr. Guilford moved that rule 11, p. 12 of the " History," be understood to mean that students coming from a college not a member of this association will not be given credit for any time spent in such institution.

The annual dues were increased from $3.00 to $5.00 on motion of Dr. Cushing, the increase to take effect in 1895-96.

On motion of Dr. Truman, the special committee on preliminary examinations was instructed to have prepared by a competent person and present at the next annual meeting a list of questions of a standard covering every branch required in the grammar schools up to the point of admission to the high schools.

On motion of Dr. Abbott, it was ordered that each college should each year present its announcement, noting any changes, the secretary to note and publish all important changes in the annual report of the association.

On motion of Dr. Morgan, all the schools were required to comply with the rule regarding dissections.

On motion of Dr. Ottofy, a committee of three was appointed to revise the constitution and by-laws, with the further instruction, on motion of Dr. Truman, to drop the qualifying term " by."

The following were introduced, and under the rules lie over till next year :

By Dr. Peirce :

Resolved,—That, in view of the recommendation of the Executive Committee, this association will require that all colleges, members of this association, shall extend the term of the session of 1896-97, and of succeeding sessions, to not less than seven months each. .

By Dr. Truman :

Resolved,—That on and after the session of 1898-99 the regular session of each of the colleges belonging to this association shall be extended to four years.

By Dr. Ottofy :

Beginning with the session of 1896-97, the examinations conducted by the colleges of this association shall be in the English language only.

By Dr. Ottofy :

Beginning with the session 1895-96, no college shall be permitted to retain membership in this association if it is conducted or managed, in whole or in part, by any person or persons who do not practise dentistry in accordance with well-recognized and generally accepted forms, generally known as dental ethics, or if they are owned in whole or in part by men or women who are engaged in disreputable dental practice, or if any college have upon its list of trustees, the faculty, demonstrators, or in any other capacity, any one who does not practise dentistry in accordance with the principles above mentioned. This shall refer to dentists only.

By Dr. Ottofy:

Beginning with the session of 1896-97, the following shall be the requirements for the admission of students to the colleges of this association:

a. A certificate of having successfully completed at least one full year's course of study in the collegiate department of any college or university registered by the regents of the State of New York as maintaining a satisfactory standard.

b. A certificate of having passed, in a registered institution, examinations equivalent to the full collegiate course of the freshman year, or to a completed three years' academic course.

c. Regents of the State of New York pass cards for any forty-eight counts.

d. A certificate of having passed the matriculation examinations of any university in Great Britain or Ireland, or of having completed a course of study recognized as an equivalent therefor.

e. A certificate of graduation from any registered gymnasium in Germany, Austria, or Russia.

f. A certificate of the successful completion of a course of five years in a registered Italian *ginnasio*, and three years in a *liceo*.

g. The bachelor's degree in arts or science, or substantial equivalents, from any registered institution in France or Spain.

h. Any credential from a registered institution, or from the government in any foreign state or country, which represents the completion of a course of studies equivalent to graduation from a registered New York high school, academy, or from a registered Prussian gymnasium.

By Dr. Gray:

Resolved,—That law 7 of the by-laws, which now reads " attendance upon three full courses of not less than five months each in separate years shall be required before examination for graduation," be amended by substituting " six " instead of " five," to take effect on and after the year 1896-97.

By Dr. Willmott:

Resolved,—That at least twenty-nine months intervene between the beginning of the freshman year and the date of graduation.

The Committee on Text-books presented the following report, which was adopted :

Your Committee on Text-books would report that only two works of this character have been presented for its consideration :

One, a work on " Dental Anatomy and Pathology," by Dr. C. F. W. Bödecker, of New York, 700 pp.; and the other, a smaller and less pretentious work of about 75 pp., on " Operative Technics," by Dr. Thomas E. Weeks, of Minneapolis.

Both of these works are in press and nearly completed. The treatment of their subjects is full, clear and concise, and the illustrations numerous, well executed, and for the most part entirely new.

Your Committee would therefore recommend these two books for endorsement as text-books.

Suitable resolutions regarding the deaths of Drs. R. B. Winder and W. H. Eames were presented and adopted, and the secretary was instructed to communicate a copy to their respective families.

The following officers were elected for the ensuing year : Frank Abbott, president ; S. H. Guilford, vice-president ; Louis Ottofy, secretary ; H. W. Morgan, treasurer ; J. Taft, B. Holly Smith and Thomas Fillebrown, executive committee ; James Truman, Truman W. Brophy and Francis Peabody, *ad interim* committee.

Dr. Abbott, the newly-elected president, was installed, and appointed the following committees :

Committee on Schools—J. A. Follett, F. J. S. Gorgas, Louis Ottofy, C. N. Peirce and Truman W. Brophy.

Committee on Text-books.—J. D. Patterson, A. O. Hunt, J. B. Willmott, T. E. Weeks and J. P. Gray.

Adjourned.

Editorial.

Splendid Work of the National Association of Dental Faculties.

If our readers were as familiar with the record on dental education of the old *Canada Journal of Dental Science* as they may perhaps be with that of its successor, the *Dominion Dental Journal*, they would realize that if the editorial views therein expressed are not admitted by our American cousins to have been influential, they were, at least, prophetic. It goes against the grain to toot one's own " bazoo ": recent controversy not only justifies the reference, but the action last month of the National Association of Dental Faculties, which we print elsewhere, is an official confirmation, by the representatives of the schools, of the position occupied in Canada for many years.

When the profession was organized in Ontario, one of the first recommendations was for the exaction of a classical and mathematical standard of entrance to study. After a while this became an accomplished fact, and to this day, in Ontario and the Province of Quebec, at least, the standard is equal to that required for the entrance to the study of medicine. This matriculation is conducted by experts beyond the control of the Dental Boards, and it is now impossible to evade it. Without an immediate prospect of establishing a college, the method of study was modelled chiefly upon the British system of apprenticeship, and compulsory attendance upon special lectures in medical schools. This indentureship had many advantages, which no college course could ever supplant. It had disadvantages which only a college course could remove. It worked uncommonly well when the student found a skilled and faithful tutor. It worked uncommonly bad when the reverse was the case. No doubt there are brilliant people around, who think that if they had been on hand, Rome could have been built in a day; but the "bazoo" is not a national instrument in Canada, and if there were such self-confident architects in our profession they did not file an appearance and our profession made haste slowly. The studentship was made to cover the twelve months of four successive years. Certified tickets of dissection and of regular attendance upon the medical lectures was demanded. When the first college was organized in Toronto, compulsory attendance was required. The difficulties in the way were gradually removed. The "bazoo" was never blown. It is not the fashion of the country. We do not expect to set the St. Lawrence on fire, but we hope to do good work in our own sphere for our Dominion, and are perfectly willing to believe that our good cousins over the border can largely supplement for our students, from their greater resources, all that we can do towards clinical and practical instruction.

One resolution in particular affects Canada as directly as any State in the American Union. We cannot too emphatically express our gratitude for the generosity of our neighbors in according to us one form of annexation, which is much more popular than the political. We refer to the admission of Canadian colleges to the privileges of the National Association of Dental Faculties. By this thoroughly kind action the degree of D.D.S. of the University of Toronto, and we hope to add some day that of the Province of Quebec, is as acceptable for practice as that of the American colleges. It widens the scope for our students, though we hope they will all find fields in our own Dominion. It will be observed that the Association now demands the approval and indorsement of the Boards of Examiners where the colleges are located, in order to secure membership. The chances of factious opposition are thus destroyed, as students will not care for degrees which are not recognized as equivalent to those of the best colleges, and the Boards will not likely indorse rival institutions founded for no other reason than miserable jealousy or spite.

The National Association of Dental Faculties has merited the utmost confidence of the profession. It has the future of Dentistry *on this continent* in its keeping. Its enemies, if there are any, must be the enemies of moral ethics, as well as of professional progress.

DOMINION
DENTAL JOURNAL.

VOL. VI.   TORONTO, OCTOBER, 1894.   No. 10.

Original Communications.

Translations.

(From Foreign Dental Journals, etc., etc.)

By CARL E. KLOTZ, L.D.S., St. Catharines, Ont.

TO REPRODUCE THE RIDGES OF THE PALATE ON A VULCANITE PLATE.—A piece of tea lead is burnished well to the model, just large enough to fit inside of the teeth after they are set up. When the case is ready for flasking, before putting it into the flask, take the tea lead plate and warm it and press it gently into the wax. Flask as usual. When flask is taken apart, remove tea lead which generally sticks to the upper part of the flask, varnish this part, and carefully burnish a piece of tinfoil on to the varnished surface. After vulcanizing you will have a polished surface underneath the tinfoil, which latter can easily be removed with a polishing brush on the lathe.

ANOTHER METHOD.—After the case is waxed up and placed into the lower part of the flask, cut out the wax close to the teeth. Soap the model and pour in plaster of Paris, but only even with the teeth. When dry, remove the block and replace wax plate, slightly warm this, as also the block of plaster of Paris, and press it into the wax. Place upper part of flask in position and pour. When flask is taken apart the block is in the upper part of the flask. Cover this with tinfoil or varnish well with waterglass. Pack as usual.—*Zahntechniche Reform.*

To prevent plaster of Paris from sticking to the palatine surface of a vulcanite plate, paint or brush the model in the flask well with soap suds.—*Zahntechniche Reform.*

UNCOMMON CASE OF SALIVARY CALCULUS.—Salivary calculus deposits at the ends of whartonian and steno ducts are easily diagnosed, through their locality as well as their consistency. The glands are generally considerably swollen, and the form of the deposits is oval. The deposit is found more frequently in the submaxillary and less in the parotid. The knowledge of their origin has not been fully brought to light. It is generally accepted to be a precipitation of uric acid salts around a foreign substance. In the majority of cases they will be found at the principal outlet of the glands, close to the buccal opening, as it is easy for a foreign substance to get into the opening of the duct. More difficult is the diagnosis if the deposit is deeper in the duct or even in the gland itself. In the latter it is scarcely probable that any foreign substance could find its way into them. It would be that it was forced in with the mucus. When such is the case, suppuration generally takes place, particularly in the parotid. The treatment is very simple ; when there is a tendency to recurrence extirpate the glands.—*Zahnärztliches Wochenblatt.*

DEATH THE RESULT OF SWALLOWING ARTIFICIAL TEETH.— G. S. Scotson, in the *Journal of the British Dental Association,* states that a woman thirty-six years of age was admitted to the Manchester Infirmary in consequence of having swallowed her artificial teeth in a fit of coughing. Patient suffered pain, dysphagia, dyspnea, and speaking was very difficult. The plate could be felt with the finger—it was wedged in behind the larynx—but all efforts failed to remove it, even under the influence of chloroform, and not until tracheotomy was performed could it be removed, but the patient died the following day.—*Deutsche Monetsschrift.*

A SIMPLE AND EFFECTIVE HEMOSTATIC.—Dr. Ramsay Smith, of Edinburgh, treats obstinate cases of bleeding where all other styptics have failed with bovist (Lycopordon giganteum) puff ball. He treated a patient who suffered with lymphadenom with several complications, one of which was profuse bleeding of the alveolus and gums. Teeth in a bad state with secession of the gums. Patient a habitual smoker, has suffered for some time, and the bleeding was periodical with intervals of three to four weeks, and sometimes lasting eight days. When patient came to him the bleeding had lasted for several hours, and streamed from the alveolus of the right side of the upper jaw, from the third molar to the central. The bovist was cut into slices and packed along the gum margin and into the interproximal spaces. Bleeding was arrested almost immediately and no recurrence. Dr. Smith trusts that ere long he will be able to explain the theory of the effects of the bovist.—*Journal fur Zahnheilkunde.*

TREATMENT OF ROOT CANALS.—Dr. Schreier, of Vienna, uses a preparation of metallic potassium and iodium for removing the patrescent particles out of root canals and for cleansing them. He bases his theory on the saponifying of the contents of the canals, and thereby easily removed with warm water. He also considers it a good antiseptic treatment of the roots, and shortens the time considerably for treatment and filling.

SMALL wooden pincers are very easily made, and are convenient for handling medicines that effect steel instruments. Take two wooden tooth picks and place between them at one end a piece of a third, and bind together with thread ; soften a little gutta percha and mould around the thread and you will have a simple pair of tweezers that will not corrode.—*Zahntechniche Reform.*

Calcification of Dental Pulps.

By A. ROSE, L.D.S., Peterborough, Ont.

The title of this paper as given in the programme would more accurately· describe the subject if written, " Calcific deposits in the dental pulp chamber," because these deposits seldom assume the appearance of a calcified pulp.

Calcific deposits, as generally found in a pulp chamber of the human tooth by the dentist in ordinary practice, vary in quantity from a very thin incrustation adhering to the surface of the pulp, to a mass of semitranslucent substance usually resembling dentine in appearance and structure and completely filling the chamber and canal. They often occur in small granular particles or spiculæ through the pulp tissue, and also either attached to the walls of the chamber or to the sheath of the pulp, as minute pearls ranged along it. Many specimens, when removed from the chamber, appear to be cone-shaped, with the base spread out towards the opening in the dentine produced by the caries. Others show very irregular shapes.

Starting from a base looking towards the approaching caries or other irritating causes, they seem to penetrate the chamber, throwing forward projections in the direction of each canal in the roots of the tooth. Also, I would mention those deposits found in the chambers of the teeth of older persons when abrasion from the work of mastication has resulted in wearing the teeth to the gums, perhaps. In this class the canal seems to be in many cases simply closed up from the deposition of calcific matter upon its walls surrounding the pulp, until the whole cavity is filled and the pulp disappears entirely. As a last class I would mention what seems to me to resemble more than any other class a real case of calcification of the pulp. These are found in the teeth of very old persons, in which I have found the pulp to assume the appearance of the pith of a goose-quill but to possess a firmer structure, being more like a piece of the quill itself.

In all classes but the last two, those specimens which I have discovered and now have to exhibit, on being removed from the chamber and canal, were enclosed or surrounded by the pulp or the sheath of the pulp, except at the base where they were perhaps attached to the dentinal wall of the chamber. The sheath seemed to remain intact, even when the deposit had penetrated the canal nearly to the apex of the root, and when inflamed from any cause whatever (which inflammation is the usual cause of the trouble leading to the discovery of the deposit), this sheath is intensely sensitive to approach and is often possessed of a very tenacious vitality, resisting the action of arsenic and cocaine, and requiring several applications to overcome its sensitiveness.

The structure of these deposits seems, according to the opinions of leading histologists and microscopists, as Miller, Black and Iszlai, to differ, sometimes being organized similar to dentine, sometimes resembling cementum and sometimes bony in structure.

It would appear to one less skilled in histological knowledge of these parts of tooth structure, that the particular formation of these deposits depends upon that portion of the odontoblastic cells retaining most vitality and receiving the necessary stimulus which may be either local or systemic in character. The writer is also led to conclude that these deposits are the result of nature's efforts to repair an injury either received or threatened, and that they are really of a physiological character, and that any irritation which may render sensitive this monitor of the dental organization, the pulp, may engage its reparative function and cause, in many instances, a deposition of calcific matter upon the walls (or within them) of its habitation somewhere in the direction of the irritation, and this matter may be organized in the shape of dentine, cementum or bone, the morphological differences between these elements of tooth structure being very slight ; and when we remember that they all originate in the cellular matter of the dental papilla, it is not unreasonable to suppose that the stimualation above referred to may as readily produce the one form of matter as the other.

A strong reason for deeming this peculiar formation of calcific matter in the pulp chamber physiological rather than pathological as to origin, is the fact that the experience of almost every observer of this formation agrees in the statement that it is found most frequently in well-developed, well-nourished and usually plethoric individuals. I have often acted upon this assumption, and on discovering one, or perhaps two, of the canals of a superior molar closed to the finest broach, and having been attacked with caries which penetrated the tooth to the position of the pulp chamber originally, the tooth had, in the words of the patient, "just rotted away and never ached at all," I have cleansed the remaining root canals, if any, and after thorough antisepting with iodoform and eucalyptus oil, or aristol and eucalyptus oil, which is less disagreeable, or perhaps with hydrarg. bi-chlor. 1-500 or 1-1000, have dried and filled just as I should have filled any ordinary case. I have several such under observation which have been thus dealt with, one two years ago, and three or four for a shorter time, all giving good satisfaction. I feel quite well satisfied myself that the real office of the ordinary "nerve stone," "nerve nodule," "pulp stone," "odontome," or "endodonthele," by whatsoever term we may choose to call it, *is not to cause* the intense pain of neuralgia, or pericementitis, or any of those terribly painful conditions which usually precede its discovery, but its work *is to prevent* this trouble, and I would just here ask, "Who knows how often this latter purpose is fulfilled to the letter?" A good idea may be formed of a proper answer to this question by filing down a hundred of those diseased teeth which have been extracted for replacement with artificial dentures, as is done by the student of the first or second year where the system of Dr. Black has been adopted in teaching "*Operative Technique.*"

Very many of these cases "never ache but just rot away," and if examined will be found to possess ample evidence of this purpose in the formation of calcific deposits in the pulp chamber.

The diagnosis of this irregularity of tooth structure is comparatively easy where the tooth has been penetrated by caries to the locality of the pulp chamber. Any effort to remove the pulp will expose the presence of the deposit ; but where this deposit exists in an apparently sound tooth, and having been produced through some irritation, perhaps of a systemic character, such as often causes loss of enamel at the gingival margin or very great sensetiveness in the same locality, its presence is suggested by extremely painful spasms, or occasional sharp piercing pain in the tooth, or perhaps a condition resembling pericementitis, which can best be ended by making forcible entrance with a good sharp bur, or a sharpened glyddon drill shank, dipped in cocaine crystals and carbolic acid or glycerine frequently while operating, and forcibly removing both pulp and the deposit. The pain above referred to often yields to cold applications, but requires several applications of arsenious acid and cocaine or morphia to effectually end the trouble when access can be got to within even a short distance of the remaining portion of the pulp.

If these few lines result in a thorough discussion of this subject, and in bringing out the experience of our senior members with this *knotty* subject, I shall have accomplished all I expected while trying to express my own. I never flattered myself with the thought that I had gained more knowledge of this subject than any ordinary practitioner of four or five years' service should have acquired, nor in fact quite so much ; but, on being asked if I would give a paper, I consented to do so, feeling it the duty of every member of our profession to aid this society as far as he is able in drawing forth what information can be gained from even an imperfect presentation of his views on any subject, and this subject being lately brought to my mind I adopted it for the occasion.

Hints.

By B.

Inspired by Dr. Beacock's interesting "dottings" in the DO-MINION DENTAL JOURNAL, I send you the following snap-shots:

1. Put a piece of linen in your impression cup to prevent the pink compound from sticking to the metal.

2. Instead of linen, use a bit of rubber dam, wet with soap and water, when you want to separate your flashes while packing.

3. Dissolve black rubber in chloroform. Paint your model two or three coats, and wait a few minutes before you pack with red vulcanite. Having no vermilion, not so likely to have sore mouth.

4. Vulcanize repairs and small plates at 195°. Full dentures, three hours and fifteen minutes at 275°. Thin vulcanite is stronger than thick.

5. Varnish teeth with glycerine before taking impression with pink compound. It will not stick.

6. Alcohol, ammonia and chloroform ; of each take equal parts to clean plates. Add pumice stone and quickly scour.

7. Burn borax before using the solder.

8. If you want a strengthener for upper vulcanite sets, solder a stiff iridium and platinum bar across the front blocks.

9. Bore a hole in your work bench and glue a cork in it.

10. Do not fail to consult a reliable physician if you feel too big for your hat. An expert in insanity preferred.

A Hint.

By G. H. Weagant, Cornwall, Ont.

Occasionally we have a corundum wheel which will not fit a chuck—the whole being too large. An easy way to remedy this fault is to make a small band, larger than the size of the hole, place it over the end of the chuck and pour in some fusible alloy. Remove the band, place the chuck in the lathe, and with a chisel, turn down the alloy to fit the wheel.

Selections.

Extent of Recuperation in Dental Tissues.*

By Dr. W. E. Burkhart, Tacoma, Wash.

In the consideration of pathological conditions we are called upon as a matter of necessity to treat them in relation to, and as a departure from, a hygienic or physiological standard. In searching for relief from pathological phases we must first acquire a full and correct understanding of the anatomy and normal functions of the part. If we trace step by step the degenerative process we shall then, by reversing the conditions, be better able to assist nature in building up again the losses that have been sustained. After making ourselves familiar with the normal conditions, and as we take in hand the work of recovery of diseased tissue, we must keep in mind that all medical and surgical treatment possesses no curative virtues of itself, but is an effort on our part to present the most favorable conditions for nature to do the work of repair. This is recuperation or recovery. In such a busy occupation as dentistry mere theorizing is profitable only for the development of latent talent, and what we need more is the discussion of theories from which we may make practical deductions. I will, therefore, confine my remarks to such as will demonstrate practical conclusions. Whatever may be our theory of dental caries in detail, we know that all destructive agents of tooth structure proceed from the external surface of the tooth. The first substance to be acted upon by the attacking forces of the oral fluids is the enamel on account of its exposed position. This is the hardest of all animal tissues and was evidently the provision

* Read before the Midwinter Dental Congress, San Francisco, by request of the Programme Committee for Washington.

of an all-wise creator, evolved in the eternal fitness of things to protect the less defensive tissue within. Nevertheless, with all this original armor so ingeniously distributed, its very coat of mail constitutes its weakest point of recuperation. Tissue originally highly organic is so heavily loaded by the deposition of the inorganic elements that it is vested with no ability to recover from injury, and only becomes a receptacle for products such as invite further destruction and more disastrous results to the newly exposed dentine beneath. Recuperative power is exercised by the more highly organized tissues and is the result of a demand from the affected part for protection, and after the condition of the part has been made known through the nervous system this is furnished largely through the vascular system. We may consider the enamel as entirely composed of inorganic material in so far as nervous impressions are concerned, and therefore lacks the first principle of recovery, and we must content ourselves with restoring lost portions of it with foreign materials entirely. With all our assistance nature cannot raise a hand to help herself. The next substance in the line of attack is the dentine, which is a very hard and ivory like formation, but less dense than enamel, and the interstices of its tubuli filled with a quasi-organic material somewhat resembling protoplasm, and possessing no definite formation justifying its classification as containing either nerves or blood vessels. Here we begin to develop attributes of organized tissues, for by irritation to the dentine there is developed sensation which clearly shows that an impression has been conveyed even though we are unable to explain the manner in which it is done. A tooth that has been prepared for filling, presenting normal live dentine, if left exposed to the action of the oral fluids for a few days will often be found to have acquired a considerable degree of sensitiveness, though it may not have been sensitive at the time of excavation. This sensitiveness must be the result of some form of irritation to the exposed portion of dentine, and is a notification that destructive agents are at work. It is the office of the nerves to convey this intelligence, but in the absence of nerves the protoplasmic material present must be regarded as conveying these impressions to the pulp from which they can be transmitted in the usual manner. When we come to the question of recuperative power in dentine we must decide yes in some respects and no in others. In dentine not actually destroyed there is this function to a limited extent, but in portions missing art must restore with foreign material the same as in enamel. And here will be noticed, in tissue not yet dissolved, defensive action against destructive agents, by notification through the medium of sensation that all is not well and there is need of reinforcements in the affected location. In tissue diseased, but still possessing a considerable degree of vitality, there is often a decided recovery to the normal standard following the insertion of a filling. The protection afforded the dentine immediately produces an alleviation of the irritation, and many times in the removal of fillings we are surprised to find such densely hand dentine exposed, which is defensive action of the pulp for its own protection. We must allow, then, that dentine under these circumstances has the power of recuperation, depending upon organic principles and general conditions localized in the pulp.

When we come to the pulp we begin the consideration of some of the most highly organized tissue in the whole economy, and within whose realm reaction is most decided and prompt. Immediately following any irritation to this organ there is a call for more blood in accordance with nature's laws, by which she intends to furnish more material for resistance. After resolution of blood to the part comes inflammation, and the blood vessels become engorged and somewhat weakened by their effort to do so much work, producing odontalgia by pressure upon the nerves of the pulp, confined as it is within unyielding walls of ivory.

This condition usually recovers very well under the influence of anodynes and sedatives ; that is they appear to do so, but the permanency of the recovery depends upon the length of time the disease has obtained and the individual recuperative power of the patient. After the pulp is reduced to an apparently healthy condition we are face to face with that ever-recurring problem of capping pulps, the success of which does not consist so much in the visual condition of the organ as it does in its relative pathological aspect. If the pulp is healthy and the capping is done in accordance with well-known scientific principles, complete success may be expected. Why then do dentists who have been all through the capping experience finally give up the practice as a general rule, and only perform the operation in the exceptionably favorable cases and as a general procedure devitalize? Of course we may say that our experience teaches us that this is the safest practice, but what scientific reasons are there which produce results at variance with our early theories? One reason, usually mistaken, why they do not live under any covering than that provided by nature is that they are not healthy when covered up. If they are not healthy, in what condition do we find them? At the point of exposure and point of former irritation, there is in all probability still a discharge of pus, indicating an effort of nature to close up the break in her ranks, or at least a discharge of serum easily degenerated. If now the discharge is limited to the ability of the power of the vascular system to carry away by absorption, all may yet be well, but if sufficient space should exist for the accommodation of these products they will soon become a very decided irritant, or, if the capacity of the vessels is over-taxed, there is certain disaster, and recuperation is not to be expected.

Disappointments along this line come thick and fast. Pulps are very obstinate things ; when you desire to save them they invite you by many pleasant smiles, and we smile to ourselves in congratulation of having discovered the key to unlock their confidence, but by the time we assure ourselves that we are master of the situation they seem to have dropped us in cold indifference, and we cast about us for consolation in approaching death. We find comfort—a mite cool—in the fact that the tendency of all pulps is toward extermination. Other things being equal a pulp would rather die than live. After maturity of a tooth, of course there is not the necessity for the preservation of the pulp that existed previously, nothing seeming to demand it but recuperative power. Nearly all recuperative power is lost with the death of the pulp. To understand the tendency of the pulps to die, let us follow the course of development. First we have all pulp, then a shell of deposited inorganic material at the periphery, gradually calcifying from here toward the centre, and co-extensive with this process is the reduction in sizes of the pulp until at mature life it remains a comparatively small organ occupying the central portion of the crown and root. After complete calcification has taken place there seems little use for it except to bestow its power of recuperation in case of disease or accident, as the gradual reduction in size is accompanied by gradually diminishing function. Some have said that the pulp is no longer needed after maturity, but I think that its value as a health-maintainer is sufficient to save it whenever that can be done.

There is always plenty of time to devitalize after a pulp will not live. Quite often the recuperative function is sufficient to bring about a state of health in the root after a portion is dead and amputated. The attenuated shape of the root portion is favorable for this, but I am of the opinion that the results' will not justify the practice to any extent. Our patients expect from us usually more permanent work than we can expect from preserving stumps, and we must keep in mind that the recovery of pulps is generally temporary in its character, and considerable allowance must be made in prognosis. Sedatives may restore a pulp to the normal condition if the inflammation is of recent origin; but it is apt in more aggravated cases to show a steady decline, and at the least irritation at a subsequent time give up life entirely though you have put an abiding faith in it.

In irritations of the gums and peridental membrane from the deposit of salivary calculus, it is remarkable what a contrast is presented in recuperative power to that of the pulp, as it is well known with what rapidity inflamed and ulcerating surfaces of these tissues will subside after removal of the irritant, many times without further treatment. And in all diseases of the gums and membrane due to local causes nature only needs a chance to do her repair work, and when this is afforded her she makes rapid strides and does all and more than we could well expect. It has been authoritatively stated by the originator of the implatation—Dr. Younger—that he has had under his observation an implanted tooth that has the attribute of " sensitiveness " when touched by an instrument.   This seems at variance to all our understanding of an implanted tooth which may have been out of the mouth for a sufficient time to have completely dessicated the tooth and adherent membrane.   A tooth out of the mouth for some time must be dead—so dead that it cannot be resurrected—neither can the dead membrane come to life again ; that is out of the question in my mind ; I mean the identical tissue that once was dead ; I do not believe that the recuperative power in the most favorable cases can approach to this length.   Though I have seen no explanation of the return of sensitiveness in the implanted tooth reported by Dr. Younger, it is clear to me how such a condition may be brought about.   You know about the sponge graft, how new tissue may be rapidly produced and extended in which granulations are induced to rapidly flow in and fill up the graft, using the sponge as a matrix.

Now the sponge is never removed except as nature cares for it and removes it through the circulation by absorption, but we do not think the sponge is left in place as a sponge nor do we think that the sponge as such is created into live tissue.   We believe that nature is able to carry away atom by atom in her mysterious way every particle of sponge according to her necessity, and replace it cell by cell with vitality, in a manner corresponding to that of petrification.   When wood is petrified the wood does not turn to stone as we thought in our boyhood days, but each tiny atom as it is dissolved out is replaced by an atom of silica, which is, to all appearance of form, the structure of wood it always had been, but in fact they are cells of an entirely new material built in the same matrix.   In the implanted tooth we are instructed to choose a tooth with a fair share of peridental membrane adherent to the root, as a necessary qualification for success, and left to infer that the membrane comes to life again.   It does this in appearance, but as this result is not reasonable to me I believe that it forms the matrix for a new peridental membrane in the same manner that the sponge does in the graft, and is not revived to life again but is replaced by new tissue vitally formed.   I see no reason why this should not be true, and that even the dental tubuli or the uncalcified portion of the cementum could not be penetrated by live matter capable of transmitting to the nerves impression in a relative manner to which it is conveyed by the protoplasmic substance originally occupying these same dental tubes.   I see in this theory an effort of nature to extend her power of recovery to original conditions made favorable by science, though it reaches beyond our usual expectations. Accepting this, we can easily see, even in the absence of a pulp, how sensation could be conveyed through the tooth substance to some of the many nerves reflected at the dental ligament. An analogous condition you may have noticed many times when a live pulp has been removed ; there is still sensation along the sides of the canal conveyed by the many filaments, penetrating through the dentine and cementum, making connection with the peridental membrane. However, this usually disappears after a day or two on account of the death of the connecting substance, especially if the canal is dressed with a medicament that would tend to destroy it.

In alveolar abscess the tendency of the surrounding tissue to rapid recovery is well known. In the usual cases the removal of the cause of disease is all that is necessary, and in the unusual cases perhaps persistent treatment and occasionally the removal of necrosed bone, but this latter is very rarely necessary considering the large number of cases presenting. The remarkable thing about alveolar abscesses is that nature is particularly tolerant of them and very often carries them along for years without any very alarming effects, when, if situated in other parts of the body, the condition would immediately become serious. In closing, I will say that I have made no effort to exhaust this subject, but only an attempt to bring before you a few of the most prominent points that have claimed my attention at various times, and will here submit a recapitulation of my conclusions that you may get them in a few condensed statements :

1st. Enamel has no recuperative power, and all loss of tissue must be restored artificially.

2nd. Dentine has no recuperative power so far as the restoration of lost tissue is concerned, but does possess such from a defensive point of view, and may recalcify softened tissue.

3rd. Pulps have recuperative power but,

4th. The tendency of all pulps is toward extermination.

5th. The peridental membrane and contiguous tissue have remarkably strong recuperative power.—*Pacific Dental Journal.*

Science in Dentistry.*

In the April issue of the *Dental Cosmos* of the present year there appeared a thoughtful editorial on " The Scientific Status of the Dental Profession," in which it was held in effect that, in this country, the art of dentistry had outgrown the science ; that our profession was tending toward a mechanical rather than a scientific

---

* Read before the Midwinter Fair Dental Congress.

excellence. It is not my intention here to combat or controvert in any sense the opinion of the writer, in which, indeed, I most fully share, but to call attention to certain aspects of the question that appear to me to have been left partly undeveloped, or, at most, merely suggested or touched upon.

Dentistry in America has, so far, been a natural growth ; it has developed from the needs of our people. The white race, not yet perhaps thoroughly acclimated to our extremes of climate, coming here as pioneers and undergoing the physical changes necessitated by the altered environment—the effects of mixture of races, new habits of diet, and especially a most rapid, and, as it were, abnormal mental stimulus—under all these new conditions, has, with the need, developed the remedy to an extent perhaps greater than in any other part of the civilized world.

The art of dentistry owes more to America than to any other country, as the standing and success of American dentists abroad during the past forty or more years sufficiently demonstrates. It is in this country also that the first systematic efforts at special dental education were made ; where the beginning of the elevation of dentistry from an art to a learned profession was first attempted ; and, whatever may be the status of dentistry here or elsewhere, so much must rightly be attributed to the credit of American dentists. The amount of human suffering that has been made unnecessary by the inventive genius of the dental profession of this country is incalculable, even when not taking into account its share in the giving of that priceless boon of surgical anæsthetics to the world.

In the natural evolution of things, however, a new state of affairs has been produced, one that requires a certain change of face on the part of the dental profession, if it is to hold what ought to be its proper place in the scientific world, and in the estimation of the public. While dentistry was only an art we easily held the lead, and it was not an unnatural presumption for us to think that progress on the same general lines that had so far lead to success would fail us no more in the future than in the past. We had created practical dentistry as an independent profession in which our pre-eminence was recognized throughout the world.

In doing this, however, we have harrowed our field and separated ourselves from those who should recognize us as co-workers in a common field of usefulness. Dental surgery is a branch of medical science ; it is really a specialty in the broader field of medicine. While this is the truth, which no one who considers it can gainsay, it is practically ignored by the public and by ourselves. There is no reason why a surgeon who limits his practice to the oral region should be less of a physician than one who confines himself to the eye, the nose or throat, or the pelvic organs ; the collateral relations of the one are not less extensive than those of the other.

Yet, at the present time, a dentist ranks lower in popular estimation, I think we must all admit, than a physician or surgeon.

If I interpret correctly a recent decision, this view has received judicial sanction, and is part of the judge-made law of the land. To-day the dentist stands, to the public, somewhere between the physician and chiropodist; his social position approaches the former; his professional rank as a specialist, outside of the lines of legitimate medicine, is nearer than we could wish to the latter.

I state these facts, as to the unsatisfactory status of our profession in certain respects, as a preliminary to what I wish to say as to its present needs, which have been so ably commented upon by the editor of the *Dental Cosmos*. The time has come, it seems to me, for us to take a higher stand to elevate our specialty, not only in popular reputation but in fact. We have one great advantage: the prestige of American dentistry from its past in good, and is only now threatened by the danger that we underestimate the importance of further progress. The world recognizes our manual skill and invention, and it is not a small matter that the leading teacher of dentistry in Germany, if not on the continent of Europe, should be an American, with all the honors that it is possible for a German university to bestow upon him. We have in this the advantage over our brethren in general medicine, for, notwithstanding what the world owes to American physicians in the progress of medical science, European writers have not yet learned to look to this country leading in the scientific branches of the profession. That this will be less the case in the future no one who observes the tendencies of American medicine at the present will doubt; and it should be our wish and our earnest effort that American dentistry should also continue the progress it has made. At the present, as Dr. Kirk says, the tendency is too much the other way; "no one who even superficially observes the matter can fail to see that our trans-Atlantic *confreres* produce an aggregate of scientific work in dentistry which far exceeds the output in this country in the same lines." This being so, and continuing to be so, it is inevitable that American dentistry must fall in the estimation of scientific men, and, as their dicta are followed invariably by the reading and thinking public, it must therefore decline still more in popular estimation.

There is no good reason why this should be so, and such reason as exists is not any defence for the actual conditions. Americans are not intellectually behind their co-workers in other lands; the ability to do scientific work is not lacking, nor are there in dentistry the deficiencies that exist in some other departments as compared to those abroad. Our clinical facilities are as extensive as those abroad, and our powers of observation certainly are not inferior. The real difficulty is the lack hitherto of the scientific spirit, and of what I may call the scientific atmosphere, which is the encourager and breeder of the spirit of scientific research. Nevertheless this is coming to us, if it is not here ; and, as Dr. Kirk says, there is, even now, "a proportion, small though it may be, of workers in the dental ranks who find or make the time to investigate problems in dental science which have a wider scope and broader application than the direct utilitarian." Were there more of these, and could they impress upon the whole of our profession a little of their spirit, the conditions of which I now complain could not exist. The trouble is that we have too much adopted what Mr. Howells says is the ideal of our country— business success—as our aim and not kept sufficiently in mind that "wisdom is the principal thing," and that with all our getting we should get understanding. We do not seem to understand what scientific work is, or how to go about getting it.

If we wish our profession to stand high in this country we should follow the lead of the regular medical profession that is now in almost every section raising its qualifications, and that has always had an ethical ideal which, although sneered at by the laity, has kept it, even at its lowest stage, within the traditions of a learned profession. At the present, in all our great centres, like New York, Philadelphia, Boston, Baltimore, etc., there is a large body of physicians acknowledged to be equals of any in the world, and their influence and example are elevating all the rest. I think I am safe in saying that, while there yet remains much to be desired, the time is coming and will probably be within the lifetime of some of us when there will be centres of medical education in this country that will turn the tide to some extent, and students will cross the Atlantic to sit at the feet of the masters on this side. The reproach that American medical science is in its "kindergarten" will not be, I think, much longer justified.

What is needed now is that American dentistry should raise its standard and make its reputation as a scientific specialty of medicine, not a manual art. Hitherto it has been one of the easiest ways to get a living—no thorough educational qualifications, no strict ethical observance, and, in short, no high grade of professional honor or feeling being universally exacted of its followers. Our cities are full of purely commercial dentists, who organize in associations, incorporate themselves for profit, and advertise without scruple or limit. To the general public we are all on one level, and that is apt to be the level of the lowest in its estimation. This is to a great extent due to the fact that some of the teachers in our colleges are men of mercantile propensities, uneducated, and in some instances not only dishonest but unprofessional. We should expect students graduated from such institutions to develop into a lower order of professional life.

To make dentistry a recognized specialty in medicine we will have to demand a medical education in the broadest sense for our dentists, and I believe that it is in this way that true reform will have to be effected. If the dental profession of some State would work for a law modelled somewhat after some of the medical practice acts that are now going into execution, requiring every one who enters the practice of dentistry after a certain date to show proofs that he has received a liberal and a medical education, and to stand an examination, not only in dental manipulation, but also in the general principles of medical science, we would elevate our profession at once. It would be but a few years until the dentists of that State were appreciated both at home and abroad ; they would take rank among their medical *confreres*, and share the advantage of wider association and a broader field of work and usefulness. With a medical education dentists could with a great advantage do a large share of the facial surgery that now passes into other hands.

With such a change the charge that American dentistry is not scientific could not long be justified. Instead of literature " replete with statements and arguments based upon mere speculation, with no foundation of fact beyond that constructed in the brain of the originator," we would begin to have reports judiciously made, original observations and scholarly criticisms upon those of others. Our people are observing and ingenious, and what they most generally lack is not the power of observation, but the education that will enable them to know what to observe. This can only be obtained by study, and can only become general with a higher grade of mental and scientific culture than we have hitherto deemed an essential for membership in our profession. However observant and ingenious a man may be, unless he knows what others have already done, he must waste his mental energies in vain in uselessly going over their work, and the publication of the results of his labors, however strenuous, instead of ranking him with the discoverers, gives him the credit only of his ignorance. There has been a vast amount of misapplied mental labor in this particular direction. I have in mind four men of ability who have contributed largely to the literature of the profession, in which hardly an original idea has been added to advance the progress of our specialty ; a lifetime having been wasted in laborious work which has not borne the fruits desired.

Even when really original observations are made, this defective knowledge stands in the way of due credit being given to their author. The world does not look for figs on what it is inclined to consider as thistles, and valuable facts may be ignored or overlooked because they are published where no one looks for them, or because they are hidden among the mass of comparatively worthless material that emanates from so many writers whose only ability is to rehash old facts or emit baseless speculations or commonplace generalities. To be sure this is also done abroad, but there is less of it and at least a reputation of more scholarship and original work. They are now learning to respect American medical science more than was formerly done, and yet "*Americana sunt, non legunter*" is too often their off-hand disposal of really meritorious contributions from this side of the ocean. Some eighteen or twenty years ago a New York physician published a paper, giving out views, based on observation that within the past few years have revolutionized opinions in regard to an important class of ailments the world over. A German author recently in alluding to them said, in excuse for the neglect they had met with in his country, that they originated in America, where medical science had been up to the present and still is in its " kinderschule." The " certain condescension in foreigners," that Lowell satirized, is often still too manifest in medical matters, and it should be the wish and endeavor of every true American to do away with any just ground on which it can be based. I say nothing of unjust ones, for I trust we are not a people who will willingly submit to injustice.

If American dentistry wishes to keep the rank it has won in the practical development of the art, in its present more scientific phases, it must raise its standards of culture, and require of its practitioners a higher grade of requirements, both general and professional, than has heretofore been its rule. I see no better ideal for it than that of being considered as a specialty in the great field of medicine. To be recognized as such we must widen our studies and be able to view our work in all its relations to the human system ; a specialist who is not also a well-educated physician is justly not in good standing in the medical profession. I care not what views are held by others in regard to the study of our specialty, if any advancement is made, it can only be accomplished (as I have said over and over again) by obtaining a broad, liberal, medical education. We must cultivate a liberal professional, rather than a commercial, spirit in our specialty. We may not be able to realize this ideal at once, but we can work toward it, and that it will be attained, if we desire it, I have no doubt. We cannot look to the medical profession to come to us ; the lesser cannot include the greater ; but it has abundant room to take us in, and there is no doubt of its good will if we only accept the conditions it imposes upon its own members. For the present we might look for a friendly appreciation only ; an organic union is only a possibility of the future. But by standing still, or following some of our present tendencies, I fear the difference between us, both as regards professional standing and public estimation, will widen instead of diminish.—*Pacific Coast Dentist.*

3

The Effect of Exercise upon the Teeth.

By A. HUGH HIPPLE, L.D.S., D.D.S., Omaha.

The action of the American Medical Association in establishing a dental section, and thereby recognizing dentistry as a specialty of medicine. has not only conferred dignity upon that calling and secured for its practitioners recognition as professional men, but it has also furnished them with an incentive to familiarize themselves with those broad principles that underlie the practice of medicine. On the other hand it has called the attention of physicians to the fact that the condition of the teeth has much to do with the condition of the general system, and patients are nowadays referred by them to the dentist quite as frequently as to the surgeon. But although physicians are beginning to recognize the seriousness of diseases of the teeth, and to impress upon their patients the importance of having them properly attended to whenever they show signs of decay, the fact that a rapid deterioration of these organs is now going on and that serious results are likely to follow this deterioration has been almost entirely overlooked. A little inquiry and investigation, however, must convince anyone that such a change for the worse is taking place. Children rarely have as good teeth as their parents had at the same age, but on the contrary their teeth are often almost hopelessly decayed before the dentures of their parents show signs of impairment. A century ago the city of New York, with a population of about fifty thousand, had only one dentist, and although much less attention was paid to the teeth then than is paid to them now, there is abundant evidence to show that our forefathers had better teeth than we have. Dr. Hammond tells us that the coming man will be hairless and toothless, and the tendency certainly seems to be in that direction. The conservation of the natural teeth is the end toward which every intelligent and conscientious dentist directs his efforts, but if the quality of the teeth continues to deteriorate the replacement of lost dental tissue must gradually give way to the replacement of lost dental organs. Every physician knows, of course, that this would not be conducive to health, but that medical men generally do not realize how important a bearing the condition of the teeth has upon the health and longevity of an individual is shown by the fact that in examining applicants for life insurance no question regarding the condition of the mouth is ever asked. The teeth may be so badly decayed that the proper mastication of food is impossible, the saliva may be vitiated, the gums and alveoli may be the seat of abscesses that are continually discharging pus, but these conditions do not concern the examining physician. Probably not one in a thousand, in reporting upon the application of a man twenty-five years of age, would think of mentioning the fact that he had lost, say, all his upper teeth and half his lower ones, although after giving it a little thought few would probably care to dispute the statement that the loss of the teeth before the twenty-fifth year will on the average shorten the life of an individual by at least several years. If this be true, no apology is needed for calling the attention of medical men to the dental deterioration that has been referred to, for discussing its probable causes, and for suggesting possible remedies.

In endeavoring to ascertain why it is that imperfect dentures are so common and dental diseases so alarmingly prevalent, it must be borne in mind that although the teeth are vital organs, developed and nourished very much like the other organs of the body, they differ from them widely in susceptibility to disease. While other organs may be delicate early in life and afterward become quite strong and healthy, or *vice versa*, the teeth, if not impaired by disease, remain the same, with the exception, perhaps, of a slight increase of density as age advances. All the other organs of the body, too, including the bones, are endowed with recuperative powers whereby injuries are to a greater or less extent repaired ; but the teeth possess no such attributes, and are apparently governed by somewhat different laws from those that regulate other parts of the animal economy. Teeth that are perfect in form and structure are rarely, if ever, attacked by decay. It is only where the enamel is defective that dental caries can obtain a foothold. As the teeth are developed early in life, it is during childhood that those influences are exerted which by interfering with their development predispose them to disease, and it is to childhood, therefore, that we must look for the causes of dental deterioration.

Scientists tell us that use and disuse have much to do with the development of organs, and that with the progress of civilization the brain has increased and the jaws have decreased in size. The wisdom teeth from disuse have degenerated and become rudimentary ; the canines, being no longer needed to tear flesh from the bone and do other heavy work, have become smaller and less prominent ; the teeth in general have become soft and chalky and very susceptible to decay. This, they say, is the result of the substitution of soft, well-cooked food for that which required vigorous use of the teeth and masticatory muscles, and as there seems to be no likelihood of civilized man going back to primeval methods of preparing food, the inference is that dental deterioration is one of the prices we are obliged to pay for a high state of civilization. But use and disuse not only modify the size and structure of organs when persisted in for a series of generations, but their effect upon the organs of any one individual are no less marked. Tie up an arm so that it cannot be used, and the muscles will soon become soft and flabby, and will eventually disappear. Lock up a child in a room by itself with nothing to occupy its thoughts, and it will in time become an imbecile. It appears that a certain amount of exercise is essential to the development of most organs. A part when performing work requires and receives more blood than when at rest, and it much work is performed the blood-vessels increase in size and the part is better nourished. That a close relationship exists between development and nourishment, and between nourishment and exercise, is a fact so well known that it need not be discussed here ; but so far as the study of the teeth is concerned the principle has been applied to the race rather than to the individual. It is undoubtedly true that what the people of a country eat for eight or ten generations will determine in a general way the size and shape of their jaws and the form and structure of their teeth at the end of that time ; but it is probably no less true that what a child eats up to the time he is eight or ten years of age will determine just as certainly what will be the condition of his dental organs for the rest of his life. If the food of the child is such as requires vigorous use of the jaws, the blood supply will be liberal, the parts will be well developed, and the teeth will not be likely to suffer from decay. On the other hand, if the child is fed on soft food, requiring little or no active mastication, the jaws and teeth will be poorly nourished, and the latter at least will be defective in structure. Erupted into the mouth in that condition, no amount of care can protect them from the ravages of decay, which will sooner or later impair their usefulness and mar their beauty.

It must be remembered in this connection that although none of the temporary teeth make their appearance in the mouth until the child is five or six months of age, their crowns are almost fully developed at birth, and that the jaws of a newly-born child also contain the germs of twenty-four of the permanent teeth in various stages of development. These permanent teeth do not begin to erupt until the child is about six years of age, but during that time the process of calcification is continually going on. ' With the first molars, the incisors and the canines, it is well started by the end of the first year ; with the bicuspids, at the end of the second year ; and with the second molars at about the fifth year. It will thus be seen that between the second and fifth years this process of calcification upon which depends the future character of the teeth is in most active progress. Nature intended that during this period the jaws and teeth should be well exercised, and to that end provided the child with a perfect temporary set of teeth, but, as a matter of fact, they are used but very little compared with the other organs of the body. The muscles of the arms, legs and head are in almost constant use, and are consequently always well supplied with blood. The brain is wrestling with the problems of life as they present themselves, and it, too, is being exercised and developed. The eye is being trained to examine every object, and the ear to catch the slightest sound, but the teeth are hardly used at all. Nine out of ten mothers feed their children of that age on soft food. Bread made from fine flour, biscuits soaked in tea or milk, meat cooked tender and cut into small bits, with potatoes and other vegetables in such a condition that they require little or no mastication, form the chief food of the little three-year-olds. Not being actively exercised, the teeth and jaws need but a small quantity of blood, and, owing to the imperfect development that results from insufficient nourishment, they are unable to resist the attacks of the pathogenic germs that are always present in the mouth, and which eventually destroy them.

The remedy is in the hands of parents. If they will see that their children, at the earliest possible age, use their first teeth vigorously, they need have little anxiety in regard to the second set. In other words, if a demand is created for sound, solid teeth, nature will be almost certain to supply them. It is by no means difficult to teach children to chew their food. Nothing pleases small children more than to be allowed to nibble a hard biscuit or bite the meat from a bone. Nature prompts them to exercise their teeth in that way, just as it prompts a puppy to spend hours gnawing at a bone which has long since been stripped of its meat. But the average mother, partly, no doubt, out of respect to dainty dresses and well-kept carpets, but more particularly from fear of possible injury to the teeth themselves, objects to the dental calisthenics in which the child would gladly indulge, and thereby unconsciously opposes the efforts of nature to develop good teeth. Since teeth that are perfect in structure rarely if ever decay, an ounce of prevention in the way of developing healthy dental organs is certainly worth more than a pound of cure after they are diseased ; and if parents will supply their children with an abundance of bone-producing food, see that the teeth are kept clean, have them examined and attended to from time to time by a competent dentist, and, above all, have them well exercised by chewing hard food, nature will do her part, and their children in after years will rejoice in the possession of that almost priceless endowment, a beautiful and complete set of teeth.

Correspondence.

Errors in Report of Union Meeting of Ontario Dental Society and Eastern Ontario Dental Association.

To the Editor of the DOMINION DENTAL JOURNAL :

SIR,—I wish to draw attention to a few errors in the report of the above meeting. While they are comparatively unimportant they are slightly misleading to those who were not present.

For instance, in the report of members present, Dr Clement, Kingston, who was ill during the forepart of the convention, and Drs. Black, Daly and Aykroyd, also of Kingston, who did not happen to be at the first meeting, attended subsequent meetings. Others arrived after the first meeting, *e.g.*, Dr. Barce, Brockville, detained in the West, Dr. Mabee, Gananoque. Dr. Weagant, Smith's Falls, and Dr. McCulloch, Perth. All these were members of the Eastern Ontario Dental Association.

I am represented as reporting Dr. Abbott to recommend Hg. Cl. " 1 to 1,000 " for disinfecting pulp canal. He says " 1 to 10,000." In the discussion, Dr. Klotz said he himself used 1 to 1,000.

The report tells us that the Eastern Ontario Dental Association did not decide upon a place of meeting next year ; while, as a fact an invitation from Smith's Falls was accepted for next year's meeting.

R. E. SPARKS.

Reviews.

Napheys' Modern Therapeutics. In two handsome volumes of 1,000 pages each. Vol. I., General Medicine and Diseases of Children. Vol. II., General Surgery, Obstetrics and Diseases of Women. Ninth edition. Edited by ALLEN J. SMITH, M.D., and J. AUBREY DAVIS, M.D. $6 per volume.

Each volume sold separately. A most complete and exhaustive *resumé* of the best methods of treating diseases, including all new remedies that have proved of practical value, and about 2,500 precise formulæ. For sale by E. M. Renouf, 2,238 St. Catharine Street, Montreal.

A Practical Treatise on Surgery. With special reference to treatment. By C. W. MANSELL MOULTIN, A.M., M.D. (Oxon.)
Second American edition. Edited by JOHN B. HAMILTON,
M.D., LL.D. 600 illustrations, over 200 of which are original,
many of which are printed in several colors. 1,200 pages.
Cloth $7, leather $8. For sale by E. M. Renouf, 2,238 St. Cath-
erine St., Montreal.

This is not only the latest, but the most complete text-book on
Surgery. Critical authorities declare that this is the best text-
book for the student and general work of reference for the practitioner, and is eminently practical. The special attention to treatment, so systematically neglected in similar works, is one of its
leading features. To the dentist it is specially useful wherein it
discusses the injuries and diseases of the head, face, nose, mouth
and jaws, tongue, salivary glands, tonsils, larynx, etc.

Special for Dental Students.

" Tomes' Dental Surgery," " Tomes' Dental Anatomy," " Stock-
en's Dental Medicine," " Gorgas' Dental Medicine," " Mitchell's
Dental Chemistry," " Sewill s Dental Surgery," " Richardson's
Mechanical Dentistry," " Essig's Dental Metallurgy," " Taft's
Operative Dentistry," " Black's Dental Anatomy," " Harris' Principles and Practice of Dental Surgery," " Harris' Dental Dictionary," " Fillebrown's Operative Dentistry," " Evan's Crown and
Bridge Work." Mr. E. M Renouf has made special arrangements
to supply dental students with the above text-books, as well as the
text-books required by medical schools. The dental works which
have been translated into French will be found specially valuable
to French students.

Editorial.

A Word to Students.

When a young man starts out in life to equip himself for a
profession, one would naturally suppose, that he would prefer to
select a college whose facilities for teaching are not only of the
best, but whose reputation is, to say the least, savory. There are
colleges and colleges, and there are students and students. We have
seen with our own eyes, and heard with our own ears, the desperate
efforts made to cheapen the curriculum, the bait of " Professor-

ships," etc., offered *ad libitum*, and the generally accepted belief that the degree of D.D.S. is an assured condition of attendance at such and such a school. Even universities under State charters, have stooped to the undignified position of truckling to that element in the dental profession who are affected with "big head," and who verily believe their clay to be a sort of which the Creator had very little to spare. The Sancho Panzas of dentistry who " think themselves fit for government," and who are the first themselves to discover it, are not disposed to bide their time and win their spurs in service. In choosing a school organized from purely factious opposition, a student reveals his own character—that it is not education he yearns for as much as for a title or tail to his name. In a visit we paid several years ago to Chicago, we were struck with this fact, from the very personal appearance of the students in a college under the government of the National Association of Dental Faculties, and one which did not seek that distinction. The latter recalled very forcibly experiences of the average dental college twenty-five years ago.

It is much wiser for a student to make sacrifices to attend the very best school than to receive the highest "honors" an inferior one has to bestow. If the student is poor and ambitious, it is all the more reason why he should endeavor to avail himself of the best. He had better wear a threadbare coat all his life than turn out a gowned fraud. It is no mystery why there are students who positively prefer to attend a cheap and inferior school. It is as clear as noonday. It is no mystery why disappointed people, who over-estimate their own abilities, oppose established colleges, and foment discord. It is as easily understood as the bite of the mad dog.

Doctors, Dentists and Druggists.

They are a drug in the market. You find them in every hole and corner, especially in our cities, many of them having all the evidence externally of hard times. In Quebec, it is the ambition of the *habitant*, who perhaps can neither read nor white, to make some of his sons priests, doctors or lawyers. It seems to us that this thing is overdone in Canada, especially in Ontario and Quebec. It is only by raising the standard that it can be restrained. Unfortunately, however, there seems to be a factious desire to cheapen education. We fully expect to see our profession reduced again to the ranks of the peddling "tooth-carpenter."

There was nothing but the diminished tail of that "same old herring" to be discovered in the last issue of the *Dental Practitioner and Advertiser. Requiescat in pace.*

DOMINION
DENTAL JOURNAL.

VOL. VI.   TORONTO, NOVEMBER, 1894.   No. 11.

Original Communications.

Little Aids in Practice.

(From St. Thomas, Ont.)

AT THE CHAIR.

Perhaps one of the safest methods of annealing sheet gold is upon a piece of mica, when the flame cannot possibly touch the gold. This method works admirably with most makes, but I find that some varieties of soft gold seem to require additional heat, and this too, by direct contact with the flame, after it has been made up ready for use.

To carry very soft mixed cement to the bottom of a cavity, remove it from the spatula on to a wee bit of paper laying at the edge of the glass slide; then, with tweezers, carry this edge-wise up between the two teeth, if an approximal cavity, and press home with an excavator.

Miniature napkins cut or torn from pure white old cotton are preferable to those from new material, and should always be thrown away when once used. I trust none of us have the heart of a certain western operator, who compelled his better-half to wash and iron an innumerable number of these requisites. One of these folded up and laid between the lip and gum, or under the tongue, wonderfully extends our time in brief operations, and makes it quite possible to perform dry work. When removing debris from a cavity, one of these little squares held in the left hand, ready to take the refuse from about the excavator is but another item of carefulness and consideration on the part of the dentist that elevates him in the estimation of the patient ; in fact, the need for these grows so rapidly that we soon find ourselves well supplied with

2

them. Not infrequently persons drop in to have one or more of the incisors ground down to match the rest ; to expedite the work hold a wet sponge against the wheel, and then you can work right along without interruption.

An especially convenient chisel is one rather broad, and the end-cutting edge ground out fish-tailed. The two sides may also be brought to a levelled, sharp edge. Try it.

Shave down silver nitrate and dust this over a freshly exposed pulp, when the patient is enduring great pain and will not tolerate the usual application at once.

When applying the cord, and it persists in slipping back into the cavity, make the knot secure, then carefully push up both it and the dam to position, when it will usually remain.

I have much faith in, and therefore disinfect every cavity immediately before filling.

Keep an oiled wool cloth to finish cleaning instruments, and they will always remain bright.

For use under anæsthetics, one pair of universal forceps should be a part of every set ; in fact, these are never to be despised, if well made, and with curving beaks so to pass well over all crowns and bring the pressure well up on neck of the tooth. I am especially successful with those weak and broken down lower molars, frequently so trying, by taking hold well down or cutting through on to the anterior root, which is the curving one if at all so.

At the Bench.

With certain varieties of flat mouths, score the model close up and around the air chamber, also several more across those soft portions of the palate, usually found on either side of the median line and back from the chamber. When smoothly done, these raises on the palate surface of plate do not seem to irritate the mucous membrane.

Occasionally a sharp, deep groove extends back along the same median line ; use soft palate rubber over this.

Hints.

By W. A. Brownlee, M.D.S.

If the rubber dam is punctured during the process of filling, dry it thoroughly and touch the spot with a thick solution of chlorapercha, such as is used for nerve canals, and allow the chloroform to evaporate before proceeding with the work. This will effectually exclude the moisture.

If you are troubled with the top plate of the flask coming off while packing, drill two holes near the rear end of the plate about half an inch apart, make a loop of heavy brass wire, insert in these holes from the inside and rivet in place. If the loop projects half an inch into the plaster it will not interfere with the denture, and will save you considerable annoyance.

Instead of soldering small strips of gold to clasps to retain them in position on rubber plates, use two platinum pins from a broken porcelain tooth. The clasp is held firmly to the plate, and the plate is not so liable to crack as if the strips are used.

A convenient rubber heater is made by taking a piece of asbestos an eighth of an inch thick and eight inches square ; put a tin rim on it to strengthen it, dip it in water, wipe the surface, lay the rubber, ready cut, upon it, and place over the vulcanizing lamp for a minute or two before packing.

Dark joints, in repairing a denture made with gum sections, are produced by the charring or burning of particles of food, etc., with which the joints have become filled. This cannot be prevented unless the sections are removed from the plate and the adjacent ends dressed on the wheel.

When filling a number of cavities with gold at the same sitting, put on the rubber dam before you begin to prepare the cavities ; remove the rough decay from all, then complete the preparation of the one you suppose will give the least pain, and fill it. By the time you have it completed the other cavities will be so thoroughly dried out that they can be excavated almost without pain. Try it.

Time as a Basis for Charging.

By W. R. WILKINSON, D.D.S., L.D.S., Elmira, Ont.

" How much do you charge to fill a tooth ? " is perhaps a question which your readers have heard before, and one which indicates to the operator that the questioner has a pre-conceived idea firmly fixed in his mind, that every dentist has an unalterable tariff of charges, and that every operation has a definite amount as payment for its performance.

I had a case not a year since where a lady who had previously never had any other work done than simple plugging of cavities, grew righteously indignant, when her account showed her that for treating and filling one tooth alone, I had charged three or four times as much as for any of the other single fillings she had hitherto had inserted. Had this patient reflected that the work in question had occupied, if the time at different sittings were summed up, about three hours, she would likely have had a little compassion on a young operator, and would not have been so swift to withdraw her patronage as she did.

On a line with this lady's action, is that where a patient expects, no charge will be made for failing to extract a root, perhaps even with the process which, it may be, an M.D. has decapitated ten minutes since, or, a frail shelled molar in a mouth which has known no other dental instrument than steel forceps. Notwithstanding the fact that the operator may work just as conscientiously on such work as upon any other, and may spend half an hour, as does happen occasionally, I presume, with some others of the profession as well as myself, there seems to be an understanding more or less widespread among the laity, that dentists charge only for extracting when they succeed in removing the offending organ.

Another patient, whose following is legion, agreed to have me remove an aching pulp and afterwards fill it and the cavity. After due medicament I began the work, and did all I could at first sitting, according to my usual practice in such cases, and dismissed the patient with instructions to call again in three days. Though a faithful promise was made, the next call was indefinitely postponed, and when the account was presented he said the tooth had not pained any since ; and as I had not extracted or filled it, he thought I should have no compensation. Sometimes we are asked to examine a mouth, and make an estimate of charges for doing what we think should be done, and if we comply, we very often find afterwards that on our first examination there was an exposed pulp we did not notice ; also, may be a distal cavity in a molar we could not see and did not probe sufficiently well to find. In these cases, though we may make only an approximate estimate of charges, we are bound by some inward feeling not to exceed it, and consequently in nine out of ten such cases we lose money by losing time.

These and many other cases in practice have caused me to wonder, if *time spent on work* should not be considered the chief basis in making charges. I cannot see my way to believe, that no other considerations should be reckoned with, as all operators do not work equally rapid, nor does the same operator work as rapidly in his first as in his fifth year of practice. Besides this, material is not of uniform price.

I do not deny that charging *by the piece* is with the majority a satisfactory system, but it does seem to me that no one should set up as his ideal of perfection to be able to insert so many sheets of foil in a day or so many amalgam fillings, or to perform any other *measure of quantity* of work; but rather to be able to say at night, "I have worked conscientiously, and have done my best with the work I have had in hand to-day."

The tendency of the fixed system of charges, seems to point to the former ideal rather than to the latter, and it seems to me that if *the time spent* were more generally considered the basis for computing our charges, more general satisfaction would result, better work would be performed, and a higher standard among the professions to-day would be accorded to ours, than which none performs what it undertakes more successfully.

Correspondence.

To the Editor of the DOMINION DENTAL JOURNAL:

SIR,—Are we drifting, or are we keeping well to some wisely selected course? To observe the manner in which Dentistry.is regulated (?) in this Province, would lead one to infer the ruling ambition, the chief *raison d'être* to be the unlimited increment of the by no means inconsiderable army of dentists already existing in this province. I think it will be granted by anyone who has given the matter even casual consideration, that we have *too many* dentists. Here is my own little town—three dental offices, whilst one dentist could do all the work alone. From an economical point of view this is not as it ought to be. When three men offer their services where there is a demand for the services of but one, what wonder that quackery and unprofessional methods become a crying evil? The condition of things is approximating to that which would obtain were there no Dental Act upon the statute book. "There is a good thing in Dentistry," say the boys to themselves, and like good patriots, at the call to arms, the plough, the counter, the forge are each deserted for the glories and emoluments of war! The efficiency of an army does not necessarily depend upon mere numbers. Give us a band of "picked men" if the campaign is to be rendered short, sharp and decisive. We, the dentists, are moving as though devoid of ordinary intelligence. We are permitting our numbers to be increased at a rate that is out of all proportion to the increase of our population, or that of the portion which avails itself of the advantages of dentistry.

Has there been a pronounced effort on the part of the College to limit the number of fresh graduates? Has all been done that could be done under the Act?

We truly seem to be at sea, without chart or compass. Were there something of organization in the dentistry of Ontario, the dental demands of every hamlet and side-line of the Province would be known. How is it with church and political organizations? They know something of the material they have to work upon, and they accomplish something definite. Such should be the learning expected in candidates, and such the strictness of the examinations, that Doctor would be no unbecoming or inappropriate title for the successful candidate to bear.   As to morality or common manliness, all else is vain without these.   Should a high degree of proficiency as a chief requisite be insufficient to limit the number of persons entering the profession, then some other means should be adopted.   That there is an undue rush into the professions, is patent to all except those who are "rushing."   Many of these men, if they knew what was before them, would remain outside of the professions.   Persons before entering a profession should have some approximate notion of what lies before them. Colleges should discourage applicants rather than encourage them, thus becoming instrumental in averting much sorrow and disappointment.   The great mass of the dentists of Ontario have not interested themselves in those matters which pertain to the general welfare of the profession and the public at large.   Apathy is the handmaid of misgovernment and disaster.   I for one must confess *peccavi* to the above charge.   Now I am ready to despair.   The conviction to me is irresistible, that we are on the wrong track. We haste to perpetuate the very evils existing in scores of other occupations.   We build with one hand while we destroy with the other.   There is a manifest want of organization.   Every man does what to himself seemeth good.   There is nothing to be gained by turning one's eyes from the evil, performing what has been called the "ostrich act."   The issue must be looked squarely in the face, and a remedy must be found.   I should like to see a general conference of the dentists of Ontario met, at some central point, and steps taken whereby the "true inwardness" of the whole dental situation in the Province might be made manifest.

Yours very truly,

Ridgetown, October 13, 1894.   A. S. VOGLER, L.D.S.

Proceedings of Dental Societies.

Royal College of Dental Surgeons of Ontario.

The twentieth session of the School of Dentistry of the Royal College of Dental Surgeons of Ontario, Toronto, Ontario, was opened on October 2, in the presence of all the members of the Faculty and about one hundred registered students.   The opening lecture was delivered by Prof. Primrose, who has joined the Faculty since the close of the last session, taking the place of Prof. Peters, who resigned.   Prof. Primrose is an honor graduate in medicine from the University of Edinburgh.   For several years he has been at the head of the Anatomical Department of the Faculty of Medicine in Toronto University.   In the Dental College he takes the chair of Physiology. In his opening lecture he referred briefly to the history of dentistry in ancient times, its more modern developments, and its association and connection with general medicine. He also enlarged somewhat on the importance of the study of comparative Dental Anatomy, pointing out the desirability of the dental student and the dentist being familiar with the dentition of the lower animals, and especially of the vertebrata. The lecture, which was well received by the class, evidenced considerable research on the part of the learned Professor, whose attention has not previously been directed to dental subjects. The class when complete will consist of 50 freshmen, 40 juniors and 45 seniors.

The financial depression and consequent scarcity of money does not seem to have deterred the young men of Ontario from directing their attention to the study of Dentistry. These numbers would seem to be out of proportion to the demand for dental practitioners in the Province. The final outcome of the inevitable competition will be but another illustration of the doctrine of the "survival of the fittest."

The Dental College of the Province of Quebec.

The regular lectures of the Dental College of the Province of Quebec began on October 17th.

The following compose the teaching staff: Medical Course, McGill—Anatomy, Prof. Shepherd; physiology, Prof. Wesley Mills; chemistry, Prof. Girdwood; materia medica, Prof. Blackader; histology, Prof. Wilkins; general pathology, Prof. Adami. Laval —Anatomy, Prof. Mignault; physiology, Prof. Duval; chemistry, Prof. Fafard; materia medica, Prof. Desrosiers; histology, Prof. Duval; general pathology, Prof. Brennan.

Dental Course—Dental pathology and therapeutics—W. Geo. Beers, L.D.S., L. J.ᵃB. Leblanc, L.D.S.; prosthetic dentistry and metallurgy, N. Fiske, L.D.S., S. Globensky, L.D.S.; dental surgery, F. A. Stevenson, D.M.D., L.D.S.; L. Franchere, L.D.S.; operative dentistry, G. W. Lovejoy, M.D., L.D.S.; J. H. Bourdon, L.D.S.; dental jurisprudence, A. Globensky, Esq., Attorney of the Board of Examiners; Crown and Bridge Work, A. McDiarmid, L.D.S.; J. Fortin, L.D.S.; operative technique, J. G. Gardner, L.D.S., Gustave Lemieux, L.D.S.

Clinical Instructors (two or more for each week day)—J. C. Nichols, L.D.S.; R. A. Alloway, D.D.S., L.D.S.; E. B. Ibbotson, L.D.S.; W. G. Throsby, L.D.S.; J. G. A. Gendreau, L.D.S.; L. P. Bernier, L.D.S.; J. S. Ibbotson, L.D.S.; T. Fitzpatrick, L.D.S.; W. S. Nichols, L.D.S; G. Maillet, L.D.S.; A. H. Beers, M.D., D.D.S., L.D.S.; R. Watson, L.D.S. (Montreal); E. Casgrain,

D.D.S., L.D.S.; T. A. Venner, L.D.S.; H. Ievers, L.D.S.; J. Paradis, L.D.S.; J. Dorval, L.D.S.; N. Lemieux, L.D.S. (Quebec); J. Lauder, D.D.S., L.D.S. (Cowansville); C. H. Wells, L.D.S. (Huntingdon); A. W. Hyndman, L.D.S.; G. W. Hyndman, D.D.S., L.D.S.; S. J. Bloomfield, L.D.S. (Sherbrooke); J. Porter. L.D.S. (Danville); J. Cleavland, D.D.S, L.D.S. (Richmond); C. H. Moulton, L.D.S. (Stanstead); J. Brassard, L.D.S. (St. John's); J. Pichette, L.D.S. (Three Rivers).

Honorary—Chas. Brewster, L.D.S.; C. F. F. Trestler, M.D., L.D.S.; J. A. Bazin, L.D.S.; H. D. Ross, D.D.S., L.D.S.; S. J. Andres, L.D.S.

The opening lecture was very largely attended, and was delivered by Dr. Beers. The following is a synopsis :

The opening of the second session of the Dental College established by the Legislature, by the unanimous vote and voice of the profession in Quebec, marks an epoch of more than immediate interest. Our sister province, Ontario, led us in the matter of legislation by one year ; but one of the earliest movements made in the English-speaking world in that direction, was a little over half a century ago in this city, when the late Dr. Bernard, the first president of our association, endeavored to get a clause regulating dentistry inserted in a medical bill then before the Legislature, almost simultaneously with the passage of the first dental law—that of Alabama. Three years previously the *American Journal of Dental Science*, the first journal of the kind in the world, had been issued in New York, and a little army of earnest men, led by Harris, opened the first dental college, that of Baltimore. Naturally enough they made some trifling mistakes, and displayed their humanity in some error ; and at once they were assailed as the foes rather than the friends of dentistry. It was a grim gratification to the iconoclasts, when they discovered weak points in the armor of the fathers of our profession. It was a wise saying of Disraeli that " the defects of great men are the consolation of the dunces "; and it is suggestive to remember, that while the names of Harris, Parmly, Baker, Brown, Hayden and others live in history, and will be ever green in our memories, every name of the obstructionists has been forgotten. The fragrance and the fruit of honest work can never die. The mischief done may have a temporary survival ; but the motives as well as the memories of the factious obstructionist will surely perish. The influence of what may be called the reform movement soon extended to Canada, and indeed to England ; for in 1841 Mr. George Waite, an eminent dentist of London, issued a pamphlet advocating the recognition of dentistry by Parliament and the medical profession, " as a legitimate branch of the science, and that no person be permitted hereafter to practise without having undergone examination by one or more censors of the Royal College of Dental Surgeons." Mr. Waite suggested not only a thorough training in the fundamental branches of medicine and surgery, but a preliminary requirement of mathematics and mechanical philosophy; and that three courses of anatomy, physiology and chemistry, together with hospital practice, should be made compulsory. It was not, however, until 1843 that any effort was made to obtain dental legislation in England, when it occurred in precisely the same manner as Dr. Bernard had attempted the previous year. France, Germany and Austria had stolen a march upon the English-speaking world of dentistry, and had several years before demanded certain legal qualifications to practise. Hunter, Fox, Blake, Bell and Kœcker in England ; Delabarre, Maury, Desirabode and Jourdain in France, had written valuable works on the teeth and their diseases. When boasting, as we sometimes do, of our professional achievements on this continent, we should not forget the original researches of the fathers and founders over the sea. We should not ignore, too, the fact that, until comparatively recent years, the dental colleges of the United States, with all their splendid practical character, drank almost exclusively at the scientific and theoretical fount of British inspiration ; and that to this day there are no text-books to surpass for original research and close reasoning the classics produced by British, French and German writers. I take pleasure in looking backward on these events, because they inspire us to look forward. As our fathers made history for us, we are making it for posterity. It may be a pride you will pardon, that some of us here this evening enjoy the retrospect in our own province of a quarter of a century, when we gathered together the disconnected elements of the profession, organized the first association, and obtained the first act of incorporation. It will be remembered that the effort of Dr. Bernard was fruitless, because, no doubt it was premature.

It is perhaps as foolish to attempt some things too soon as too late. It was reserved for Dr. Chas. Brewster to take the helm at the opportune time. Aided by the generous and sympathetic encouragement of Drs. Bazin, Trestler and the late Dr. Webster, the movement began in earnest, by a successful professional protest to the Committees of Exhibitions, against the bestowal of prizes for mechanical dentistry. In the document Dr. Brewster then (1860) issued to the dentists of Upper and Lower Canada, he revived the proposal for legislation in the interests of the public and the profession, and his chief correspondent in the Upper Province was Dr. B. W. Day, of Kingston, who was thus inspired to start the ball rolling, and who became the father of dental legislation in Ontario seven years afterwards. On September 2, 1868, the first meeting was held in this city to organize the Dental Association of the Province of Quebec, at which the following were present: Messrs. Brewster, Bernard, Bazin, Trestler, Cantwell, Alloway and Beers. On the 17th of the same month another

meeting was held, which met with a heartier response. The following were present: Messrs. Brewster, Bernard, Bazin, Trestler,
Leblanc, Webster, Belle, Alloway, Valois, Nichols and Beers, of
Montreal ; McKee, of Quebec ; Lefaivre, of St. John's ; Dowlin, of
Sherbrooke, and Brodeur, of St. Hyacinthe. There were a few
men who believed they had encompassed the limits of dental
knowledge, and that the best education was to be sought for at
the bench of the jeweller, or, at best, in the laboratory. They
opposed the Dental Act of Incorporation, as they would, had they
lived in the days of Moses, have opposed the passage of the Ten
Commandments, as an arbitrary piece of legislation. The proposal
made at that remote date, that the student should embrace in his
curriculum certain of the medical and surgical branches, was considered as preposterous as a suggestion that he should study
Sanscrit. The cry went forth that the only knowledge a dentist
needed was practical, that a dentist had no more need of a
knowledge of the anatomical and histological structures of the
teeth and adjacent tissues, than a barber had of the physiology
of the hair in order to cut it, or a butcher of the comparative
anatomy of the cow, in order to serve the public with a sirloin
or a fillet. This conviction of the exclusive importance of practical knowledge, no doubt, originated the sarcastic expression that
the dentist was nothing but a "tooth carpenter;" and yet it
seems to animate some otherwise enlightened members of our
profession to-day. And, indeed, no inconsiderable portion of the
public are not only led by the same opinion, but voluntarily invite
all sorts of imposture from advertising humbugs. Even to-day
it would seem as if a portion of the public, and not alone in the
townships, revel in the prospect of their own deception, and
measure men not by their professional or collateral education, but
by the loudness of their pretensions. I am sure that no sensible
practitioner depreciates practical skill. None of us can succeed
without it. It would be a gross incongruity to pretend to ignore
the importance of a branch which this college and the Board of
Examiners so emphatically enforce. It would be foolish to
disparage any branch of the mechanical arts, especially when in
this city, by the munificence of Mr. W. C. McDonald, the University of McGill has now in operation the most complete course of
instruction on this continent in Applied Science, embracing the
finest workshops and museums, as well as perfectly equipped
laboratories in mathematical, chemical, physical, electrical, mag-
netic and testing branches. I look forward to the time when the
curriculum of our own college will be privileged to embrace some
of these branches in this magnificent institution. The supersti-
tion that a man cannot be both theoretical and practical was
founded upon ignorance. No better annihilating retort can be
made to such an assumption, than the record of the best thinkers

and operators in our own profession, as well as the theoretical
and practical courses required for graduation in our dental
colleges, and in such an institution as that of the Applied Science
of McGill.

At the same time, we must recognize with imperative force,
that the dentist whose education does not embrace to-day the
fundamental subjects of anatomy, physiology, chemistry, materia
medica, histology, part of pathological anatomy, oral surgery and
microscopy, is an imperfectly educated man, "a fractionally qualified being." It is not an impossible educational feat to take an
average boy out of the gutter, and in a year or two produce a
fair and sometimes a first-class mechanical dentist. It is quite
probable that a very fair practical operator may be made out of a
man who can neither write, read nor spell his mother tongue.
Such a man may even rise to a high pinnacle in public opinion,
because public opinion asserts its right to judge for itself in
matters it does not understand. Technical and manual skill are
indispensable ; but they are so much more easily attained that
students are apt to slight the preliminary branches upon which
they are founded. As dentists, we have frequent experience of
the ignorance medical men display of the direct and indirect
diseases of the teeth. Having abandoned the teeth to the dentist,
they are apt to overlook the relations of dental lesions to diseases
of other parts. Cases are not infrequent of serious diseases
originating direstly in diseased teeth ; of reflex ocular and aural
disorders induced by dental irritation ; of neuralgic affections of
the most intense character ; epilepsy and paralysis caused by
carious teeth. The extensive sympathetic connections of the
trigeminal nerve easily explain why the neck, face, throat or any
of the parts associated that are supplied by the nerve itself, may
be the seat of reflex trouble. Dental abscesses have been mistaken for scrofula. If there is one thing more than another which
marks the highest dental standard to-day, from what it was a
quarter of a century ago, it is not, by any means, the advancement in the mechanical and purely practical, but the closer connection established between the sciences embraced in bacteriology
and pathology ; the study of the relation of fermentation to
caries, and the knowledge that just as the brain is dependent
upon the heart and lungs for its supply of arterial blood, as the
heart is dependent upon the brain for nervous energy, and upon
the lungs to purify its blood ; as the action of the lungs cannot
be sustained without the influence of the nervous system and the
propelling action of the heart, so is the dependence and inter-
dependence of the dental organs upon their immediate neighbors,
and frequently upon distant organs. We should therefore enjoy
the legitimate pride in the reflection that, while we claim to be a
distinct profession, dealing with the most prevalent disease of the

age, we are or should be governed by the same fundamental
principles of medicine and surgery as the general practitioner;
and that the exclusively practical man, who wilfully ignores or
who is content to remain ignorant of these principles, can no
more claim rank as a scientific dentist, than the manufacturer of
orthopedic appliances can claim rank as a surgeon. Every
province of our Dominion is infested with the "local anæsthetic"
fiend, whose office is converted into a dental abattoir. Every city
and many a town has its professional charlatan, and it is only by
the influence which will emanate from our educated and ethical
members that the public will learn to detect deception, even if
true "science be dragged at the heels of sensation."

Referring to the College Dr. Beers said : When by the unanimous vote and voice of the dentists of this province, at the largest
meeting ever held, the desire was repeated for the third time in
their history, and finally put into a resolution to seek for affiliation
with one French and one English University—Laval and McGill
—it was done in no selfish or offensive spirit. It was simply a
matter of business ; a conviction that concentration was desirable
in the interests of the students ; that it was not as desirable to
enter into the wholesale and retail manufacture of Doctors of
Dental Surgery, as a collateral boost to impecunious institutions,
as it was desirable to place our profession under the ægis of
eminent universities, whose degree would be respected wherever
it was displayed, and of which the sneer could never be made, as
was said of a foreign college, that it "hoped to get rid of its debt
—by Degrees." The question of affiliation was not one of precipi-
tate haste. It is not generally the custom among the universities
of our Empire to advertise inducements for affiliation, much less to
affiliate a college which exists only on paper. We could not
decently ask consideration for such a matter, until by at least one
scholastic year's work we had given a *raison d'être* for our existence.
The Montreal Veterinary College was nearly twenty-five years old
before it was created a Faculty of McGill. The dentists of the
province have for over twenty-five years elected that their interests
and the interests of dental education should be governed and
guided by the Dental Board. The public must have educated
dentists, as well as physicians, but the dentists must be governed
by dentists and physicians by physicians. The highest medical
authorities in the world would not presume to dictate the purely
practical demands of dentistry. It would be as foolish as futile, to
fritter our small force through several disconnected and discordant
channels, when concentration of effort, under the most experienced
dental practitioners, and under the most eminent universities, is
within our grasp.

Just a word to the students. It was Goethe who said, that if
a man does one good thing in the world, society forms a league to

prevent him from doing another.   In choosing to make your future in the ranks of a very arduous and not a very lucrative profession, it seems to me that if you realize the seriousness of the work before you, you will help rather than hinder the unselfish labors which the teachers and demonstrators voluntarily offer to place within your reach.   This business of study is no fool's play.   Genius, it has been said, is nothing but constant attention.   You will often feel weary and perhaps discouraged, but surely if gray-haired men can face discipline and difficulties, youth has no excuse for fear.   By and by we hope to welcome you into the ranks of the profession ; but you can never enter except by diligence.   If you knew what was before you, you would never wish to enter, unless you were well prepared.   To-day is the day of education.   The ignoramus must step to the rear.   " What will you charge to educate my son ? " said a rich Athenian to one of the early philosophers.   A large sum was mentioned.   " By Hercules ! I could buy a slave for the money."   " Do so," calmly replied the philosopher, " and you will then have two."

Dr. S. Globensky, the President of the Board of Examiners, gave the following address :

Gentlemen,—The opening of the third session of the Dental College of the Province of Quebec produces a twofold but very different effect.   To me, it offers the pleasure and the honor of addressing you ; on you it imposes the *onus* of listening to my words.

The pleasure afforded me is not without a tinge of remorse, when I reflect on the task I am called upon to perform, and on my very poor eloquénce.   You will, therefore, allow me to excuse myself beforehand, and to beg your kind indulgence.   Rest assured that if I am obliged to put you on the rack, it is my intention to keep you there but for the briefest space possible.

And to begin with, let me express my very profound gratitude to the numerous and distinguished audience which favors this young and promising institution with its presence.   All, no doubt do it, remembering that this college has undertaken to dispense to the young student the means of science necessary in the practice of an art, which ranks amongst the most important and most useful to humanity.   Who can deny the importance of the Dental Art, when one stops to consider how intimately it is connected with the enjoyment of those two great boons of life, health and beauty ?   Is it not, indeed, by the resources found in our art that the dentist repairs alike the ravages of time and those of disease, and is enabled to replace the ivory pearls which Nature has given man, as an ornament, and as the indispensable instruments of mastication ?   Where are, I ask you, the charms of ruby lips, when from behind them glisten no more the pure, snowy, polished gems ?   It would be superfluous to undertake to prove that perfect health is impossible, when the double row of useful servants which a kind Providence has set in our mouths are gone for ever.

Is it to be wondered at, then, that men of serious talent have ever studied the means of helping Nature and of remedying to its defects? Such is the useful art, Gentlemen, students of this college, to which you devote your time and your talents. It is to facilitate your studies and to make them more profitable that those who are your elder brothers in the profession, have undertaken the establishment of this institution. Here, the experience of your professors offers you the learned lessons which will enable you to advance, with honor and success, in your chosen career. I will not stop to develop the programme followed in this college nor the lessons given to our pupils. I will say, though, that in future our curriculum and our lectures will be more complete than ever.

The trials inseparable to all foundations are happily things of the past for this college. It is now of age for the affiliation allowed it by law. It is with pleasure, mingled with not a little pride, that I am able to announce the conclusion of all necessary arrangements with our great educational institutions, McGill and Laval, and to state that before many days the affiliation of the Dental College of the Province of Quebec shall be *un fait accompli.* Our college is highly gratified by the work accomplished since its birth. What will we not do when we advance, hand in hand, with those great schools of learning in the paths of scientific progress ; yes, with those schools, the glory of the land.

To the lessons of your professors the eminent men of McGill and Laval will now add their own lore, in order to perfect your education. You will learn anatomy, physiology, pathology and surgery. The study of these different branches of human science, which treat of the body and of health, will prove to you the importance they have in the practice of the Dental Art. " For," as writes Mr. Pierre Sébilean, the learned professor of the Medical Faculty of Paris, " it is not enough to extract, plant, graft, garnish and pivot. Learn a little anatomy. Without it how can you understand dental cysts, mandibulæ, adenitis in caries, carodital adenitis in lingual cancer? Have some knowledge of physiology. Otherwise, how can you explain the stomatitis which appears under the influence of mercurial intoxication or the syncope under that of chloroform? Have an insight into the general laws of pathology. It will make you acquainted with the different evolutions of syphilis and cancer of the tongue. Do not neglect pathological surgery. You cannot afford to ignore the nature, etc., of ulceration of the tongue ; they have too close an affinity with diseases of the teeth. I hear some of you say, you ask too much. Yes, it would be too much if you were left to yourselves.

But the different studies prescribed you are but little, because at your sides are your professors, who have prepared programmes and have learned and studied for you. For you, they have made choice of and prepared the morsel of food, and have cut away the thorns which grew along the road. In your turn, make some efforts to show yourselves worthy of the interest borne you. Remember, also, that your work must prove you worthy sons of a college, which has already done so much for the Dental Art. This institution educates you ; reward it by your devotedness to your studies. After all your efforts shall come the crowning. As we have been, so shall you be calumniated and ill-treated. The whole clan of ignorants, sorcerers, charlatans, and men *ejusdem farinae* shall rise against you. But, say, did you ever dream of such glory ? "

Truly, one is tempted to believe that the lines I have just read were written for the present occasion, and for the actual state of things. But of this, enough ; I do not wish to make further allusion to the subject. According to the promises made us, and I doubt not but that they shall be fully realised, the students of the Dental College, who already have nothing to envy others from an educational point of view, shall receive from McGill and Laval the degree of Doctor in Dental Surgery. Such will be, gentlemen, the crowning of your studies, if you strive for it.

Another word before I take my seat. There is no doubt but that the Dental College of the Province of Quebec has opened a new era, and offers to its students advantages unknown to those who studied for the profession before them. Its progress and success in the past as well as in the future, must be attributed to its clinical dispensary, and to the ever-increasing number of patients to which the college gives its attendance in the interests and for the instruction of its pupils. It is with very legitimate satisfaction that I make the following satement : During the past session months the college has fully done its duty towards poor and suffering humanity, having treated more than 2,000 patients.

I invite those interested in our art to come forward and help us to thoroughly regenerate, by new reforms, the study and teaching of the Dental Art, a profession destined to occupy a high rank among those which render the greatest services to humanity.

Selections.

The Treatment and Filling of Pulpless Teeth as Learned from Papers Read at the World's Dental Congress, A.D., 1893.*

By J. D. BANES, D.D.S., Chicago, Ill.

MR. PRESIDENT AND GENTLEMEN,—The object of this paper. is to bring before this society for discussion the methods of treating and filling pulpless teeth, which were presented in papers or exhibited in clinics at the World's Dental Congress, of 1893.

Upon the second day of the session Dr. J. H. Woolley prepared and filled the roots of a superior second molar for a crown. The tooth was decayed very high up, so that the pulp chamber was fully open and all the canals accessible. Dr. Woolley cleaned out the canals with his broaches. He then volatilized alcohol in them by means of a Small's canal dryer. He then thoroughly dried the tooth with Richmond's hot air dryer, and tested the dryness of the canals by inserting the probe of a root canal dryer of his own design, with which you are probably familiar. Next he pumped eucalyptol into the canal, and volatilized it with hot air, so as to drive it to the end of the tubuli, or fill them with vapor. Finally he flooded the canals with eucalyptol, the pulp chamber with chloroform, and inserted some cones. After driving off the chloroform by hot air he dismissed the patient.

The trouble with that kind of a filling is that there is too much liquid used. I question whether the eucalyptol passed to the apical foramen, and I do not believe that the gutta-percha, upon which we must depend to stop those passages permanently, passed so far. When the cone reached the small portion of the canal it would act as a piston and drive the liquid through the foramen, producing pain, the operator concluding therefrom that his filling was complete; but we think in time, and in a short time at that, the eucalyptol will diffuse away, leaving the apical portion of the canal above the cone unfilled.

On the third day Dr. W. H. Richards exhibited his method of filling tortuous canals with a metalic fiber. He cleaned out the canal and moistened. the walls with oil of cassia, pumping it in with a broach. He picked up the metallic fiber on the moistened broach and passed it into the canal, working it up until by the sense of touch he determined that it had reached the apical foramen.

---

* Read before the Odontographic Society, May, 1894.

This method seems to me to be open to many and very serious objections. First, I do not believe any man can be sure when he has reached the apex with his metallic fiber. In ninety-nine cases he will force it through the foramen, or stop before reaching it, to one where the fiber would just pass to the foramen and stop there. Second, the fiber does not fill the canal, and the tooth is left only a little better off than it would be if the canal were entirely empty. Third, if you can get a probe, into a canal you can file a gold wire as fine or finer than the probe and after pumping in the chloro-percha you can drive in your gold wire. The chloro-percha will fill in around the wire and you thus have a more perfect filling than is afforded by a loose metallic fiber in the canal. Still further, if you can pass a probe part way into a canal, with patient effort you can fill that canal to the end with solid Hill's stopping.

In the discussion of the question " Can apical pericementitis result about a root that has been thoroughly sterilized and filled ? " some valuable points were brought out. Dr. Fernandez said that he hoped the time would come when arsenic would no longer be used to devitalize the pulps of teeth. He dwelt upon the fact that we are using a very strong and uncontrollable poison, that we do not know how far its energy extends, or exactly how it acts in devitalizing the organ. He advocated some mechanical method, giving gas, if necessary, to avoid the pain. If obliged to use arsenic he would use only enough to devitalize the body of the pulp and desiccate the rest with tannin and glycerine or tannic acid in glycerol. If he could not then remove all of the tissue he would digest it in pepsin and wash it out. Dr. Fernandez said he thought a large number of cases of pericementitis were caused by the action of the arsenic or the poisonous medicaments used in the destruction of pulps.

Dr. I. P. Wilson pointed out the way in which the arsenic pro-bably caused the pericementitis. If you will notice a longitudinal section of a tooth you will see a small portion at the apex of the root that is entirely composed of cementum ; this small portion of cementum is undoubtedly nourished by blood vessels from the pulp, and if the pulp is devitalized by the arsenic beyond this point its nourishment is cut off. It then acts as a source of irritation, causing that permanent uneasy feeling at the end of the tooth. That portion of the tooth is prone to become necrosed after the death of the pulp, as is shown by the number of cases of chronic abscesses, which cure up nicely after drilling in and cutting off the end of the root.

During the same discussion, Dr. A. O. Rawls, of Lexington, Ky., said that to protect the teeth perfectly it was necessary to fill the canals to the end, and also the tubuli of the dentine to their extremities. In order to do this he advocated drying the entire tooth from crown to apex with hot air. Then applying some ethereal solution as a varnish, that will fly like a flash to the farthest extremity of the tubuli.

I would want to try a good many experiments with teeth in plaster and wet plaster, so that I could test the method by microscopical examination, before adopting the method in the mouth.

On the fourth day of the session, the paper of Dr. Poinsot, of Paris, France, upon the subject of the " Extraction of the pulps of teeth in a calcified state by trepanning," was read by the chairman of Section IV. The Doctor claims that physiology teaches us that the teeth receive their nourishment from two different sources. viz : the external and the internal ; the external life of the teeth through the peridental ligament, and internal through the pulp, the function of which consists in securing the calcification of the organ in the internal part of the periphery, diminishing the pulp chamber in a progressive way. Calcification is generally complete at the age of thirty-five or forty years, and no matter what the cause may be, either local or general, when once calcification is complete he considers it advantageous to perform the operation of trepanning, which he accomplishes by drilling through the axis of the central pulp chamber, using a small drill for single rooted teeth, and a large drill for teeth with more than one root, carefully removing the enamel at the spot where the drill acts, by the use of drills made from small diamond chips. The way to extract the dental pulp with muscular fillet attached is by the use of a nerve broach, which is used after obtunding the tissues with cocaine phenate, or if root canal is mechanically inaccessible, by the use of electro-cautery. Finally, by filling the canals and remainder of cavity in the usual way. He suggests two ways of indicating when calcification is complete. First, when the gum following the peridental ligament surrounds and enclasps the crown of the tooth. And second, by a careful examination by means of an electric light.

The Doctor's patients have the sympathy of the author of this paper at least, if not of my auditors, inasmuch as his ideas as set forth in the paper presented, necessitates the wholesale slaughter of pulps, without any exception, as soon as the calcification is complete—which is claimed to be from thirty-five to forty years—in order to preserve their usefulness and longevity. Such a method of treatment may possibly be excusable in Paris, but for the sake of humanity keep the Doctor and his trepanning on the other side of the water.

The first of the two papers on the treatment of root canals was that sent by Dr. Miller, of Berlin, Germany. It was read in the general session of the third day. The paper reports his experiments with methods to avoid the removal of dead pulps from the canals of bicuspids and molars. The method is one of mummification. The object sought is to find some substance with which to impregnate the remaining portion of the pulp, so that it will not decompose in the future. He points out seven characteristics or qualities, which are briefly :

1. It must be a strong antiseptic.
2. It must be soluble and diffusible.
3. It must not be too soluble and diffusible.
4. Coagulating action is desirable.
5. It must not be irritating to the pericementum.
6. It must not discolor the tooth.
7. Solids are better than liquids.

The only substance that I know of that meets all these conditions is gutta-percha in a clean, aseptic canal.

The first method used by Dr. Miller was to remove the body of the pulp after completely devitalizing it by the application of a small tablet containing

Sublimate (Hy. Clo.) .... 0.01 gram.
Boracic Acid...................................... 0.02 "

Or,

Sublimate .... 0.01 gram.
Sodium Chloride .... 0.02 "

The tablets were applied, crushed slightly and moistened, then covered with a layer of gold foil and the cavity filled. But in about 30 per cent. of the cases this method caused violent pain because of the rapid diffusion. The painfulness resulting from the use of the first compound led to the use of

Sublimate. .... 0.0075 gram.
Thymol.. 0.0075 "

The thymol was used to prevent the too rapid diffusion of the sublimate. He also used

Sublimate .... 0 005 gram.
Thymol.... .... 0 005 "
Tannin... 0.005 "

But the tannin discolors the tooth. He also used the cyanide and the salicylate of mercury, but expressed himself as having achieved the best results from using diaphtherin (oxychinaseptol), a new antiseptic recently introduced by Emmerich. The Doctor reports that in over two hundred cases at the University of Berlin, where this method had been used, only one failure had come to his knowledge, which we are constrained to admit is a good record if he, in fact, heard of all that failed.

As Dr. Miller observes, such a method can only be fairly tested by time, and in any case should be used very seldom, and only in teeth that would otherwise be treated by the forceps.

I think we had all looked for a valuable paper from Dr. Miller, but I must confess I was very much disappointed in it. I think that as with the mastery of geometrical science, no royal road to an easy solution of the most difficult problems has yet been blazed out for the student's guidance, so with root filling in dentistry, no absolutely perfect and easy method capable of universal application has yet been discovered.

And as Dr. Miller admits the present method of filling the anterior teeth is not likely to be improved upon, and can be trusted to give success in a respectable number of cases, is it not fair then to say that the greater number of failures in filling the molars and bicuspids are due to the carelessness or impatience of the operator? In my opinion two things are absolutely necessary in the treatment of a root canal. First, it must be aseptic. Second, it must be sealed at the apex and the pulp chamber. I believe it would make little difference if the canals were absolutely empty if the apical foramen and the crown cavity were positively sealed. But to seal the foramen all the rest of the canal must be filled. Dr. Miller's method does not provide the second condition, and so long as the apical foramina are open so as to make the canals receptacles for serum, trouble is sure to follow sooner or later. I think for myself I would sooner extract a tooth than to make such an operation simply to save time and expense. If the tooth could be temporarily saved by this method it would surely be saved longer by a careful filling.

In the discussion of this paper Dr. Frank Abbott, of New York, brought out his method of filling root canals. In the first place, he said that he very seldom used arsenic to devitalize a tooth pulp, and when he did so it was only to relieve pain.

When a tooth comes to him for treatment, with the remains of a dead pulp in it, he opens into the pulp chamber so that he can have easy access to the canals. He then uses a one in ten thousand solution of the bichloride of mercury (one grain to twenty ounces), syringing out all the canals as thoroughly as possible. With a broach he probes into the canals so as to stir up the contents, and syringes again, repeating the process until the canals are clean, and the solution in coming out will not stain a white napkin. When he has thoroughly washed it out he fills it with oxychloride of zinc, to which he adds one drop of a one in two thousand bichloride solution. He said this is the material that mummifies or holds the substance which remains in the root of the tooth in such a condition as to give no trouble. He cleans out the canals and fills at the same sitting, before dismissing the patient, painting over the gum with aconite and iodine, as a counter-irritant.

The paper on this subject which has created the greatest amount of interest was that presented by Dr. Emil Schreier, of Vienna. He has given us a positively new method for removing dead and putrescent pulps, and all operators are interested in it because the value of such a new method can only be tested by a large amount of clinical experience.

I presume you are all familiar with his method. He prepares a mixture of metallic sodium and potassium (about two parts sodium and one part potassium) of such a consistency that when a platinum broach is plunged into it, through the parafine coating, a film of the alloy will adhere and be carried on the broach, and the broach thus laden is passed into the moist canal. The metal decomposes the watery contents, liberating the hydrogen and forming the hydroides of the metals (caustic potash and caustic soda), which in the nascent state actively decompose the organic matter of the pulp, saponifying it (if that is a proper term to apply, as there is little or no fat in the tissue). At any rate, the tissue is actively decomposed and rendered soluble, so that it is readily washed out with water.

The substance destroys the germs present partly by the heat evolved and partly by the chemical products. Of course this method is only applied with the rubber dam in position to protect adjacent tissues.

The questions which arise in connection with this method, some of which were suggested by Dr. Schreier, are:

1. Is there danger of forcing septic matter through the apical foramen, when the broach is first plunged into the canal?

2. Is the heat evolved too great?

3. Is there danger of an explosion?

4. Is there danger that the substances formed will pass through the foramen and set up irritation of the peridental membrane?

The latter is far the greatest danger. I would be very much afraid that in case of an open foramen, some of the caustic substance might get into the apical space, and if it should, trouble would doubtless manifest itself.

In connection with Dr. Schreier's paper, I have consulted some fifteen dentists in good practice regarding the Doctor's method, and found only two of that number who have ventured its use since Congress adjourned, and one of the gentlemen was very much gratified with the results, whilst the other's experience was quite the reverse.

I have since been advised that other gentlemen present have used this method in their practice before the meeting of the World's Dental Congress last year, and some of them with much satisfaction, and we should certainly be pleased to hear from any such parties.

Through the courtesy of Mr. Fred Noyes, I am enabled in this connection to submit the following letter from Prof. Noyes, of the Rose Polytechnic Institute, of Terre Haute, Ind., a prominent chemist in our sister State, regarding the chemical action of the compound used by Dr. Schreier. Prof. Noyes' letter is as follows:

"I do not see how anything could be gained by the use of metallic sodium and potassium in the manner you indicate, which would not be gained equally as well by the use of sodium hydroxide, or potassium hydroxide, and with far less danger. The metals I should think likely to lead to ugly accidents in such a use. The hydroxides would, I think, have little effect on bony tissue, fats would be saponified, and other organic matter in general would be disintegrated by them."

We had hoped to have access to the official publication of the entire transactions of the Congress, but owing to delays of various kinds it has not yet been published —*Dental Review.*

Editorial.

The Horace Wells Celebration.

A very interesting meeting in honor of the memory of Dr. Horace Wells will be held in Philadelphia on the 11th of next month. Prof. Thos. Fillebrown, of Boston, is to read a paper on the "History of Anæsthesia," and Prof James E. Garretson on the "Benefits of Anæsthesia to Mankind." A banquet, at which there will be appropriate addresses, will be held, and a souvenir volume of the event will be issued. It is further proposed that at the meeting, subscriptions will be invited for a permanent memorial.

We venture to draw attention to the fact that Dr. Wells did not "*discover* the anæsthetic properties of nitrous oxide," though we must admit that, like many others, we have been under the misapprehension that he had the claim of priority. In the *Canada Journal of Dental Science,* in September, 1871, we wrote editorially under this belief, instigated by a meeting of dentists at Hartford, Conn., and the request of the late Dr. J. H. McQuillen. At that time the widow of Dr. Wells was in very poor circumstances, and she had declared that "the discovery of her husband had been to her and her family an unspeakable evil, for it cost the life of her husband, and substituted the *res augusti domi* (scanty fortune) in place of a lucrative profession and a happy home."

Unquestionably, to Horace Wells, then a dentist at Hartford, Conn., is due the inestimable blessing to mankind of the practical application of nitrous oxide. On the evening of December, exactly fifty years ago, Dr. Wells witnessed its administration by Mr. Colton, and observing that one of the patients was unconscious of severe bruises he sustained during the excitement of the anæsthetic, he there and then stated that he believed it could be used for painless extraction. The following day he inhaled it, and the late Dr. J. M. Riggs extracted a molar. Upon his recovery, Wells exclaimed, "A new era in tooth-pulling!" Wells carried it into general surgery as well as dental practice. No one can deny to his memory the lasting tribute of applying nitrous oxide as an anæsthetic.

However, historical accuracy and the correct use of words demand that there shall be no mistake as to the "discovery." Sir Benjamin W. Richardson, in an article in *Longman's Magazine*, proves that "by every rule of justice and of truth, Sir Humphrey Davy deserves the credit of the discovery, and that Horace Wells is entitled to the credit of the practical application of the discovery by a test performed upon himself." In 1759, Sir Humphrey tried the effects of nitrous oxide upon himself, and has left us a graphic description, and suggested in the following words its practical use : "As nitrous oxide, in its extensive operation, appears capable of destroying physical pain, it may probably be used with advantage during surgical operations in which no great effusion of blood takes place.' His "Researches on Nitrous Oxide," published early in the present century, prove, moreover, that he used it to relieve himself of violent attacks of toothache.

Harris' "Principles and Practice" : "The anæsthetic effects of nitrous oxide was first suggested by Sir Humphrey Davy in 1776, and practically demonstrated by Dr. Horace Wells." Harris' Dictionary of Dental Science : "Sir Humphrey Davy, in 1799, first discovered its anæsthetic properties upon inhalation, and in 1844, Dr. Horace Wells, of Connecticut, applied it to dental purposes."

Dr. James E. Garretson's "System of Oral Surgery" : "Nitrous oxide owes its discovery to Priestley, 1776. Credit for its use as a pain-obtunding agent is due both to Sir Humphrey Davy and Dr. Horace Wells ; to the latter particularly."

"The History of American Dentistry," prepared under direction of the American Academy of Dental Science. 1876 : "This gas, as such, was discovered by Priestley in 1776. Its exhilarant and anæsthetic properties were first noticed in 1800 by Sir Humphrey Davy."

Dental Cosmos, June, 1860, page 594 : "With regard to priority in suggesting the use of nitrous oxide in surgical operations, the credit undoubtedly belongs to Sir Humphrey Davy," and . . . "the credit of first making a practical application of this suggestion unquestionably belongs to Horace Wells."

Dr. J. F. B. Flagg, in his work on "Ether and Chloroform," refers to the history of the introduction of nitrous oxide by Dr. Wells, but recognizes Sir Humphrey Davy's claim of first suggestion.

However, that is a very unimportant matter in comparison with the value of Dr. Wells' share. The dental and medical professions recognize the great blessing which followed the unselfish and self-sacrificing efforts of the latter. The monument to his memory in the public park of Hartford was contributed to by Britishers and Canadians, and the engrossed testimonial from England to Mrs. Wells referred to her late husband as one "to whom the world is indebted, not only for the introduction of nitrous oxide gas as an anæsthetic, but also for giving that impetus to the study of anæsthesia, which has resulted in the introduction of chloroform, bichloride of methylene and various other agents for affecting that purpose."

We appreciate most heartily the duties assumed by the Committee who have undertaken to commemorate the fiftieth anniversary of Dr Wells' share; but with all possible good-will we would suggest that the word "discovery" be omitted, and that the resolution passed by the American Dental Association in 1864 be adhered to, "That to Dr. Horace Wells (now deceased) belongs the honor of *the introduction* of anæsthesia in the United States of America." He could not have greater glory if he had really been "the discoverer" of nitrous oxide.

Obituary.

Whereas, the members of the British Columbia Dental Association have learned with deep regret that Divine Providence, in His inscrutible ways, has seen fit to remove, by death, our late brother, Dr. C. E. C. Brown, of New Westminster;

Whereas, the professional character of the deceased was such as to command the love and respect of his professional brethren at large; therefore

Resolved,—That in the death of Dr. C. E. C. Brown, the Dental profession has been deprived of one of its most active, efficient and honorable members.

Resolved,—That we, the members of the British Columbia De tal Association, deplore the grievous loss which the family have sustained, and cordially sympathize with them in their bereavement.

Resolved,—That the Secretary be instructed to forward a copy of these resolutions to Mrs. C. E. C. Brown, and furnish a copy to the DOMINION DENTAL JOURNAL.

J. M. McLAREN, L.D.S.,
A. J. HOLMES, D.D.S., } *Committee.*
LEWIS HALL, D.D.S.,

Victoria, B.C., October 4th, 1894.

Two rooms, ground floor, best locality in Toronto, used as medical office for ten years, vacant about February. This is a splendid chance for a student expecting to remain in city. For particulars apply to DOMINION DENTAL JOURNAL, Box 418.

DOMINION
DENTAL JOURNAL.

| VOL. VI. | TORONTO, DECEMBER, 1894. | No. 12. |

Original Communications.

Pulp Canal Filling.

By Mark G. McEelimney, D.D.S., Ottawa.

Almost every dental journal contains an article, and every dental association has a section, pertaining to the filling of root canals.

It is through this interchange of ideas that we arrive at the best methods for accomplishing our objects.

While my way of doing this is by no means new, I think that a description may be interesting.

After destroying the nerve, the first and most important thing is cleanliness. Every possible particle and fibre of dead tissue must be removed, and the canals made thoroughly antiseptic.

I say every possible particle, because it is impossible for the most skilful operator to remove everything, except in very accessible cases. The difficulty increases with the remoteness and tortuousness of the canal.

There is a tendency amongst dental writers to forget the practical limitations, and construct a very fine theory of perfect work on paper.

While I recognize fully the absolute necessity of a high standard of excellence, toward which we should constantly struggle, there is also present to me the fact, that the very best work in the treatment of canals depends upon the forms of the canals themselves.

I have split open many extracted teeth, and in a comparatively large proportion have found, that the canals were so constricted that theoretically, perfect treatment would be a very difficult matter.

2

In cases where nerve broaches cannot be used with full satisfaction, it is necessary to depend for success upon thorough medication of the remaining debris.

For removing debris from canals, the prepared nerve bristles are very unsatisfactory. They are either too soft or too brittle, or the barbs rub off very easily.

It is a wonder that so many firms keep on making, and so many dentists buying, articles that are of no earthly value to anyone who wishes to do thorough work.

A broach must be stiff, springy, and of even taper. It must also be cheap and adaptable to various circumstances. Broaches for lower molar roots should be somewhat flattened to suit the canals. The points must be very sharp to avoid pushing debris ahead ; while the butt must be of sufficient thickness to give strength.

To make nerve broaches that will do reasonably satisfactory work, take No. 18 piano wire, and draw the temper a little.

A little experience will enable one to draw to any desired temper for any particular case. A Bunsen flame will do very well. The wire should be left sufficiently stiff to come back straight when the point is deflected thirty or forty degrees. Place a piece of hard wood end up in the vise, and with the corner of a file cut a light groove parallel with the jaws. This groove is to keep the wire from slipping while it is being filed.

Place the piano wire in a pin vise and file it taper with a square section, or slightly flattened for some cases. Care must be taken to make the taper even from butt to point, or the broach will be liable to break.

With a sharp graver nick the square corners of the broach, and the result is a series of barbs that will stand a great deal of use. The barbs may be placed on one, any, or all corners, according to requirement. The butt must be adapted to the particular kind of broach-holder used. For a screw chuck-holder the butt should be made square. For a sliding ring-chuck the butt will stay better if slightly flattened.

A foot of piano wire will make nine broaches, and costs less than a cent. One of these broaches will do more work than three ordinary ones at fifty cents a dozen.

Having now a serviceable broach, it is necessary to use it rightly. It should not be sent to the apex at first, but the debris must be carefully removed as one goes up, care being taken to avoid wadding the narrower portion with debris, as it is very difficult to remove and may get solid enough to be taken for the apex. To properly cleanse a root requires time and patience, for it is a really tedious operation.

Having removed all dead matter that will come out, the next step is the thorough medication of the root. A few fibres of cotton twisted around a fine broach makes a most efficient pump. Each dentist has a favorite preparation for roots—suffice it to say that whatever is used must be used thoroughly.

Having the canals clean and ready to fill, I do not dry them; but rather leave them full of root preparation, which is forced into every crevice by the filling.

The most important question is, What material for filling? When a tooth is healthy and the indications favorable, I use silver.

Even where there has been periosteal trouble, now cured, or even an abscess that has yielded to treatment, I recommend silver as the most impervious and safest material. Silver can be got into more difficult situations, and is surer to stay, than any other material. Silver is less likely to be affected by adverse circumstances in the canal; moisture and constriction do not prevent it from reaching its place.

In the case of cement, moisture is fatal to the proper pumping up of the material, and I doubt if one dentist in a hundred can get one canal in a hundred fit to hold cement.

Another objection to cement is that subsequent leakage through the apex must eventually disintegrate it in the immediate vicinity, and, once disintegration is set up, there is an end to all confidence.

The silver can be put into position by means of pluggers of various sizes made of piano wire and used in the broach-holder.

Filling a canal with silver is at first somewhat difficult, and never becomes really easy. The best way is to put a pellet in the pulp-chamber, and with a burnisher press it gently against the canal openings, then send it up the canal with the probe-like plugger, the end of which should be cut off square. This cuts a cylinder out of the pellet and carries it ahead right up the canal. Whatever small space is beyond is forced full of root preparation, which should be crystallizable, astringent and antiseptic.

In cases where there has existed chronic abscess, and a recurrence is feared, where it may some day be necessary to reopen the canal, I insert a gutta-percha point dipped in chloroform. These points I make by rolling gutta-percha pellets on a glass slab with a warm spatula. They can be rolled to any required length, thickness or angle. While I do not regard gutta-percha as equal to silver, yet it is the next best material where a non-removable filling is distinctly contra-indicated.]

It has been suggested to saturate the dead pulp with some powerful agent, and leave it in the tooth. This is little less than criminal.

The use of cotton saturated with preservatives as a canal-filling I regard as unscientific, careless, and the invention of a lazy man, whoever he may be. If there is such a thing as leakage through the apical opening, the preservative must in time wash out; then the canal is left filled with unprotected organic matter. Disintegration, irritation and abscess are only a matter of time. At college I learned that cotton-filling was good for roots. For the first few months all went well with the few teeth that a cold and unsympathetic public allowed me to fill. Then the chickens "came home to roost." Those chickens are all disposed of some time ago, and I have learned a valuable lesson, and that is, that a nice, easy way of doing a difficult operation is generally no good. There is no royal road to successful root-filling; it is a test of ability.

Selections.

A New Era in Dental Practice.

By PROF. FLAGG, Philadelphia.

Through your courtesy* I am with you again, to reveal the silence of years which has culminated in what I am pleased to call " A New Era in Dentistry." Forty-five minutes is but a moment, which you accord me to condense forty years of active labor and practice. I cannot blame you for the restriction, as I have always written exhaustively and hours have been consumed by me, leaving no chance for discussion at the same meeting. I will hold to your order, and leave for the future other chances for details and the consummation of the work, that my efforts may not have been in vain.

The great Master once said, " Neither will they be persuaded, though one rose from the dead." The profession of dentistry, as that of medicine, is demanding, " What shall we do to be saved?" We are in the light of the waning days of the nineteenth century, asking each other for some system by which we can be saved the humiliation of failure in dental practice to save the human teeth, one upon which each and all can rely.

Before we can attain to any true system that shall work universally, as in the laws of interchangeable mechanics, we must accord to someone the right from a life of precedents to be umpire in his line of work.

The title of this paper is an assumption, and all I ask is to follow, and for once get out of the old ruts and walk upon the broad plane of liberality and common sense, and with unselfish eye and charity

---

*New York Odontological Society.

calmly act and show that something good can come out of Nazareth.

Every journal bears upon its pages the desire of men to flee to a practice that will bring universal good results. Let us ask, where are our failures? Are they in men or things or materials? Are they in false education? Is it that new difficulties arise to baffle every past partially-successful effort? Have we really been successful in anything we have done to insure us in following the same old cause? The cry is for new light and new methods. If the world knew how few teeth are saved by us for any number of years they would not spend time, health and money, but give up to the juggernaut of destruction, and extraction would be the rule, even with the wealthier classes. The poor and medium classes have had to give up their teeth in early life because of failure upon failure of even the best men. Then it is a fact, dentistry of the present hour is not near the goal of perfection in practice we long for. Why is it? Is there any relief? When shall we commence in our declaration of failure?

THE PRIME NECESSITY.

First. Men. With all the vaunted advantages of colleges everywhere, how few who enter their sacred precincts are fitted by nature, general education, special talent, surroundings, or by long family precedents! Could we but be as true to principles and bold to assert as was Plato when he had inscribed over the garden-gate to his studio, " Let none enter here who know not geometry," we would then have some hope for the future.

Anyone can be taught to fill a cavity with the instruments and material at our disposal, but when to do it and how it should be shaped to insure its future usefulness is quite another consideration. We must not teach men that our art is solely to allow teeth to decay and fill our coffers from Nature's weakness. Are you prepared to-night to lay down your life as the missionary, and for the good of humanity attempt to save a tooth in its purity whether fortune in gold favor you or not?

Are you ready to ignore self and be the benefactors of your race, and adopt a system that promises to save more teeth, more pulps, give greater beauty, and more usefulness? If not, then step aside.

Medical men can well ask for " preventive medicine," for every honest M.D. soon learns to give less and less medicine, and rely not only on Nature, but in knowing the laws of hygiene, even if he be dethroned for his empiricism.

We, as dentists, have an entirely different field, for we have millions coming to us where no law of prevention can be applied. We can only save and restore the lost structure by our cunning and art.

With the rising generation, we can do, if we have a system to prevent the ravages so universally found in the human race, that which will preserve a much greater number in their purity and also check decay without filling with gold and other materials, and drive from our practice artificial substitutes in the majority of cases.

This leads us to a most important matter—ignoring the "greed for gold." If we are ever so perfect in our manipulation and able to preserve, yet if we do not have that charity to purge ourselves from the "lust for gain," and do for others as we would do for our own families, it will not bring us success at the end of our journey.

GENERAL CAUSES OF FAILURE.

Let us take up the general causes of failure. We cannot ignore the almost utter worthlessness of tooth-structure. This we will call the "predisposition." My experience is that we are more degenerate every year, and the fight is harder to save teeth. It requires wisdom, foresight and skill to dare attempt the anticipation of caries. I have attempted to make the effort. *True, anticipation, as a general rule, cannot be relied on* by the average dentist. But there is much that can be done to check caries in its very incipiency and that without filling.

The materials as substitutes for lost structure we will now take up. Gold is acknowledged by the profession generally to be pre-eminently the best, and we want no better testimony than to look into any and every mouth and behold gold, gold, gold. Fillings no larger than pin-points and heads dotting every valley. Men talk and write gold, and yet they deplore it does not save. They ask for the reason, why? The "New Departure" said "*never use it.*" Here are two extremes, and neither has shown why either should be practised. You ask for testimony. I refer you to the many kinds of gold and preparations or forms of gold, each manufacturer claiming special features for success; the immense quantity of it used; the cases that have been filled and refilled. I filled a superior central incisor last week with Abbey's gold that had been filled fifteen times before. There was left for me a tooth with living pulp with the palatal surface one-half gone and both mesial and distal surfaces involved to the cervix. Think of it! None of you can deny that gold is the idol of the profession, and a man who talks against it is risking his reputation.

Gold, *per se*, is good for preserving tooth-structure. Compatibility has nothing to do with it. Adaptability is all of it! If tooth-structure is worthy as a base and a man knows how to line the walls of the cavity, it will preserve, provided the cavity is rightly shaped and the contour is given such form as to preclude any possibility of the active causes of caries. There is no greater error made than to suppose it is necessary to have various qualities and forms of this metal.

IDOLIZE IT.

Make to yourself an idol in this metal, and, in spite of the manufacturers, follow it ; learn to manipulate one kind, and you have all you can ask, and there will be less failures. But the sin is not only in seeking for some better form of gold, but in learning how to use but one or two, and have the conscience and honor to confess that the fault is in yourself, and discriminate when and where it should be used. They tell us it quite always fails at the cervix, and, to attest this, they reproach the gold and use amalgam or gutta-percha at this point. It is not the gold, but it lies in you and your judgment and conscience. Franklin showed he was a philosopher when he said he "would not give much for a mechanic who could not bore with a saw and saw with a gimlet."

Some dentists have piled up around them every new instrument that comes out,—every new plugger-point with serrations of greater or less depth and extreme fineness and all sizes,—every form of mallet from the thud blow to the most approved power mallet. And withal, they fail, but few recognizing the fact that perfectly smooth points will do the whole business perfectly in adapting one fold of gold to another though perfectly burnished.

Tin and gold and hand-pressure is another proof of gold's failure when used alone. I could multiply proofs of failure, but enough, —gold is a failure !

THE PLASTIC CRUTCH.

Take amalgam. Look at the tons of it used; yet, so many men say they do not have it in their office.

Do you ask for proof of failure ?

Take the craze for "copper amalgam." What a curse it has been to the profession and their patients ! I never used it once ! I saw what it was when I looked into patients' mouths when I was abroad. Had they known what proper contouring was they would never have used it so universally in all cavities.

It has been a stench in the nostrils of nearly every American dentist.

Has amalgam any good qualities in itself ? Have we any good alloys ?

How many men know how to use it and get the best results ? What curses have been heaped upon its hallowed head ? Where is the man who dares say he uses it ? Anathemas come thick and fast from the M.D.'s of both old and new school as if they were the Supreme Court to sit upon its merits.

Several years ago, at one of the first meetings of our Odontological Society of Pennsylvania, one of its oldest and most prominent members went so far as to place on record in the Proceedings,—

" All men, falling away from manipulative ability, lean on plastics."
To-day he is experimenting to find an ideal alloy to help him out
in his failures with gold. How sad such a record! Who among
you so mean as to deny using it and without "apologizing"?

I say it is one of the grandest filling materials we have,—and
while I have spent nearly thirty years in inventing power mallets
and special smooth oval points for gold work, I confess I throw all
aside very quickly, and while I delight to wield the electric or
mechanical mallet in distancing time and space with gold, yet I use
more amalgam to-day than ever before in my life.

I am thankful I had the courage and principle to stand by it,
and recommend and show how much could be done when condensed under Japanese bibulous paper. To me it is a sheet-anchor
for the class of cases every day coming to me from others. If you
use amalgam and wish to make your practice a success with it,
learn how to manipulate it and prepare your cases for its adaptation.

ANOTHER.

Oxyphosphate,—what of it?

Is it good as a permanent filling alongside of gold or amalgam?
Is it a failure also?

What does the profession say of it?

Everywhere you hear the cry, it gives way at the cervix in all
cases and soon wears away, and is not fit for contour or permanent
work. It is not to be relied upon!

If this be true, then it is useless to place it in carious teeth.

That it will preserve tooth-structure from further decay admits
of no doubt whatever.

That it will preserve the contour of the tooth is certain in the
bulk of cases.

That it will not destroy the pulp in near contact with it is equally
sure.

That it will preserve tooth-structure with nearly all the decay left
in the cavity and without much or really any shaping is incontest-
able, which, further on, I will show for a fact that I am willing to
stand by and from a part of the new era of which I am here to
speak. It is beyond value when you know how to mix it, how to
manipulate it, how to shape it; how to treat it before you remove
the dam or allow it to get wet; how to treat the phosphoric acid,
to keep it from crystallizing, insuring you thereby a better result in
every way; and when proper precautions are taken with these
fillings, how inestimable are the results, and beyond cavil and
doubt!

I cannot say too much for it,—a good article. But, just here let
me say that, when you can get a good article, use no other kind in
the mouth; as I forgot to tell you of amalgam, as with gold, use

one kind only, that will work as well under water as above the surface. The oxyphosphate, of course, will have to be kept absolutely dry to be a perfect success.

AN IDEAL MATERIAL.

In nearly every sense I know of nothing so important as pink base-plate gutta-percha.

To teach you how I use it for the preservation of the human teeth, both temporary and permanent, will be the foundation of a system that, if I have had any success at all, I can attribute to this one article as much as or more than any other filling-material.

In conjunction with this I cannot overestimate the value of the discovery of the laws of articulation and the articulator that bears my name, and of which I am more proud than of all my other productions. Without knowing what I do of articulation, the gutta-percha might never have been seen in the same light by me.

Let us review, now, before I enter upon this simple revelation of truth, what and wherein are our failures.

LIST OF FAILURES.

I told you, poor elements in tooth-structure as the grand predisposing cause of failure.

Worthlessness of tooth-structure as a very great cause of failure, let us be ever so competent and with the best of materials for restoration.

The materials as substitutes for lost structure,—gold, amalgam, oxyphosphate, gutta-percha and tin,—and how failure comes from each and all.

The failure that comes from not understanding the laws of articulation, and which shows how the loss of one tooth affects all the teeth of both jaws.

The failures that result from the indiscriminate cutting of approximal surfaces in filling, and the great change of relationship between the upper and lower dentures.

And the failures that ensue from the want of a definite system in knowing what to do in the keeping of the original articulation, and, when lost from bad dentistry, restoring it again to its proper relations that each tooth will bear its exact burden and no undue pressure be brought to bear upon any one.

The importance, finally, of those laws and this system in the prevention of recurrent caries and the blotting out of the greatest cause for pyorrhœa alveolaris,—which comes largely from undue pressure and use of the teeth thrown out of arrangement by non-restoration of contour.

I cannot enumerate all the causes as now acknowledged by the profession. Look into every journal, go into every depot, talk with every dentist you meet, scan the proceedings of every society, go where you will, and we can infer from it all.

Dentistry is a failure, because it can neither anticipate nor prevent decay superficially or arrest it when substitutes are made to take the place of lost tooth-structure.

We have labored in vain, and I am invited here to tell you whether I am satisfied with the practice I have instituted after forty years of servitude.

To say that I am really satisfied is not true. But I am conscious that my practice shows that I not only anticipate successfully, but preserve teeth superficially decayed without filling, and, when too far gone for this practice, then the conscientious use of the materials we have at hand enables me to snatch from the ravages of the " tooth of time."

Yes, I am happy to tell you how much can be done to rescue our profession from its perilous practice. But, I know you will not adopt what I tell you ! Or at least the bulk of dentists will not, for they will fear starvation.

BRAINS A BIG ITEM.

If you can have the courage to charge a patient as much for tin, amalgam, oxyphosphate, gutta-percha or beeswax,—which is a valuable material to save trouble,—then you have accepted the highest creed I offer you in my " New Era." Unless you can dare to face the public and say to them brains must be paid for, and all our operations are upon brain work as the standard of price, then do not accept my creed,—go on as aforetime. Hobbs, the celebrated locksmith and maker of the first complicated bank-locks, which were marvels of ingenuity, was brought before a bank committee to have him show cause why he asked such high prices for his inventions. They had him take the lock to pieces, and inquired what each piece would cost to duplicate it. When the sum total was made they found it did not foot up the price Hobbs asked for the completed lock. How is this, Mr. Hobbs? He then looked over all the items and said to them, " Gentlemen, there is one item you have left out." They could not tell what it was,—when, to their chagrin, he said, " Brains."

But with this blot upon my career, " high charges," I am proud ; and, if any one thing has added to my success above all else, it has been in daring and boldness to make people pay what I believed my brain, as a machine, was worth.

I often say to my patients now, when speaking of prices and they want an estimate made, I cannot do it, for " I have no more right to cheat myself than to cheat you."

Then, I am sure you will agree with me that this first article of my creed is worthy of following. If not, then do no listen to my simple system of practice.

It is not as manual laborers we can show our highest skill! No : one piece of timely advice—the extraction of one tooth ; the teaching how to use a brush and what kind to use ; and in many ways, where no labor at all is performed—is worth hundreds of dollars, and besides, a deep gratitude for the salvation from vandalism and sacrifice of Nature's most beautiful pearls and God's grandest piece of architecture.

Let us all dare to do right, even if we get no immediate compensation further than our own approving conscience.

Let us all dare to stop when we are in doubt, and the kindly consultation with another brother practitioner may be of the greatest value to us and our patient.

If we must link ourselves at all to the medical men, let us emulate their example in one thing at least,—anticipative medicine, or, as they have it, "preventive medicine."

As I have previously told you in this article, I have held opinions for many years that with every disadvantage impeding our course we can anticipate and cheat the "tooth of time" of its ravages. Yet it is a dangerous remedy in the hands of ignorance.

Must Have Sole Charge.

Unless we can have sole charge of patients from the second year on, and no one else to interfere, we cannot hope to do our fullest duty and found a practice for all men to follow.

Ignorance, stupidity and downright dishonesty give us more trouble than we like to admit.

I have told you only of a few of the causes of our failures. One, above all the rest, faces us, and a wail is sent up everywhere. " Recurrence of decay at the cervical border ; " no man yet has dared to say he was conqueror.

The next most treacherous is what is known as pyorrhœa.

I never use gold in the temporary teeth, seldom amalgam or tin, save on grinding surfaces, where cavities are very small or very large and no pulp involved in the part, and oxyphosphate very seldom, and only where I can keep it perfectly dry. Not that any of these articles are not valuable, but the preparation of cavities and the situation of decay, the near approach to the pulp of nearly every proximal decay and the age of the subject preclude their use. Never demoralize any youthful client by much excavation or formidable show of instruments, or by slow, sluggish movements. My aim is expedition ; as few minutes in the chair as possible ; inflicting but little pain and inconvenience,—gentleness, kindness, and yet positiveness.

My greatest ally as the filling-material is pink gutta-percha, such as is used for base-plate, and further on you will see how far I use it in the treatment of the permanent teeth. Aside from its use for a stopping on all approximal surfaces, there is one grand object in view to be ever held in mind, the importance of the position of the first permanent molar when it emerges. Unless this base column, or abutment if you please, is not kept well back towards the ramus, then *irregularity will come to the incisors*. It is not enough to merely stop decay and stuff in amalgam or oxyphosphate; we must keep the temporary molars from approaching each other more than normal, and prevent the alveolar processes from encroachment and absorption from direct pressure of the roots of the temporary molars, which is invariably the case when the approximating surfaces are cut by caries and allowed to trespass on each other. We cannot use a separator here to gain space; we dare not cut or shape the cavities for a metal filling for fear of the pulp. What is to be done?

If possible, as soon as the least decay is noticed on the approximal surfaces and you can get in from the crown or on the buccal sides with the least excavating, by hand or machine, if it must be used, whether you can keep the cavity dry or allow it to remain moist, stuff in the gutta-percha forcibly between the teeth, smooth, and let alone to watch every three or six months. Where the cavities are large when you first see them, remove no decay over the pulp. Break down all superfluous walls, saturate with carbolic acid or creosote, force in a lump of the gutta-percha by filling all space as one filling, and let it go until the teeth have become so far separated by the act of mastication—not by expansion of the material—as to have replaced with another or a patch on the surface. Now, here is the point I wish to make that you have never recognized as a factor, because you have ignored the laws of articulation.

By this means I save from future decay and the risk of pulp exposure; but, above all else, I give a condition that enables the child to use with impunity every part of the jaws with hard or soft food, and no pain or fear of it, which no other plan could offer. And, above all this, I drive the first permanent molar so much farther back upon the ramus that, the nearer it is to the condyle or point of motion, the wider it keeps the jaws apart at the incisors, and prevents absolutely the too great encroachment of the lower upon the palatal surfaces of the superior incisors, which, if allowed, would destroy normal articulation,—make too deep an overbite and underbite, and, withal, cause an overlapping of the inferior incisors and the full use of the jaw teeth, because, in the lateral movements of the lower jaw, the incisors would strike first too long before the molars could come in contact, and really only the up-and-down movement would be attained.

Must Grasp Articulation.

This you could never know, nor can you appreciate now, unless you fully grasp the laws of articulation. This has never been taught, and, save a few followers of my special friends, is not practised.

This was a revelation to me when, in 1858, the articulator was born. And, as soon as the pink gutta-percha made its appearance, with rubber plates for trial or base plates, before they were brought forth, I struck upon this treatment and have followed it ever since; and the results have proved I have but few cases of irregularity in my own immediate practice, and those but simple ones, and seldom a pulp exposed for treatment, and but few demoralized subjects, and a brighter future for the permanent set, with plenty of room and to spare for them to come in. Should decay occur on the anterior approximal surface of the first permanent molar, I prevent its spread and in many cases anticipate or treat it superficially; and, if to fill, do so when I have all the room I want,—but seldom with gold even then, as I do not know the exact position the second bicuspid will take; besides, most of the cavities are very small and not susceptible of contouring over all the approximal surface, which has to be done if we contour at all on any surface. From the temporary incisors of children I generally remove caries when small, and do not scruple to fill with amalgam if they need filling. I have never used the dam for any child except when the permanent molars required filling.

Lastly, to detect the incoming permanent tooth when the temporary one shows no sign of its approach, I, at the proper time, use an exploring needle under, or in some cases directly through, the gum to feel for it. It is the precursor of events, and saves much irregularity and fear. Without this precaution many temporary molars that become fastened between the permanent molars and first permanent bicuspids would remain in for years too long. So much for the treatment to the twelfth year. Gutta-percha is my sheet-anchor.

In the permanent incisors anticipation is generally adopted; if decayed, oxyphosphate or pink gutta-percha is used, never gold. I seldom have any fillings at all in these teeth. The sixth-year molars on buccal surfaces are generally smoothed and decay arrested, or, if to be filled, pink gutta-percha. It is impossible to save every tooth without filling; yet, even with the worst of these cases, *superficial* decay can be arrested and thousands of fillings saved, and our art made a comfort and a blessing.

RECURRENCE OF DECAY AT THE CERVIX.

You all admit that recurrence of decay at the cervical border gives you the greatest difficulty to surmount, and as yet you have not reached the cause nor the remedy. It must be admitted that, if this one thing alone can be mastered, we have overcome our most powerful foe.

It is a fact not to be denied that every dentist cries out for some method to prevent recurrence at the cervix. This is positive proof that everyone has hands full of proximal cavities from the cuspid back. Everyone must admit that contour fillings alone have been the only help or partial cure, although it has to be repeated or requires oft patching.

A case presents where caries have run wild. Not an approximal surface scarcely but is involved. No pulps quite exposed, but threatening. Every tooth has been filled and refilled, and by more than one dentist. Contour has been attempted. Where the fillings of gold remain they are so undermined there is nothing but utter annihilation unless all are removed. The teeth from their loss of proximate surfaces are all out of articulation, which can be best seen by taking an impression and putting the casts in my articulator. Look closely at the cervix, and you will find the root of each so close that no thread can be forced through, and the decay is far up under the cervix. Look further and probe for the alveolar process, and not a vestige of it remains for a quarter of an inch up. Look also to the second molar where the first has been extracted, and on that side the process is gone far down and nothing but loose gum tissue remains, and is constantly receding, and whenever a tooth has been lost the process about the cervix absorbs as the body of the jaw absorbs.

In this state of affairs you put on your dam and separator, and you obtain a slight widening and at once fill permanently the excavated tooth. No attention is paid to the articulation of the teeth. You have no desire to wait, and you rush on headlong to fill and get your pay. The rest of the teeth are left without anything in them until one by one you have had your patient at least twice a week for months, two hours or more at a sitting, until they are exhausted and condemn dentistry, and while you are rushing through to complete every cavity with a filling you have done nothing to prevent further rapid decay, and pulps become exposed and the patient has to suffer.

Now, I know this is the case with nearly every man's practice. I see it every week, and I know from personal contact in conversations with patients of others who have not come to me for treatment.

Now, you can do better than this and not only retain your patients, but bridge over time as well as space and fill and treat at your leisure.

I will take the same mouth just illustrated, and without placing in one single permanent filling of any kind of metal treat it with pink gutta-percha alone, with a little of the white as a facing, where necessary. I cut out only partially the cavities on one side of the jaw or jaws, always exposing every grinding surface where the approximal is gone and make compound by running all of the cavities into one, seldom leaving any approximal cavity to stand alone, but opening it into the grinding surfaces. This is a cardinal principle with me.. There is one surface or border I complete at once, and that is the cervical, so that I never have to touch it again, and this I cut so far up as to not only remove all caries, but where I know the gum and process will grow up and over it. This is finished, and to enable me to do so I forgot to say I never put on the rubber dam in any case until I fill permanently, when the cervix is firm and will admit of its adjustment. It is easy to stop the blood with perchloride of iron, creosote, or any styptic.

TREATMENT.

And now for the further treatment. Into all the spaces I have made on one or more sides in one or more teeth I place great pieces of pink gutta-percha, and, with no separation between them in any case, stuff the whole intervening space, trim, and let alone. This I do until every place is filled in. I dismiss the patient, and have him call in three or six months or a year, as I may please ; and, as I find the teeth wide enough apart for a plus-contour filling, and the alveolar gum border and process is in perfect health, and the process has grown up to the gutta-percha, then I fill only those that show that they are far enough apart at the cervix to permit a healthy, full process to grow in order that the gum will have proper substance, and cleave to the root and cover up and over the margin of the filling at the cervix. In this, I tell you, is your future security at the alveolar border.

No one has ever called attention to the difference in width of the approximal spaces at the cervix for the bicuspids and molars. The gutta-percha should remain in until double the width or space is gained between the molars than the bicuspids, on account of the greater size of the molars, where more proximal surface is in contact and no room left for cleansing, unless the spaces are very much greater than normal, and the contour made to suit this issue. Here is where you will say, " You will destroy the articulation and cause greater strain on the fillings and also the teeth." No, you are mistaken. When the whole of these proximal surfaces are filled with the semi-elastic stopping, and the act of mastication set up, the teeth that at first are out of the normal position and only touch on part of their crown surfaces are now allowed to readjust themselves ; as the gutta-percha will give where the greatest pressure is brought to bear, and where least resistance is offered, no change occurs. I am not mistaken in this. Try it, and watch a few cases if you cannot believe me.

COMPENSATION.

This method is a test for any further treatment, which, if needed, can so easily be done. It permits of weeks, months and years before the permanent filling need be introduced. No danger of decay, none of loss of structure from fracture. And, in fact, you can dismiss the patients thus treated with the greatest indifference as to the issue. Do you ask whether I charge for all this work, and when I send in my bill? I charge for even my thoughts as well as my work. My patients never object, but often beg me to leave in the gutta-percha.

Thus I practice with all; and I am happy in this, knowing that I do far more good, am not troubled about immediate root filling, —fillings falling out,—"conservative treatment of dental pulp." Nor does pyorrhœa ever invade upon my domain of original work, because I know the value of articulation, and how to make every tooth perform its individual and collective function, and no undue pressure given it to press or work its life out of it and give rise to the denudation of the peridental membrane; nor is the food ever found pressing up into the cervical border and remaining, nor the cervix so weakened by want of contact with firm alveolar processes, and the gum is left to hug the root at this vital portion so tightly that nothing ever creeps in to cause recurrence at the cervix.

SHOULD BE SUED.

Any dentist who allows his original patient who follows orders to have pyorrhœa should be sued for damages. See that no food presses on the gum border; see that no tooth is unduly pressed and contorted by false articulation, caused by improper width and contouring; allow no biting of threads, cracking of nuts, biting of ice upon one tooth only; or, when a tooth, or teeth, has been lost, see that the articulation is restored, and my word for it gout or no gout, syphilis or disease, pyorrhœa will not come, except filth and malaise of one or more teeth.

Gutta-percha used as matrices for gold, amalgam, or oxyphosphate fillings I will not dwell upon; you need nothing better. For holding teeth in position after correction where there are cavities in both, I need only mention it. As for assistance on the temporary and permanent teeth, to keep the ligature from slipping down on the cervix by carrying the ligature through it; for fastening pins into roots for crowns; as a medium between crowns and roots to prevent further caries; as a protection to all roots when a gold crown is used; and, in fact, as a factor in our practice, there is nothing to fill its place.

In only one instance it will not do. Never place it in contact with an amalgam filling, especially when it is covered up over a nearly exposed pulp, for it will oxidize the amalgam and discolor it and make it valueless at the margins. White gutta-percha is not so. The sulphur in the pink will do the work; hence, I say, this contact with amalgam is a failure. I am in love with it, and without it I would be lost.—*International.*

Alveolar Abscess.*

By E. Herbert Adams, M.D., D.D.S., Toronto.

Alveolar abscess is a term applied to any abscess having its origin in the alveolar process of either of the maxillæ. It is generally due to a pericementitis occurring at the apex of the root of the tooth, and caused by the death of the dental pulp. The first pus is pent up in the apical space by bony walls, and the pressure being very great results in the rapid destruction of the surrounding osseous tissue. The pus burrows where there is least resistance, and on account of the cancellous nature of the bone surrounding the root, and the denser nature of the bone nearer the surface, a larger pus cavity is formed.

The pericemental membrane surrounding the apex of the tooth is even yet not perhaps destroyed ; but its fibres become elongated and their meshes filled with pus ; the swollen tissue forming the shreddy bag-like mass so often seen attached to the end of a root of an abscessed tooth after extraction.

Should the outer lamina of bone be perforated, the pus has then ready exit through the soft tissues. The pain now lessens, and the symptoms abate somewhat. This may, however, be only a temporary cessation. The whole side of the face may swell up, the eye be distorted, or the jaws be so stiffened or swollen that they cannot be separated sufficiently for feeding purposes.

An examination will show a large swelling over the affected root. The swelling will usually show signs of fluctuation, and if left to itself will generally open just above the root. It is better, however, to anticipate nature by opening with a bistoury. After the discharge of pus, the swelling and pain usually subside.

Unless the affected tooth is removed, or the diseased pulp removed from the interior of the tooth by a dentist and the pulp cavity rendered aseptic, a chronic source of irritation is kept up, and the abscess assumes the chronic type.

In acute alveolar abscess there may be seen, occasionally, a considerable elevation of temperature, even as high as 103° or 104°. During abscess formation, and before the pus has found exit, a peculiar dull, throbbing pain is often present, and the lymphatics at the angle of the jaw are sometimes sore and swollen.

An abscess, if left to itself, usually assumes the chronic form, the pus continuing to be discharged, but in lessened volume. In the chronic form of alveolar abscess the burrowing of pus may cause a fistulous opening in the cheek, chin or neck, though the most usual

*Read before the Toronto Medical Society.

place for the abscess to discharge is on the gum over the roof of the affected tooth.

Abscesses associated with the wisdom teeth, or third molars, sometimes pass in the direction of the parotid region. In these cases it is not uncommon to find the orifice of the fistula as low down as the clavicle. This is due to the unyielding character of the parotid fascia, which is a continuation of the deep cervical.

On account of the close relation of the roots of the teeth of the upper jaw to the antrum abscesses may open in the maxillary sinus, and thence be discharged through the nares. These cases are frequently mistaken for a diseased condition of the nasal passages, and treated accordingly, and, of course, invariably without success. The relation of the roots of teeth to the antrum is variable. In some cases the floor of the antrum is perforated by the first and second molars, so you can readily see how an abscess can open in this way.

The habit of applying hot fomentations, poultices and counterirritants to the cheek and face is often to blame for abscesses pointing on the face and neck.

One of the most common places for abscessed teeth of the upper jaw to open on the face is just beneath the malar bone, and just in front of the anterior border of the masseter muscle. A disfiguring scar often results, if the abscess is allowed to open in this or any other facial region. Such abscesses may discharge anywhere below the region of the eye

Occasionally, abscesses of the superior incisors discharge directly into the nasal cavity, and an abscess of an anterior tooth has been known to pass back beneath the mucous membrane of the hard palate, and discharge at the junction of the hard and soft palate.

The greater number of abscesses discharging on the face are in the lower jaw. This is probably due to gravitation. Frequently these abscesses open first on the gum, but during the healing process this opening becomes closed. Little pus perhaps remains as the abscess becomes chronic, but the slow burrowing of this, according to the law of gravitation, causes it finally to find exit through the lower jaw. There may be no pain nor other symptoms until this opening has occurred, much to the surprise and annoyance of the patient ; the pus in some cases passing directly downward through the bone, but more frequently passing outward into the soft tissues, and then following these downward to point at the lower margin of the jaw.

Blind abscesses may occur, the pus being small in quantity, and being apparently absorbed without any external opening being formed for its exit.

Occasionally, alveolar abscesses have been known to cause extensive necrosis of the bones of the face. This is more especially the case in strumous or syphilitic patients.

Abscesses may also form osseous cysts on the side of the jaw. The pus, instead of being absorbed, is provided for by the expansion of the outer plate of the bone. These cysts form somewhat rapidly, and are sometimes half the size of a hazelnut. The rapid growth of these cysts is an important point in diagnosis.

In persons with an abnormally small jaw, the eruption of the wisdom teeth often cause severe inflammation and abscess, the jaw being too small to accommodate the new tooth. These abscesses generally discharge at the margin of the gum, but the swelling is often so severe as to cause almost complete immobility of the jaw. In a recent case where it was impossible to open the jaw sufficiently to extract the offending wisdom tooth, the second molar was removed, and of course the third molar had now a chance to come forward and the inflammation soon subsided.

Imprisoned teeth may be a cause of alveolar abscess. The diagnosis of these forms is rather obscure. A probe passed into the sinus, if one has been formed—if not, a bistoury passed through the softer parts and bone—will often assist in the diagnosis of such cases. Abscesses of temporary teeth require especial care, and if they are not readily amenable to treatment the diseased tooth should be extracted.

The *diagnosis* in most cases is comparatively simple ; but from what has been said it will be seen that the diagnosis, of some forms at least, of alveolar abscess is not an easy matter for the general practitioner. And it is these unusual and anomalous cases that most frequently come under the observation of the physician and surgeon, and the ignorance displayed in treatment renders matters often uncomfortable for the patient, and not infrequently so for the surgeon.

A simple means of testing whether a tooth is abscessed is by rapping the tooth with an instrument. If it should prove tender on pressure, the apical pericemental membrane is inflamed, and the root of the tooth probably abscessed.

Abscesses most frequently occur on teeth with dead pulps. In such teeth the natural translucence of the tooth is gone, the dentinal tubuli being filled up with dead matter, due to the disintegration of the pulp. The dark color and opacity is often very marked, but is occasionally so slight as to escape notice. If, however, the patient is placed in the sunlight and the rays of light reflected on the teeth by means of a mirror, a slight opacity will be noticed.

The patient's notice is often directed to a painful tooth as a possible cause of the trouble, but it must be remembered that neither a decayed tooth nor pain need necessarily be present. The pulp may have died from some other cause, and the diagnosis can be made by the opacity of a tooth and its tenderness on pressure.

The following are some of the cases which have been recorded in dental and medical literature as cases of mistaken diagnosis:

Dr. Otto Arnold (*Dental Review*) mentions a case where a patient was confined to her bed by what her physician supposed to be diphtheria. After being treated for about a week, she began to suspect that her teeth were in some way implicated. The pharynx and tonsils were severely inflamed, but after some difficulty the diagnosis of an impacted wisdom tooth was made, and on its extraction she got well.

Dr. C. R. Butler (*Items of Interest*, 1891) mentions a case diagnosed by the patient's physicians as carbuncles, but which proved to be due to alveolar abscesses from three dead teeth. On their extraction a cure was effected.

J. P. Wilson (*Items of Interest*, 1888) mentions a case of alveolar abscess of eight years' standing, where there was a fistulous opening over the clavicle, near the place of origin of the platysma myoides muscle. The disease had been pronounced by a council of physicians to be of a strumous character. He removed the roots of a diseased first molar and the discharge soon ceased, and the abscess healed without further treatment.

Dr. Tees (*Items of Interest*, 1886) mentions a case where death occurred from a surgeon performing a surgical operation on a case of alveolar abscess with much facial swelling, the patient sinking gradually after the operation. He states that the abscess differed in no way from an ordinary alveolar abscess, the three roots of the first left superior molar being diseased, and the swelling of a sudden and recent nature.

A case recently occurred which had the following history : A boy had a swelling of the face. His family physician applied poultices and hot fomentations to the side of the face, and afterwards opened into the pus cavity with a lancet. A running ulcer formed, which lasted for about a year and three months. The school authorities refused to admit the boy to school during this time on account of the disease. The boy was examined by a couple of physicians from the civic health department, who also recommended his detention from school. He would probably be absent from school still and the abscess still discharging had not another physician made the diagnosis of an abscessed tooth. On the extraction of the tooth, the abscess healed readily, and the sinus closed of its own accord.

The *treatment* is comparatively simple in most cases, and consists in the evacuation of the contents of the pus cavity, and in injections of antiseptics until it is rendered thoroughly aseptic.

In the more simple cases this is readily accomplished by a dentist drilling through the root canal and thus allowing an exit for the pus, and an opening through which antiseptics can be injected. It is rare, indeed, that a skilled dentist cannot successfully treat even the worst cases by this means. Of course, if the offending tooth is for any reason considered of no value, the simplest method of cure is its removal, when the abscess will, as a rule, heal without any medication.

In some cases a simple way is to drill through the alveolus, just above the root of the tooth, and thus give an exit for the pus, and an opening for antiseptic medication. If it is desirable to keep the sinus open, a simple method is to place a pledget of cotton, soaked in a strong solution of carbolic acid, in the sinus.

In acute alveolar abscess where there is much swelling of the face, it is often well to endeavor to cause the abscess to point on the buccal surface of the gum over the root of the abscessed tooth. This can often be accomplished by the application of a counter-irritant, such as capsicum or cantharidine, to the gum overlying the root of the affected tooth. A roasted fig or raisin is said also to accomplish the same result.

All applications of hot tomentations, or poultices or counter-irritants to the external surface of the face should be religiously avoided, and if the abscess seems to have a tendency to point externally a free incision for the pus should be made *in* the mouth, and the counter-irritants or other medicaments applied *in* the mouth. This will prevent many an opening on the face, and its consequent scar.

Constitutional treatment should not be neglected where indicated. A saline cathartic will often assist in hastening the removal of an acute abscess.

In those cases where there is a fistulous opening on the face, it is always well to direct, if possible, the discharge into the mouth. If this is done the sinus will heal of its own accord, and the abscess can then be treated in the usual manner. As a rule, the sinus needs little attention after the abscess has healed.

Often considerable disfigurement results from the scar due to a fistulous opening on the face. If under the chin, the scar does not show much, and in a male can be covered by a beard. If on the neck it may be hidden by the clothing; but on the cheek, especially in a female, little can be done to hide the disfigurement.

And here let me give a note of warning. A great many cases have come under my observation where surgeons have made external facial incisions simply because the abscess showed a tendency to point on the face. In one case where the simple extraction of the tooth would have been all that was required to heal the abscess (though even that was not necessary), a prominent surgeon made a crucial incision in the cheek, thrust in a couple of his fingers as an exploratory procedure, and then ordered a lotion of ac. carbol., 1 in 20, to be applied externally.

It is needless to state that such treatment is very reprehensible· There are cases where an external incision is indicated, but these are the exception and not the rule. In such cases, if the knife is used in a conservative manner, the healing process is speedy on account of the vascularity of the facial tissues, and often no perceptible scar remains.

From an æsthetic point of view, the surgeon should always endeavor to give vent to the pus by an incision inside the mouth, and not by an incision on the surface of the face.

One of the hardest tests to which my powers of argument were ever put was in persuading a fellow-practitioner from making a great gash in the cheek of a lady who had an alveolar abscess, which any good dentist could successfully treat by drilling through the root canal, and giving vent to the pus in that manner.

In regard to antiseptic medication any reliable antiseptic will do. Carbolic acid, peroxide of hydrogen, listerine and camphophenique are perhaps the favorites with dentists. Thymol, creasote, oil of cloves, oil of cinnamon, sanitas, salicylic acid, iodine, and various other antiseptics, all have their advocates.

In this paper I have purposely omitted going into the detail of treatment of the simpler forms of alveolar abscesses, as they belong to the domain of the dentist and not of the surgeon. I would also strongly recommend that in all cases of doubtful diagnosis a competent dentist or oral specialist be called into consultation. These abscesses respond speedily to proper treatment, and the diagnosis, too, is, as a rule, simple to the dentist or oral specialist ; and yet there are innumerable cases where the patient has been disfigured or inconvenienced for years by this disease simply through the ignorance of their family physician, who has failed to make a correct diagnosis. Later on, perhaps, a correct diagnosis is made by a dentist, or someone who is familiar with the disease, and the patient is cured in a few days or a week. Naturally, the patient is much embittered against the medical man whose ignorance allowed such a foul ulcer to remain on their face for such a long time.

Prophylaxis is of importance in the prevention of alveolar abscesses, but this belongs largely to the domain of the dentist. It should, however, be the duty of every physician, whenever he finds decayed or offensive teeth present in any patient, to impress on them the importance of visiting their dentist and having their teeth attended to.

Editorial.

Wanted, more Original Communications.

We have seven provinces in Canada, and seven dental organizations, and there is no reason but that of absolute laziness why we should not have a steady stream of original communications flowing in two directions, from Halifax and Vancouver. This journal has no fault to find on the score of subscribers in Canada and the border States, as well as elsewhere; but it is a shame that we have so many able pens that are so indifferent to the duty they owe to our own dental literature. With many it is a sensitiveness to personal criticism. They can avoid that if they wish by writing impersonally. Our college graduates seem to have largely subsided into silence. We should be glad to hear more from them. Then we have a large number of first-rate men whose experience of twenty years' or more practice is better than all the books. If we could afford it, we would like nothing better in the interest of the journal than visiting every dentist from Halifax to Vancouver, taking notes of new ideas. It would be a feast of reason.

Questions and Answers.

In the January number Dr. R. E. Sparks, of Kingston, Ont., will kindly begin the editorship of a department of "Questions and Answers." All correspondence in this department should be sent directly to him. It is desirable to use brevity both in asking and answering questions, and the busy man—we have none other in dentistry—who cannot make time to write a longer article ought to be able to find time to write a post card.

The following queries have been received, to which we hope answers will be sent before the 25th of the present month :

Ques. 1.—How would you take an impression of lower maxillary, very flat ridge ; muscles risen almost to surface ; hypersecretion of saliva ?

Ques. 2.—Explain difference of cohesiveness and discoloration as occurring in one or two sheets, or in pellets, of same book or bottle ?

Ques. 3.—When, where and how would you trim models for full upper dentures ?

Public Perversity.

There are people whose philanthropy is never excited but by the crime of some hardened scoundrel. They have never a sympathetic affection aroused for a fellow-being struggling manfully against temptation to do wrong ; but let the same man murder his mother, and they turn up the whites of their eyes in morbid pity, and become tutelary saints to the brute who has been sentenced to hang. They not only decorate his cell with the white flowers symbolical of purity, but their sickening sentimentality runs to such excess that, had they the power the day before the execution, they would incarcerate the jury and let the criminal go free.

It is no surprise, then, that dental quacks should find friends to deny or extenuate their quackery. In every community there are men who instinctively ally themselves with whatever is morally and legally wrong. They fly to it as the steel to the magnet. They are not only communistic but iconoclastic, and are never so happy as when they throw mud at organized society. It is a wonder to many how these frauds sometimes manage to woo the sympathy of respectable people. There is no mystery about it. We know how it is with the practice of medicine. We know that the Canadian cities are frequently infested with a perambulating syndicate of inferior medical men, headed by an ostentatious humbug, and that even in such University centres as Toronto and Montreal, they repeatedly gull and defraud the public, and leave with a rich harvest. Even the pulpit is not free. Smooth hypocrisy and sleek intrigue sometimes impose for a long time upon a godly people. The dental quack draws sympathy—First, by lying about himself and his " superior abilities ; " second, by lying about the conduct of his confreres. He pretends to mistake their contempt for malice, and would be in the seventh heaven of satisfaction if some confrere would notice him—or kick him. The class who expend their pity upon a condemned criminal, are instinctively led to sympathize with the dental outlaw. The people who swallow the falsehoods and prescriptions of the medical humbug, are as likely to believe the dental liar who declares he can perform miracles upon dead bones. The public must suffer because respectable practitioners dislike to show any appearence of opposition, which gullible people think to be jealousy. A quack has no "reputation " to lose, but everything to gain in a conflict with respectable men. It is by lying that he "prospers," and no respectable dentist would enter into a competition in that line. However, in spite of the flowers of a mistaken sympathy, the murderer hangs. He may die in the odor of roses, but not of sanctity. A quack's "reputation," too, is remembered by his contemporaries, and passed on to posterity.

This book must be returned to
the Dental Library by the last
date stamped below.   It may
be renewed if there is no
reservation for it.

MAY - 7 1965

Lightning Source UK Ltd.
Milton Keynes UK
UKHW012221110219
337137UK00006B/1341/P